Clinical Teaching Strategies in Nursing

Marilyn H. Oermann, PhD, RN, ANEF, FAAN, is the Thelma M. Ingles Professor of Nursing and director of evaluation and educational research at Duke University School of Nursing, Durham, North Carolina. She is author or coauthor of 19 nursing education books and many articles on teaching and evaluation in nursing and on writing for publication. She is the editor of *Nurse Educator* and *Journal of Nursing Care Quality* and past editor of the *Annual Review of Nursing Education*. Dr. Oermann received the National League for Nursing Award for Excellence in Nursing Education Research, Sigma Theta Tau International Elizabeth Russell Belford Award for Excellence in Education, the American Association of Colleges of Nursing Scholarship of Teaching and Learning Excellence Award, and the Margaret Comerford Freda Award for Editorial Leadership from the International Academy of Nursing Editors.

Teresa Shellenbarger, PhD, RN, CNE, ANEF, is Distinguished University Professor and doctoral coordinator at Indiana University of Pennsylvania, Indiana, Pennsylvania. Dr. Shellenbarger is an experienced nursing faculty member and administrator. She is widely published and a frequent presenter on nursing education issues such as professional development, technology use in education, and the faculty role. Dr. Shellenbarger has been the recipient of several teaching awards. She currently serves as secretary and member of the Board of Governors of the National League for Nursing.

Kathleen B. Gaberson, PhD, RN, CNOR, CNE, ANEF, is the owner of and nursing education consultant for OWK Consulting, Pittsburgh, Pennsylvania. She has over 35 years of teaching and administrative experience in graduate and undergraduate nursing programs. She is a coauthor of nine nursing education books and an author or coauthor of numerous articles on nursing education and perioperative nursing topics. Dr. Gaberson presents and consults extensively on nursing curriculum revision, assessment and evaluation, and teaching methods. The former research section editor of the *AORN Journal*, she currently serves on the *Journal* Editorial Board.

FIFTH EDITION

Clinical Teaching Strategies in Nursing

MARILYN H. OERMANN, PhD, RN, ANEF, FAAN

TERESA SHELLENBARGER, PhD, RN, CNE, ANEF

KATHLEEN B. GABERSON, PhD, RN, CNOR, CNE, ANEF

SPRINGER PUBLISHING COMPANY

No part of this publication may be reproduced, stored in a retrieval system, or transmitted in any form or by any means, electronic, mechanical, photocopying, recording, or otherwise, without the prior permission of Springer Publishing Company, LLC, or authorization through payment of the appropriate fees to the Copyright Clearance Center, Inc., 222 Rosewood Drive, Danvers, MA 01923, 978-750-8400, fax 978-646-8600, info@copyright.com or on the web at www.copyright.com.

Springer Publishing Company, LLC
11 West 42nd Street
New York, NY 10036
www.springerpub.com

Acquisitions Editor: Margaret Zuccarini
Composition: diacriTech

ISBN: 978-0-8261-4002-9
ebook ISBN: 978-0-8261-4003-6
Instructors' Manual: 978-0-8261-4023-4
Instructors' PowerPoints: 978-0-8261-4024-1

Instructors' Materials: Instructors may request supplements by emailing textbook@springerpub.com

17 18 19 20 / 5 4 3 2 1

The author and the publisher of this Work have made every effort to use sources believed to be reliable to provide information that is accurate and compatible with the standards generally accepted at the time of publication. Because medical science is continually advancing, our knowledge base continues to expand. Therefore, as new information becomes available, changes in procedures become necessary. We recommend that the reader always consult current research and specific institutional policies before performing any clinical procedure. The author and publisher shall not be liable for any special, consequential, or exemplary damages resulting, in whole or in part, from the readers' use of, or reliance on, the information contained in this book. The publisher has no responsibility for the persistence or accuracy of URLs for external or third-party Internet websites referred to in this publication and does not guarantee that any content on such websites is, or will remain, accurate or appropriate.

Library of Congress Cataloging-in-Publication Data

Names: Gaberson, Kathleen B., author. | Oermann, Marilyn H., author. |
    Shellenbarger, Teresa, author.
Title: Clinical teaching strategies in nursing / Marilyn H. Oermann, Teresa
    Shellenbarger, Kathleen B. Gaberson.
Description: Fifth edition. | New York, NY : Springer Publishing Company,
    LLC, [2018] | Kathleen B. Gaberson's name appears first in the previous
    edition. | Includes bibliographical references and index.
Identifiers: LCCN 2017034207| ISBN 9780826140029 | ISBN 9780826140234
    (instructors' manual) | ISBN 9780826140036 (e-book) | ISBN 9780826140241
    (instructors' powerpoints)
Subjects: | MESH: Education, Nursing | Teaching
Classification: LCC RT73 | NLM WY 18 | DDC 610.73071—dc23 LC record available at
    https://lccn.loc.gov/2017034207

Printed in the United States of America by McNaughton & Gunn.

Contents

SECTION III: EVALUATION STRATEGIES IN CLINICAL TEACHING

Contributors to Previous Editions

Eric Bauman, PhD, RN

Suzanne Hetzel Campbell, PhD, WHNP-BC, IBCLC

Mickey Gilmore-Kahn, CNM, MN

Debra Hagler, PhD, RN, ACNS-BC, CNE, CHSE, ANEF, FAAN

Susan E. Stone, DNSc, CNM, FACNM

Diane M. Wink, EdD, FNP, ARNP

Contributors to the Fifth Edition

Kimberly Day, DNP, RN
Clinical Assistant Professor
College of Nursing & Health Innovation
Arizona State University
Phoenix, Arizona

Debra Hagler, PhD, RN, ACNS-BC, CNE, CHSE, ANEF, FAAN
Clinical Professor
Coordinator, Scholarship of Teaching and Learning
College of Nursing & Health Innovation
Arizona State University
Phoenix, Arizona

Elizabeth Speakman, EdD, RN, FNAP, ANEF, FAAN
Associate Provost of Interprofessional Education
University of the Sciences
Philadelphia, Pennsylvania

Preface

Teaching in clinical settings presents nurse educators with challenges that are different from those encountered in the classroom and in online environments. In nursing education, the classroom and clinical environments are linked because students must apply in clinical practice what they have learned in the classroom, online, and through other experiences. However, clinical settings require different approaches to teaching. The clinical environment is complex and rapidly changing, with a variety of new settings and roles in which nurses must be prepared to practice.

The fifth edition of *Clinical Teaching Strategies in Nursing* examines concepts of clinical teaching and provides a comprehensive framework for planning, guiding, and evaluating learning activities for prelicensure and graduate nursing students. It is a comprehensive source of information for full- and part-time faculty members whose responsibilities center largely on clinical teaching and for adjuncts and teachers whose sole responsibility is clinical teaching. The book also is useful when teaching nurses and other health care providers in the clinical setting. Although the focus of the book is clinical teaching in nursing, the content is applicable to teaching students in other health care fields.

The book describes clinical teaching strategies that are effective and practical in a rapidly changing health care environment. It presents a range of teaching strategies useful for courses in which the teacher is on site with students, in courses using preceptors and similar models, in simulation, and in distance education environments. The book also examines innovative uses of technologies for clinical teaching.

A continuing feature in the fifth edition is an exhibit in each chapter that highlights sections of the Certified Nurse Educator (CNE®) Examination Test Blueprint that relate to the chapter content; the entire test blueprint is reprinted as an appendix. **In addition to the book, we have prepared an instructor's manual with a course syllabus, chapter-based PowerPoint presentations, and materials for an online course (with chapter summaries, student learning activities, discussion questions, and assessment strategies). To obtain an electronic copy, contact Springer Publishing Company (textbook@springerpub.com).**

The book is organized into three sections. The first section, Foundations of Clinical Teaching, comprises six chapters that provide a background for clinical teaching and guide the teacher's planning for clinical learning activities. Chapter 1 discusses the context for clinical teaching and presents a philosophy that provides a framework for planning, guiding, and evaluating clinical learning activities. Chapter 2 discusses outcomes of clinical teaching; it emphasizes the importance of cognitive, psychomotor, and affective outcomes that guide clinical teaching and evaluation. Chapter 3 focuses on how to identify and develop appropriate clinical learning sites. It includes a discussion of underused sites, community-based clinical sites, online delivery and clinical education, and clinical learning in international sites. In Chapter 4, strategies for preparing clinical teachers, staff members, and students for clinical learning are discussed. This chapter includes suggestions for selecting clinical settings and preparing faculty, staff, and students for clinical learning. Chapter 5 discusses the process of clinical teaching, including identifying learning outcomes, assessing learning needs, planning learning activities, guiding students, and evaluating performance. Various clinical teaching models are described, including traditional, in which one teacher guides the learning of a small group of students; preceptor; and dedicated education units and other partnerships. This chapter also addresses important qualities of clinical teachers as identified in research. Chapter 6 addresses ethical and legal issues inherent in clinical teaching, including the use of a service setting for learning activities, the effects of academic dishonesty in clinical learning, incivility between students and clinical teachers, and appropriate accommodations for students with disabilities.

The second section of the book focuses on effective clinical teaching strategies. One important responsibility of clinical teachers is the crafting of appropriate learning assignments. Chapter 7 discusses a variety of clinical learning assignments, in addition to traditional patient care activities, and suggests criteria for selecting appropriate assignments. In Chapter 8, the use of clinical simulation is discussed, including suggestions for using simulation as a teaching–learning strategy. Prebriefing, as a component of simulation, is examined, and debriefing after simulation is also discussed. Chapter 9 examines different technologies that can be used in clinical education. The chapter includes suggestions for selecting these technologies and the importance of matching the choice of technology to the intended type of learning. Chapter 10 discusses the use of case method, case study, and grand rounds as clinical teaching methods to guide the development of problem-solving and clinical judgment skills. In Chapter 11 the role of discussions in clinical learning and clinical conferences is explored. Effective ways to plan and conduct clinical conferences, questioning to encourage exchange of ideas and higher level thinking, and the roles of the teacher and learners in discussions and conferences are presented.

Chapter 12 describes effective strategies for using preceptors in clinical teaching. The selection, preparation, and evaluation of preceptors are discussed, and the advantages and disadvantages of using preceptors are explored. This chapter also discusses the use of learning contracts as a strategy for planning and implementing preceptorships.

Chapter 13, a new chapter in this edition of the book, examines interprofessional education and collaborative practice. Opportunities to develop skill in teamwork should be integrated in nursing programs for students to gain the confidence needed to practice collaboratively and deliver patient-centered care. Providing students with deliberate interprofessional clinical opportunities has the greatest potential to move beyond the current practice of silo education and practice in health professions. The chapter presents the competencies to be developed and clinical activities for preparing students to work and function in interprofessional health care teams.

The final section contains two chapters that focus on clinical evaluation and grading. Chapter 14 discusses written assignments for clinical learning, including short written assignments, reflective journals, concept maps, and electronic portfolios, among others. Suggestions are made for selecting and evaluating a variety of assignments related to important clinical outcomes. Chapter 15 describes the process of clinical evaluation in nursing, rating scales and other methods for evaluating clinical performance, and how to grade students in clinical courses. For a more extensive discussion of those topics, readers are referred to Oermann and Gaberson's *Evaluation and Testing in Nursing Education*, fifth edition (Springer Publishing Company, 2017).

We acknowledge Margaret Zuccarini, our editor at Springer, for her enthusiasm and continued support. We also thank Springer Publishing Company for its support of nursing education and for publishing our books for many years.

Marilyn H. Oermann
Teresa Shellenbarger
Kathleen B. Gaberson

Foundations of Clinical Teaching

CHAPTER 1

Contextual Factors Affecting Clinical Teaching

Effective clinical teaching and learning is influenced by a number of factors. Clinical teaching is performed by a faculty within a curriculum that is planned and offered in response to professional, societal, environmental, and educational expectations and demands, using available human, intellectual, physical, and financial resources—the context of the curriculum.

However, considering that educational context is not enough for clinical teachers, they must also consider the health care context so that they are adequately preparing qualified nurses to be capable of responding to the needs and challenges of a rapidly changing health care environment. Clinical teaching is also impacted by trends and issues beyond the clinical setting and the nursing program. Issues such as diversity, health care financing, globalization, technology development, and other trends also influence health care and clinical teaching. Curricula must be aligned with the ever-changing practice setting (Veltri & Barber, 2016). Faculty members face a rapidly changing health care system burdened with financial pressures, consumption of services by patients with complex needs, delivery of care with expanding technology, and staff shortages. The context of the higher education environment is also a consideration for nursing faculty. Within the educational environment nurse educators feel the pressures of tightening resources, increased workload demands, and changes in student characteristics. Adjunct or part-time teachers are being employed as clinical teachers. They may not have the understanding of the full scope of the academic nurse educator role and may need guidance to understand the nursing curriculum, program, requirements, and students. These clinical teachers need to know how a clinical course is positioned within the curriculum so they can build upon previous knowledge and position clinical learning appropriately.

Because the context is different for each nursing education program, each curriculum is somewhat unique (Iwasiw, Goldenberg, & Andrusyszyn, 2015). Therefore, the practice of clinical teaching differs somewhat from program to program. It is not possible to recommend a set of clinical teaching strategies that will be equally effective in every nursing education program. Rather, the faculty must make decisions about clinical teaching that are congruent with the planned curriculum and relevant to its context (Iwasiw et al., 2015).

THE CURRICULUM PHILOSOPHY

In the sense that it is used most frequently in education, a philosophy is a system of enduring shared beliefs and values held by members of an academic or practice discipline that help to guide actions and curriculum implementation. Philosophy as a comprehensive scientific discipline focuses on more than beliefs, but beliefs determine the direction of science and thus form a basis for examining knowledge in any science.

Philosophical statements serve as a guide for examining issues and determining the priorities of a discipline (Iwasiw et al., 2015; Valiga, 2016). Although a philosophy does not prescribe specific actions, it gives meaning and direction to practice, and it provides a basis for decision making and for determining whether one's behavior is consistent with one's beliefs. Without a philosophy to guide choices, a person is overly vulnerable to tradition, custom, and inconsistencies (Valiga, 2016).

A curriculum philosophy includes statements of belief about people, society, health, the goals of education, the nature of teaching and learning, and the roles of learners and teachers (Keating, 2015; Valiga, 2016). It provides a framework for making curricular and instructional choices and decisions based on a variety of options. The values and beliefs included in a curriculum philosophy provide structure and coherence for a curriculum, but statements of philosophy are meaningless if they are contradicted by actual educational practice or incongruent with the parent institution (Valiga, 2016). In nursing education, a curriculum philosophy directs the curriculum development process by providing a basis for selecting, sequencing, and using content and learning activities while aligning with the mission, vision, and values of the academic institution.

Although traditional views of curriculum development hold that a philosophy is essential as the foundation for building a curriculum, some nursing education leaders have suggested that a set of assumptions or one or more theories could be used instead (Iwasiw et al., 2015; Valiga, 2016). When used as a curriculum foundation, learning theories such as behaviorism, cognitive theories, and interpretive pedagogies reflect a faculty's beliefs about learning, teaching, student characteristics, and the educational environment. Nursing theories, frameworks, or models such as Rogers's Unitary Person Model, Newman's Model of Health, and Watson's Theory of Human Caring may also serve as both theoretical and philosophical contexts for a curriculum and help to organize the curriculum. However, these nursing models, theories, and frameworks have fallen out of favor and are less frequently used for an entire curriculum; instead they are more often used in select courses (Iwasiw et al., 2015).

Contemporary nursing curriculum philosophies are often a blend of philosophy, nursing theory, and learning theory. Among others, these blended philosophical approaches include:

- Adult learning
- Apprenticeship or cognitive apprenticeship
- Cognitive constructivism
- Critical social theory
- Feminism
- Humanism
- Phenomenology
- Pragmatism
- Transformative learning (Iwasiw et al., 2015)

While helpful in providing a guide for clinical education these philosophies, if not embraced by educators may not always provide a focus on the learner, the nurse educator, and those they care for in clinical practice. They may be forgotten, inconsistently used, disregarded, or misunderstood, thus resulting in several philosophical approaches (Iwasiw et al., 2015). Learners exposed to these differences may then experience confusion as they move from course to course.

These clinical courses comprise an important part of the overall curriculum offering opportunities for students to link the philosophy to their clinical learning and experiences. These courses based upon the philosophy provide a scaffold or structure for the program and directs course sequencing and clinical learning experiences. Course configuration must logically build and offer learning opportunities that will enable students to achieve outcomes. Clinical teachers are therefore urged to engage in faculty development opportunities to understand the underlying framework of the curriculum so that clinical teachers can operationalize the program consistently and align their work with the program mission, philosophy, and organizing framework (Iwasiw et al., 2015).

This book provides a framework for planning, guiding, and evaluating the clinical learning activities of nursing students and health care providers based on the authors' philosophical approach to clinical teaching. That philosophical context for clinical teaching is discussed in the remainder of this chapter.

A PHILOSOPHICAL CONTEXT FOR CLINICAL TEACHING

Every clinical teacher has a philosophical approach to clinical teaching, whether or not the teacher realizes it. That philosophical context determines the teacher's understanding of his or her role, approaches to clinical teaching, selection of teaching and learning activities, use of evaluation processes, and relationships with learners and others in the clinical environment. These beliefs serve as a guide to action, and they profoundly affect how clinical teachers practice, how students learn, and how learning outcomes are evaluated. Reflecting on the philosophical basis for one's clinical teaching may evoke anxiety about exposing oneself and one's practice to scrutiny, but this self-reflection is a meaningful basis for continued professional development as a nurse educator (O'Mara, Carpio, Mallette, Down, & Brown, 2000).

Readers may not agree with every element of the philosophical context discussed here, but they should be able to see congruence between what the authors believe about clinical teaching and the recommendations they make to guide effective clinical teaching. Readers are encouraged to articulate their own philosophies of nursing education in general and clinical teaching in particular to guide their clinical teaching practice.

A Lexicon of Clinical Teaching

Language has the power to shape thinking, and choice and use of words can affect the way a teacher thinks about and performs the role of clinical teacher. The following terms are defined so that the authors and readers will share a common frame of reference for the essential concepts in this philosophical approach to clinical teaching.

Clinical

This word is an adjective, derived from the noun *clinic. Clinical* means involving direct observation of the patient. Like any adjective, the word clinical must modify a noun. Nursing faculty members often are heard saying, "My students are in clinical today" or "I am not in clinical this week." Examples of correct use include "clinical practice," "clinical instruction," and "clinical evaluation."

Clinical Teaching or Clinical Instruction

The central activity of the teacher in the clinical setting is clinical instruction or clinical teaching. The teacher does not supervise students. Supervision implies administrative functions such as overseeing, directing, and managing the work of others. Supervision is a function that is more appropriate for professional practice situations, not the learning environment.

   The appropriate role of the teacher in the clinical setting is competent guidance. The teacher guides, supports, stimulates, and facilitates learning. The teacher facilitates learning by designing appropriate activities in appropriate settings and allows the student to experience that learning.

Clinical Experience

Learning is an active, personal process. The student is the one who experiences the learning. Teachers cannot provide the experience; they can provide only the opportunity for the experience. The teacher's role is to plan and provide appropriate activities that will facilitate learning. However, each student will experience an activity in a different way. For example, a teacher can provide a guided observation of a surgical procedure for a group of students. Although all students may be present in the operating room at the same time and all are observing the same procedure, each student will experience something slightly different. One of the reasons teachers require students to do written assignments or to participate in clinical conferences is to allow the teacher a glimpse of what students have derived from the learning activities.

ELEMENTS OF A PHILOSOPHICAL CONTEXT FOR CLINICAL TEACHING

The philosophical context of clinical teaching that provides the framework for this book includes beliefs about the nature of professional practice, essential nurse educator competencies, the importance of clinical teaching, the role of the student as a learner, the need for learning time before evaluation, the climate for learning, the essential versus enrichment curricula, the espoused curriculum versus curriculum-in-use, and the importance of quality over quantity of clinical activities. Each of these elements serves as a guide to action for clinical teachers in nursing.

Clinical Education Should Reflect the Nature of Professional Practice

Nursing is a professional discipline. A professional is an individual who possesses expert knowledge and skill in a specific domain, acquired through formal education in institutions of higher learning and through experience, and who uses that knowledge and skill on behalf of society by serving specified clients. Professional disciplines are differentiated from academic disciplines by their practice component.

Clinical practice requires critical thinking and problem-solving abilities, specialized psychomotor and technological skills, and a professional value system. Practice in clinical settings exposes students to realities of professional practice that cannot be conveyed by a textbook or a simulation (Oermann & Gaberson, 2017). Schön (1987) represented professional practice as high, hard ground overlooking a swamp. On the high ground, practice problems can be solved by applying research-based theory and technique. The swampy lowland contains problems that are messy and confusing, that cannot easily be solved by technical skill. Nurses and nursing students must learn to solve both types of problems, but the problems that lie in the swampy lowlands tend to be those of greatest importance to society. Most professional practice situations are characterized by complexity, instability, uncertainty, uniqueness, and the presence of value conflicts. These are the problems that resist solution by the knowledge and skills of traditional expertise (Schön, 1983).

Because professional practice occurs within the context of society, it must respond to social and scientific demands and expectations. Therefore, the knowledge base and skill repertoire of a professional nurse cannot be static. Professional education must go beyond current knowledge and skills to prepare for practice in the future. Thus, clinical teaching must include skills such as identifying knowledge gaps, locating and using new information and technology, and initiating or managing change. Additionally, because health care professionals usually practice in interdisciplinary settings, nursing students must learn teamwork and collaboration skills to work effectively with others (Institute of Medicine, 2011).

Thus, if clinical learning activities are to prepare nursing students for professional practice, they should reflect the realities of that practice. Students must be exposed to the demands and issues confronting nursing and health care. Clinical education should allow students to encounter real practice problems in the swampy lowland. Rather than focus exclusively on teacher-defined, well-structured problems for which answers are easily found in theory and research, clinical educators should expose students to ill-structured problems for which there are insufficient or conflicting data or multiple solutions (Oermann & Gaberson, 2017).

Clinical Teaching Is More Important Than Classroom Teaching

Because nursing is a professional practice discipline, what nurses and nursing students do in clinical practice is more important than what they can demonstrate in a classroom. Clinical learning activities provide real-life experiences and opportunities for transfer of knowledge to practical situations (Oermann & Gaberson, 2017). Some learners who perform well in the classroom cannot apply their knowledge successfully in the clinical area.

If clinical instruction is so important, why doesn't all nursing education take place in the clinical area? Clinical teaching is the most expensive element of any nursing curriculum. Lower student-to-teacher ratios in clinical settings usually require a larger number of clinical teachers than classroom teachers. Students and teachers spend numerous hours in the clinical laboratory; those contact hours typically exceed the number of credit hours for which students pay tuition. Even if the tuition structure compensates for that intensive use of resources, clinical instruction remains an expensive enterprise. Therefore, classroom instruction is used to prepare students for their clinical activities. Students learn prerequisite knowledge in the classroom and through independent learning activities that they later apply and test, first in the simulation laboratory and then in clinical practice.

The Nursing Student in the Clinical Setting Is a Learner, Not a Nurse

In preparation for professional practice, the clinical setting is the place where the student comes in contact with the patient or consumer for the purpose of testing theories and learning skills. In nursing education, clinical learning activities have historically been confused with caring for patients. In a classic study on the use of the clinical laboratory in nursing education, Infante (1985) observed that the typical activities of nursing students center on patient care. Learning is assumed to take place while caring. However, the central focus in clinical education should be on learning, not doing, as the student role. Thus, the role of the student in nursing education should be primarily that of learner, not nurse. For this reason, the term *nursing student* rather than *student nurse* is preferred, because in the former term, the noun *student* describes the role better.

Sufficient Learning Time Should Be Provided Before Performance Is Evaluated

If students enter the clinical area to learn, then it follows that students need to engage in activities that promote learning and to practice the skills that they are learning before their performance is evaluated to determine a grade. Many nursing students perceive that the main role of the clinical teacher is to evaluate, and many nursing faculty members perceive that they spend more time on evaluation activities than on teaching activities. Nursing faculty members seem to expect students to perform skills competently the first time they attempt them, and they often keep detailed records of students' failures and shortcomings, which are later consulted when determining grades.

However, skill acquisition is a complex process that involves making mistakes and learning how to correct and then prevent those mistakes. Because the clinical setting is a place where students can test theory and apply it to practice, some of those tests will be more successful than others. Faculty members should expect students to make mistakes and not hold perfection as the standard. Therefore, faculty members should allow plentiful learning time with ample opportunity for feedback before evaluating student performance summatively.

Clinical Teaching Is Supported by a Climate of Mutual Trust and Respect

Another element of this philosophy of clinical teaching is the importance of creating and maintaining a climate of mutual trust and respect that supports learning and student growth. Faculty members must respect students as learners and trust their motivation and commitment to the profession they seek to enter. Students must respect the faculty's commitment to both nursing education and society and trust that faculty members will treat them with fairness and, to the extent that it is possible, not allow students to make mistakes that would harm patients.

The responsibilities for maintaining this climate are mutual, but teachers have the ultimate responsibility to establish these expectations in the nursing program. In most cases, students enter a nursing education program with 12 or more years of school experiences in which teachers may have been viewed as enemies, out to get students, and eager to see students fail. Nurse educators need to state clearly, early, and often that they see nursing education as a shared enterprise, that they sincerely desire student success, and that they will be partners with students in achieving success. Before expecting students to trust them, teachers need to demonstrate their respect for students; faculty must first trust students and invite students to enter into a trusting relationship with the faculty. This takes time and energy, and sometimes faculty members will be disappointed when trust is betrayed. However, in the long run, clinical teaching is more effective when it takes place in a climate of mutual trust and respect, so it is worth the time and effort.

Clinical Teaching and Learning Should Focus on Essential Knowledge, Skills, and Attitudes

Most nurse educators believe that each nursing education program has a single curriculum. In fact, every nursing curriculum can be separated into knowledge, skills, and attitudes that are deemed to be essential to safe, competent practice and those that would be nice to have but are not critical. In other words, there is an essential curriculum and an enrichment curriculum. No nursing education program has the luxury of unlimited time for clinical teaching. Therefore, teaching and learning time is used to maximum advantage by focusing most of the time and effort on the most common practice problems that graduates and staff members are likely to face.

As health care and nursing knowledge grow, nursing curricula tend to change additively. That is, new content and skills are added to nursing curricula frequently, but faculty members are reluctant to delete anything. Neither students nor teachers are well served by this approach. Teachers may feel like they are drowning in content and unable to fit everything in; students resort to memorization and superficial, temporary learning, unable to discriminate between critical information and less important material. Faculty members must determine what content is critical and necessary and what information is nice to know but may not be necessary to include. Nurse educators in prelicensure programs should focus on what knowledge is appropriate for the novice nurse, attend to the basic competencies, and ensure the provision of safe patient care while making the tough decisions about what content and clinical activities should remain and which can be removed (Sullivan, 2016).

The traditionally designed curriculum, using blocks of content structured around clinical specialties (i.e., pediatrics, medical–surgical, community health), is one curriculum approach used in nursing education. However, many programs are shifting to a concept-based curriculum that uses core nursing concepts to offer a more flexible approach to clinical teaching and learning (Sullivan, 2016). Concepts frequently used include oxygenation, pain, nutrition, quality and safety, and teamwork as well as other broad concepts. Clinical activities in a nursing program using a concept-based curriculum align with concepts discussed in the classroom; thereby expanding student understanding of the concepts, developing clinical judgment, and enhancing knowledge of the broader health care organization (Giddens, Caputi, & Rodgers, 2015).

Every nurse educator should be able to take a list of 10 clinical objectives or learning outcomes and reduce it to five essential objectives or learning outcomes by focusing on what is needed to produce safe, competent practitioners. To shorten the length of an orientation program for new staff members, the nurse educators in a hospital staff development department would first identify the knowledge, skills, and attitudes that were most essential for new employees in that environment to learn. If faculty members of a nursing education program wanted to design an accelerated program, they would have to decide what content to retain and what could be omitted without affecting the ability of their graduates to pass the licensure or certification examination and practice safely.

Making decisions like these is difficult, but what is often more difficult is getting a group of nurse educators to agree on the distinction between essential and enrichment content. Not surprisingly, these decisions are often made according to the clinical specialty backgrounds of the faculty; the specialties that are represented by the largest number of faculty members are usually deemed to hold the most essential content. These beliefs may explain why a group of nursing faculty members who teach medical–surgical or adult health nursing would suggest that a behavioral health clinical practice session should be canceled so that all students may hear a guest speaker's presentation on arterial blood gases, or why many nursing faculty members advise students to practice for a year or two after graduation in a medical–surgical setting before transferring to the clinical setting in which students initially express an interest, such as behavioral health, community health, or perioperative settings.

This is not to suggest that the curriculum should consist solely of essential content. The enrichment curriculum is used to enhance learning, individualize activities, and motivate students. Students who meet essential clinical objectives can quickly select additional learning activities from the enrichment curriculum to satisfy needs for more depth and greater variety. Learners need to spend most of their time in the essential curriculum, but all students should have opportunities to participate in the enrichment curriculum as well.

The Espoused Curriculum May Not Be the Curriculum-in-Use

In a landmark guide to the reform of professional education, Argyris and Schön (1974) proposed that human behavior is guided by operational theories of action that operate at two levels. The first level, espoused theory (the "paper curriculum"), is what individuals say that they believe and do. This is also referred to as the official or legitimate curriculum. Espoused theory is used to explain and justify action. The other level, theory-in-use (the "practice curriculum" or operational curriculum), guides what individuals actually do in spontaneous behavior with others. Individuals are usually unable to describe their theories-in-use, but, when they reflect on their behavior, they often discover that it is incongruent with the espoused theory of action. Incongruity between espoused theory and theory-in-use can result in ineffective individual practice as well as discord within a faculty group.

Similarly, a nursing curriculum operates on two levels. The espoused curriculum is the one that is described in the self-study for accreditation or state approval and in course syllabi and clinical evaluation tools. This is the curriculum that is the subject of endless debate at faculty meetings. However, the curriculum-in-use is what actually happens. A faculty can agree to include or exclude certain learning activities, goals, or evaluation methods in the curriculum, but when clinical teachers are in their own clinical settings, they often do what seems right to them at the time, in the context of changing circumstances and resources. In fact, one of the competencies included on the National League for Nursing (NLN) Certified Nurse Educator (CNE®) Examination Detailed Test Blueprint is "Respond effectively to unexpected events that affect clinical . . . instruction" (NLN, 2016). In other words, every teacher must interpret the espoused curriculum in view of circumstances and resources in the specific clinical setting and the individual needs of students and patients at the time. In reality, a faculty cannot prescribe to the last detail what teachers will teach (and when and how) and what learners will learn (and when and how) in clinical settings. Consequently, every student experiences the curriculum differently; hence the distinction between learning *activity* and learning *experience*.

When the notion of individualizing the curriculum is taken to extremes, an individual faculty member can become an "academic cowboy" (Saunders, 1999), ignoring the curriculum framework developed through consensus of the faculty in favor of his or her own "creative ideas and unconventional approaches to learning" (p. 30). Because a curriculum philosophy is designed to provide clear direction to the faculty for making decisions about teaching and learning, the integrity of the program of study may be compromised if the practice of an individual clinical teacher diverges widely from the collective values, beliefs, and ideals of the faculty. Academic freedom is universally valued in the educational community, but it is not a license to disregard the educational philosophy adopted by the faculty as a curriculum framework (Saunders, 1999). Thus, the exploration of incongruities between espoused curriculum and curriculum-in-use should engage the faculty as a whole on an ongoing basis while allowing enough freedom for individual faculty members to operationalize the curriculum in their own clinical teaching settings.

Quality Is More Important Than Quantity

Infante (1985) wrote, "The amount of time that students should spend in the clinical laboratory has been the subject of much debate among nurse educators" (p. 43). More than 30 years later, this statement still holds true for clinical teaching. Infante proposed that when teachers schedule a certain amount of time (4 or 8 hours) for clinical learning activities, it will be insufficient for some students and unnecessarily long for others to acquire a particular skill. The length of time spent in clinical activities is no guarantee of the amount or quality of learning that results. Both the activity and the amount of time need to be individualized.

Most nursing faculty members worry far too much about how many hours students spend in the clinical setting and too little about the quality of the learning that is taking place. A 2-hour activity that results in critical skill learning is far more valuable than an 8-hour activity that merely promotes repetition of skills and habit learning. Nurse educators often worry that there is not enough time to teach everything that should be taught, but, as noted in the previous section, a rapidly increasing knowledge base assures that there will never be enough time. There is no better reason to identify the critical outcomes of clinical teaching and focus most of the available teaching time on guiding student learning to achieve those outcomes.

USING A PHILOSOPHY OF CLINICAL TEACHING TO IMPROVE CLINICAL EDUCATION

In the following chapters, the philosophical context for clinical teaching articulated here will be applied to discussions of the role of the clinical teacher and the process of clinical teaching. Differences in philosophical approach can profoundly affect how individuals enact the role of clinical teacher. Every decision about teaching strategy, setting, outcome, and role behavior is grounded in the teacher's philosophical perspective.

The core values inherent in an educator's philosophy of clinical teaching can serve as the basis for useful discussions with colleagues and testing of new teaching strategies. Reflection on one's philosophy of clinical teaching may uncover the source of incongruities between an individual's espoused theory of clinical teaching and the theory-in-use. When the outcomes of such reflection are shared with other clinical teachers, they provide a basis for the continual improvement of clinical teaching.

Nurse educators are encouraged to continue to develop their philosophies of clinical teaching by reflecting on how they view the goals of clinical education and how they carry out teaching activities to meet those goals. A philosophical approach to clinical education will thus serve as a guide to more effective practice and a means of ongoing professional development (Valiga, 2016).

SUMMARY

The context in which clinical teaching occurs is a major determinant of its effectiveness. The context of the curriculum comprises internal and external influences, expectations, and demands that ground the curriculum and make it unique. The internal contextual factors include the faculty's shared beliefs about the goals of education, the nature of teaching and learning, and the roles of learners and teachers—the philosophical context of the curriculum.

Nursing education philosophies today are often a blend of philosophy, nursing theory, and learning theory. A philosophical context for clinical teaching influences one's understanding of the role of the clinical teacher and the process of teaching in clinical settings. This philosophy includes fundamental beliefs about the value of clinical education, roles and relationships of teachers and learners, and how to achieve desired outcomes. This philosophical approach to clinical teaching is operationalized in the remaining chapters of this book.

Terms related to clinical teaching were defined to serve as a common frame of reference. The adjective *clinical* means involving direct observation of the patient; its proper use is to modify nouns such as *laboratory, instruction, practice,* or *evaluation.* The teacher's central activity is *clinical instruction* or *clinical teaching* rather than supervision, which implies administrative activities such as overseeing, directing, and managing the work of others. Because learning is an active, personal process, the student is the one who experiences the learning. Therefore, teachers cannot provide *clinical experience*, but they can offer opportunities and activities that will facilitate learning. Each student will experience a learning activity in a different way.

The philosophical context of clinical teaching advocated in this book contains the following beliefs: Clinical education should reflect the nature of professional practice. Practice in clinical settings exposes students to realities of professional practice that cannot be conveyed by a textbook or a simulation. Most professional practice situations are complex, unstable, and unique. Therefore, clinical learning activities should expose students to problems that cannot be solved easily with existing knowledge and technical skills.

Another element of the philosophy of clinical teaching concerns the importance of clinical teaching. Because nursing is a professional practice discipline, the clinical practice of nurses and nursing students is more important than what they can demonstrate in a classroom. Clinical education provides opportunities for real-life experiences and transfer of knowledge to practical situations.

In the clinical setting, nursing students come in contact with patients for the purpose of applying knowledge, testing theories, and learning skills. Although typical activities of nursing students center on patient care, learning does not necessarily take place during caregiving. The central activity of the student in clinical education should be learning, not doing.

Sufficient learning time should be provided before performance is evaluated. Students need to engage in learning activities and practice skills before their performance is evaluated summatively. Skill acquisition is a complex process that involves making errors and learning how to correct and then prevent them. Teachers should allow plentiful learning time with ample opportunity for feedback before evaluating performance.

Another element of this philosophy of clinical teaching is the importance of a climate of mutual trust and respect that supports learning and student growth. Teachers and learners share the responsibility for maintaining this climate, but teachers are ultimately accountable for establishing expectations that faculty and students will be partners in achieving success.

Clinical teaching and learning should focus on essential knowledge, skills, and attitudes regardless if using a traditional curriculum model or a concept-based curriculum. Because every nursing education program has limited time for clinical teaching, this time is used to maximum advantage by focusing on the most common practice problems that learners are likely to face. Educators need to identify the knowledge, skills, and attitudes that are most essential for students to learn. Learners need to spend most of their time on this *essential curriculum.*

In clinical settings, the espoused curriculum may not be the curriculum-in-use. Although most faculty members would argue that there is one curriculum for a nursing education program, in reality, the espoused curriculum is interpreted somewhat differently by each clinical teacher. Consequently, every student experiences this curriculum-in-use differently. A faculty cannot prescribe every detail of what teachers will teach and what learners will learn in clinical settings. Instead, it is usually more effective to specify broader outcomes and allow teachers and learners to meet them in a variety of ways. Individual faculty members are cautioned not to take individualizing the curriculum as a license to ignore the shared philosophy that guides curriculum development and implementation.

Finally, the distinction between quality and quantity of clinical learning is important. The quality of a learner's experience is more important than the amount of time spent in clinical activities. Both the activity and the amount of time should be individualized.

CNE EXAMINATION TEST BLUEPRINT CORE COMPETENCIES

1. **Facilitate Learning**
   A. Implement a variety of teaching strategies appropriate to
      1. content
      2. setting
      3. learner needs
      4. learning style
      5. desired learner outcomes

(continued)

    B. Use teaching strategies based on
      1. educational theory
    C. Create a positive learning environment that fosters a free exchange of ideas

2. Facilitate Learner Development and Socialization

    A. Create learning environments that facilitate learners' self-reflection, personal goal setting, and socialization to the role of the nurse

3. Participate in Curriculum Design and Evaluation of Program Outcomes

    A. Actively participate in the design of the curriculum to reflect
      1. institutional philosophy and mission
      2. current nursing and health care trends
      3. community and societal needs
      5. educational principles, theory, and research

4. Engage in Scholarship, Service, and Leadership

    A. Function effectively within the organizational environment and the academic community
      1. Identify how social, economic, political, and institutional forces influence nursing and higher education.
      2. Consider the goals of the nursing program and the mission of the parent institution when proposing change or managing issues.

Note: This exhibit and the CNE Core Competency exhibits in subsequent chapters identify selected competencies that relate to content in each chapter. The lettering and numbering of competencies correspond to the structure of the Certified Nurse Educator (CNE®) Examination Detailed Test Blueprint.

Source: National League for Nursing (2017). Copyright by National League for Nursing. Reprinted with permission.

REFERENCES

Argyris, C., & Schön, D. A. (1974). *Theory in practice: Increasing professional effectiveness.* San Francisco, CA: Jossey-Bass.

Giddens, J. F., Caputi, L., & Rodgers, B. (2015). *Mastering concept-based teaching: A guide for nurse educators.* St. Louis, MO: Elsevier.

Infante, M. S. (1985). *The clinical laboratory in nursing education* (2nd ed.). New York, NY: Wiley.

Institute of Medicine. (2011). *The future of nursing: Leading change, advancing health.* Washington, DC: National Academies Press.

Iwasiw, C. L., Goldenberg, D., & Andrusyszyn, M. (2015). *Curriculum development in nursing education* (2nd ed.). Sudbury, MA: Jones & Bartlett.

Keating, S. B. (2015). *Curriculum development and evaluation in nursing.* New York, NY: Springer Publishing.

National League for Nursing. (2017). *Certified nurse educator (CNE) 2017 candidate handbook.* Retrieved from http://www.nln.org/certification/handbook/cne.pdf

Oermann, M. H., & Gaberson, K. B. (2017). *Evaluation and testing in nursing education* (5th ed.). New York, NY: Springer Publishing.

O'Mara, L., Carpio, B., Mallette, C., Down, W., & Brown, B. (2000). Developing a teaching portfolio in nursing education: A reflection. *Nurse Educator, 25,* 125–130.

Saunders, R. B. (1999). Are you an academic cowboy? *Nursing Forum, 34,* 29–34.

Schön, D. A. (1983). *The reflective practitioner: How professionals think in action.* New York, NY: Basic Books.

Schön, D. A. (1987). *Educating the reflective practitioner.* San Francisco, CA: Jossey-Bass.

Sullivan, D. T. (2016). An introduction to curriculum development. In D. M. Billings & J. A. Halstead (Eds.), *Teaching in nursing: A guide for faculty* (5th ed., pp. 89–117). St. Louis, MO: Elsevier.

Valiga, T. M. (2016). Philosophical foundations of the curriculum. In D. M. Billings & J. A. Halstead (Eds.), *Teaching in nursing: A guide for faculty* (5th ed., pp. 118–129). St. Louis, MO: Elsevier.

Veltri, L., & Barber, H. (2016). Forces and issues influencing curriculum development. In D. M. Billings & J. A. Halstead (Eds.), *Teaching in nursing: A guide for faculty* (5th ed., pp. 73–88). St. Louis, MO: Elsevier.

CHAPTER 2

Outcomes of Clinical Teaching

In a study of the status of and proposed solutions for the global nursing faculty shortage, Nardi and Gyurko (2013) found that:

> In many ways, nursing education appears to be stuck in the 19th and 20th centuries' apprentice model of a small group of nursing students following a clinical instructor around a hospital ward of inpatients for instruction and experience. In the real world of outpatient and nontraditional settings, quick and fragmented encounters, and high-tech delivery systems, this process is anachronistic and inefficient. It also makes nursing education, with its additional clinical practice component, a very expensive and time-consuming endeavor. (p. 320)

To justify the enormous expenditure of resources on clinical education in nursing, teachers must have clear, realistic expectations of the desired outcomes of clinical learning. What knowledge, skills, and values can be learned only in clinical practice and not in the classroom or through independent learning activities?

Nurse educators have traditionally focused on the *process* of clinical teaching. Many hours of discussion in faculty meetings have been devoted to how and where clinical learning takes place, which clinical activities should be required, and how many hours should be spent in the clinical area. However, current accreditation criteria for higher education in general and nursing in particular focus on evidence that the nursing education program is producing important intended outcomes of learning. Therefore, the effectiveness of clinical teaching should be judged on the extent to which it produces such outcomes.

This chapter discusses broad outcomes of nursing education programs that can be achieved through clinical teaching and learning. These outcomes may be operationally defined and stated as competencies and specific objectives in order to be useful in guiding teaching and evaluation. Competencies and specific objectives for clinical teaching are discussed in Chapter 5.

INTENDED OUTCOMES

Since the 1980s, accrediting bodies in higher education have placed greater emphasis on measuring the performance of students and graduates, holding faculty and institutions accountable for the outcomes of their educational programs. Outcomes are the products of educational efforts—the behaviors, characteristics, qualities, or attributes that learners display at the end of an educational program. Teachers are responsible for specifying outcomes of nursing education programs that are congruent with the current and future needs of society. Changes in health care delivery systems, demographic trends, technological advances, and developments in higher education influence the competencies needed for professional nursing practice. A nursing faculty must take these influences into account when designing a context-relevant, evidence-informed curriculum (Iwasiw & Goldenberg, 2014).

In the curriculum development process, after the faculty agrees on the philosophical context for the nursing education program, it formulates curriculum outcome statements (Iwasiw & Goldenberg, 2014). The desired outcomes for clinical teaching contribute to the achievement of the overall curriculum outcomes and therefore should be congruent with them.

In nursing education, a number of different terms are used to refer to professional abilities that learners are expected to demonstrate at program completion. *Outcomes* can be used to indicate the actual abilities demonstrated by program graduates or the intended or expected results of the education program. The latter connotation is more accurately referred to as *outcome statements*. Other terms used to denote such outcomes are *terminal objectives* (usually associated with a behaviorist philosophical approach) and *goals* (more broadly stated). Expectations of performance at the end of a curriculum level or course are often termed *competencies*. In this book, we use the term *outcomes* to refer to the intended or expected results of clinical teaching.

The curriculum reform movement of the 1980s focused on the importance of outcomes rather than process in improving the quality of teaching and learning in nursing education. This approach suggests that an orderly curriculum design does not take into account each learner's individual needs, abilities, and learning style and that learners can reach the same goal by means of different paths. Development of an outcome-driven curriculum begins with specifying the desired ends and then selecting content and teaching strategies that will bring about those ends.

Thus, planning for clinical teaching should begin with identifying learning outcomes that are necessary for safe, competent nursing practice. These outcome statements are derived from the philosophical approach chosen to guide curriculum development and are related to the three domains of learning: cognitive (knowledge and intellectual skills), psychomotor (skills and technological abilities), and affective (professional attitudes, values, and beliefs) (Oermann & Gaberson, 2017). They also include outcomes that incorporate more than one of these domains.

Cognitive Domain Outcomes

Clinical learning activities enable students to transfer knowledge learned in the classroom and through other learning activities to real-life situations. In clinical practice, theory and scientific evidence is translated into practice. By participating in clinical activities, students extend the knowledge that they acquired in the classroom, simulation lab, and in self-directed learning. To use resources effectively and efficiently, clinical learning activities should focus on the development of knowledge that cannot be obtained in the classroom or other settings.

As discussed in Chapter 1, new content is added to nursing curricula frequently, reflecting the growth of new knowledge in nursing and health care. If the faculty is not willing to delete content that is no longer current or essential, the potential exists for creating a congested, content-saturated curriculum in which both students and teachers lose focus on the essential knowledge outcomes. Nurse educators thus need to develop evidence-based teaching skills that will help them to critically evaluate the evidence for content additions and deletions and decide what knowledge is essential for students to acquire. For nursing education programs that prepare candidates for licensure or certification, consulting the licensure or certification examination test plans will help the faculty to focus attention on essential program content. The National Council of State Boards of Nursing (NCSBN®) test plans for the National Council Licensing Examinations (NCLEX®) (NCSBN, 2015) and the American Association of Colleges of Nursing (AACN) publications *The Essentials of Baccalaureate Education for Professional Nursing Practice* (AACN, 2008), *The Essentials of Master's Education in Nursing* (AACN, 2011), and *The Essentials of Doctoral Education for Advanced Nursing Practice* (AACN, 2006) are helpful resources for selecting and organizing essential content in undergraduate and graduate programs in nursing.

Knowing how to practice nursing involves high-level cognitive abilities such as problem solving, critical thinking, decision making, clinical reasoning, and clinical judgment. Traditional pedagogies that emphasize memorizing content and applying it in clinical practice are not sufficient for teaching the high-level thinking abilities necessary to ensure high-quality nursing care and patient safety in the complex environments of the contemporary health care system. Newer approaches such as narrative pedagogy promote teaching the process of thinking instead of content. Shifting emphasis away from covering content to engaging students in understanding the evolving context for nursing practice promotes development of thinking from multiple perspectives. When faculty members intend to teach high-level thinking, they should use approaches that engage students as participants in questioning, interpreting, and thinking about significant issues from multiple perspectives.

Problem Solving

Clinical learning activities provide rich sources of realistic practice problems to be solved. Some problems are related to patients and their health needs; some arise from the clinical environment. As discussed in Chapter 1, most clinical problems tend to be complex, unique, and ambiguous. The ability to solve clinical problems is thus an important outcome of clinical teaching and learning, and the nursing process itself is a problem-solving approach. Most nurses and nursing students have some experience in problem solving, but complex problems of clinical practice often require new methods of reasoning and problem-solving strategies. Nursing students may not be functioning on a cognitive level that permits them to solve clinical problems effectively. To achieve this important outcome, clinical activities should expose the learner to realistic clinical problems of increasing complexity.

Many nurse educators and nursing students believe that problem solving is synonymous with critical thinking. However, the ability to solve clinical problems, while necessary, is insufficient for professional nursing practice, because it focuses on the solution or outcome instead of a more complete understanding of a situation in context. Problem solving involves identifying and defining the problem, collecting relevant data, proposing and implementing solutions, and evaluating their effectiveness. Students cannot solve problems for which they lack understanding and a relevant knowledge base. Only when students have a deep understanding of the problem in its context can they apply their knowledge and previous experience with similar patients as a framework for solving it (Oermann & Gaberson, 2017).

Critical Thinking

Critical thinking is an important outcome of nursing education. Early emphasis on developing critical thinking skills was stimulated by previous criteria for accreditation of prelicensure nursing education programs, but it is no longer an accreditation standard. However, current standards, competencies, and recommendations from the Institute of Medicine (2011), Quality and Safety Education for Nurses (QSEN) Institute (QSEN, 2014a), AACN (2006, 2008, 2011), and American Association of Colleges of Nursing QSEN Education Consortium (2012) address the importance of nurses who can think critically to promote patient safety and achieve cost-efficient, quality patient outcomes. The complexity of patient needs, the ever-expanding amount of health care information that nurses need to process in clinical settings, and multiple ethical issues faced by nurses require the ability to think critically to arrive at sound judgments about patient care (Oermann & Gaberson, 2017).

Because critical thinking is integral to the ability to practice professional nursing, most employers of new nursing graduates expect them to demonstrate this competency. However, it is important to remember that while discipline-specific critical thinking skills may be formed during the nursing education program, experience in nursing practice refines and strengthens them (Newton & Moore, 2013). Nurse educators face the challenge of developing true critical thinkers who will be comfortable practicing in the ever-changing health care environment of the future (Newton & Moore, 2013). This challenge suggests that clinical learning activities must focus intently on developing students' critical thinking skills and dispositions throughout the nursing education program, so that students can build on their experiences to begin to refine these skills before they enter the professional nursing workforce.

Many definitions of critical thinking exist, and the faculty must agree on a definition that is appropriate for a given program to provide direction for teaching and assessing this outcome as well as communicating the construct effectively to students. Critical thinking is a process used to determine a course of action involving collecting appropriate data, analyzing the validity and utility of the information, evaluating multiple lines of reasoning, and coming to valid conclusions. It is purposeful, outcome directed, and evidence based (Alfaro-LeFevre, 2017).

Students who think critically:

- Ask questions and are curious and willing to search for answers
- Consider alternate perspectives and explanations
- Question current practices
- Are open-minded (Oermann & Gaberson, 2017)

Although most educators would classify critical thinking as a cognitive domain outcome, some definitions of critical thinking characterize it as a composite of attitudes, knowledge, and skills. It involves the ability to seek and analyze truth systematically and with an open mind as well as attitudinal dimensions of self-confidence, maturity, and inquisitiveness. Critical thinking is not restricted only to clinical situations. Professionals in every discipline use critical thinking, and this often results in uncertainty about how to measure and evaluate this important outcome. However, clinical learning activities help learners to develop discipline-specific critical thinking skills as they observe, participate in, and evaluate nursing care in an increasingly complex and uncertain health care environment.

Clinical Reasoning

Clinical reasoning is an essential feature of nursing competence that is often demonstrated by experienced nurses. Clinical reasoning is "a complex process that uses cognition, metacognition, and discipline-specific knowledge to gather and analyze patient information, evaluate its significance, and weigh alternative actions" (Simmons, 2010, p. 1151). The result of clinical reasoning is *clinical judgment*, the inference or conclusion arrived at through clinical reasoning (Alfaro-LeFevre, 2017; Simmons, 2010). Like critical thinking, clinical reasoning is a poorly defined construct that is therefore difficult to measure (de Menezes, Corrêa, e Silva, & da Cruz, 2015).

Clinical reasoning is discipline specific and applied in clinical settings. In nursing, clinical reasoning involves the process of evaluating the quantity, quality, and reliability of available evidence; analyzing and evaluating patient information; and making professional judgments about patient management. Effective clinical reasoning, like the more general process of critical thinking, is dependent on a deep understanding of the context of a particular patient. It is the ability to reason as clinical situations change, grasping the nature of patients' needs as they change over time (Benner, Sutphen, Leonard, & Day, 2010). Clinical experience of appropriate duration, diversity, and quality is crucial for developing nursing students' clinical reasoning (de Menezes et al., 2015).

Clinical Decision Making

Professional nursing practice requires nurses to make decisions about patient care involving problems, possible solutions, and the best approach to use in a particular situation. Other decisions involve managing the clinical environment, care delivery, and other activities (Oermann & Gaberson, 2017). The decision-making process involves gathering, analyzing, weighing, and valuing information in order to choose the best course of action from among a number of alternatives. However, nurses rarely know all possible alternatives, benefits, and risks; thus, clinical decision making usually involves some degree of uncertainty.

Clinical decision making should be guided by national standards of nursing practice such as the American Nurses Association *Scope and Standards of Practice* (2015b), specialty organization evidence-based practice (EBP) guidelines such as the Association of periOperative Registered Nurses *Guidelines for Perioperative Practice* (2017), and health care organization standards of care, policies and procedures, and critical paths (Alfaro-LeFevre, 2017). However, an essential element of decision making is recognizing when such standards and guidelines are not relevant to the particular clinical context (Alfaro-LeFevre, 2017). Decisions are also influenced by an individual's values and biases and by cultural norms, which affect the way the individual perceives and analyzes the situation. In nursing, clinical decision making is mutual and participatory with patients and staff members so that the decisions are more likely to be accepted. Clinical learning activities should involve learners in many realistic decision-making opportunities to produce this outcome.

Psychomotor Domain Outcomes

Skills are another important outcome of clinical learning. Nurses must possess adequate psychomotor, communication, technological, and organizational skills to practice effectively in an increasingly complex health care environment. Skills often have cognitive and attitudinal dimensions, but the skill outcomes that must be produced by clinical teaching typically focus on the performance component.

Psychomotor Skills

Psychomotor skills are integral to nursing practice, and any deficiency in these skills among new graduates often leads to criticism of nursing education programs. Psychomotor skills enable nurses to perform effectively in action situations that require neuromuscular coordination. These skills are purposeful, complex, movement-oriented activities that involve an overt physical response. The term *skill* refers to the ability to carry out physical movements efficiently and effectively, with speed and accuracy. Therefore, psychomotor skill is more than the capability to perform; it includes the ability to perform proficiently, smoothly, and consistently under varying conditions and within appropriate time limits. Psychomotor skill learning requires practice with feedback in order to refine performance until the desired outcome is achieved. Thus, clinical learning activities should include plentiful opportunities for practice of psychomotor skills with knowledge of results to facilitate the skill-learning process.

However, psychomotor skill development involves more than technical proficiency. While performing technical skills, nursing students and staff members must also perform caring behaviors, critical thinking, clinical reasoning, problem solving, and clinical decision making. However, the ability to integrate all of these competencies at once is not usually achieved until the technical skill component is so well developed that it no longer requires the nurse's or nursing student's conscious attention for successful performance. It is only at this point that the learner sees the whole picture and is able to focus on the patient as well as the technical skill performance.

Interpersonal Skills

Interpersonal skills are used throughout the nursing process to assess patient and family needs, plan and implement care, evaluate the outcomes of care, and record and disseminate information. These skills include communication abilities, therapeutic use of self, and using the teaching process. Interpersonal skills involve knowledge of human behavior and social systems, but there is also a motor component largely comprising verbal behavior, such as speaking and writing, and nonverbal behavior, such as facial expression, body posture and movement, and touch. To encourage development of these outcomes, clinical learning activities should provide opportunities for students to form therapeutic relationships with patients; to develop collaborative relationships with other health professionals; to document patient information, plans of care, care given, and evaluation results; and to teach patients, family members, and staff members individually and in groups.

Organizational Skills

Nurses need organization and time management skills to practice competently in a complex environment. In clinical practice, students learn how to set priorities, manage conflicting expectations, and sequence their work to perform efficiently.

One organizational skill that has become an important job expectation for professional nurses is delegation. In most health care settings, patient care is provided by a mix of licensed and unlicensed assistive personnel, and professional nurses must know how to delegate various aspects of patient care to others. "When certain aspects of nursing care need to be delegated beyond the traditional role and assignments of a care provider, it is imperative that the delegation process and the state nurse practice act . . . be clearly understood so that it is safely and effectively carried out" (NCSBN, 2016). Nurses need to know both the theory and skill of delegation—what to delegate, to whom, and under what circumstances—and to understand the legal aspects of empowering another person to carry out delegated tasks. However, students will not learn these skills unless they are given opportunities to practice them with faculty guidance. They need to learn to communicate clearly what is to be done; why, when, and how it should be done; and expectations for response or report back to the delegator. As discussed in Chapter 7, if clinical learning assignments focus exclusively on total patient care activities, students will not gain enough experience in carrying out this delegation responsibility to perform it competently as graduates.

Nursing faculty members, clinical teachers, and administrators and staff members in clinical facilities should provide opportunities for nursing students to understand delegation as a skill set that must be practiced to be performed competently (American Nurses Association and NCSBN, n.d.). These skills may be initially developed in simulation activities. Debriefing after the simulation should focus not only on students' performance of delegation skills, but also on the clinical judgment process that resulted in the decision to delegate the work of others during the simulation and the effect that the simulated delegation would have had on clinical and financial outcomes (Weydt, 2010).

Depending on the level of the learner (graduate or undergraduate student), clinical activities also provide opportunities to develop leadership and management skills. These skills include the ability to manage the care of a group of patients, to evaluate the performance of self and others, to allocate and coordinate resources, to work as part of a health care team, to ensure patient safety and quality of care, and to manage one's own career development. Clinical teachers may model these skills to students as well as encourage staff members in the clinical setting to do so. Examples of modeling opportunities include serving on a unit or institution-wide practice committee, demonstrating how to deal with a safety concern or health care error (Adelman-Mulally et al., 2012), and how to delegate effectively, as previously described. Because such activities are not always visible to nursing students in clinical settings, clinical teachers and staff members should discuss aloud the rationale for their decisions and actions with students, intentionally making the thinking process more apparent (Adelman-Mulally et al., 2012).

Affective Domain Outcomes

Clinical learning also produces important affective outcomes—beliefs, values, attitudes, and dispositions that are essential elements of professional nursing practice (Oermann & Gaberson, 2017). Affective outcomes represent the humanistic and ethical dimensions of nursing. Professional nurses are expected to hold and act on certain values with regard to patient care, such as respect for the patient's uniqueness, supporting patient autonomy and right to choose, and the confidentiality of patient information. The values of professional nursing are expressed in the American Nurses Association *Code of Ethics for Nurses* (2015a), and the nursing faculty should introduce the code early in any nursing education program and reinforce its values by planning clinical learning activities that help students to develop them.

Additionally, professional nurses must be able to use the processes of moral reasoning, values clarification, and values inquiry. In an era of rapid knowledge and technology growth, nursing education programs must also produce graduates who are lifelong learners, committed to their own continued professional development.

According to Benner et al. (2010), professional nursing role formation is the process of developing a professional identity and sense of self as a member of the profession, taking on the social role and responsibility, and accepting the nurse's moral agency and advocacy role. Professional role formation occurs at every level of nursing education: in initial preparation for nursing, when entering into the work setting as a new graduate, when returning to school for an advanced degree, and when changing roles within nursing.

Students form the role of professional nurse in the clinical setting, where accountability is demanded and the consequences of choices and actions are readily apparent. The clinical setting provides opportunities for students to develop, practice, and test these affective outcomes. Clinical education should expose students to strong role models, including nursing faculty members and practicing nurses who demonstrate a commitment to professional values, and it should provide value development opportunities that serve to support role formation.

Integrated Domain Outcomes

Although in the previous discussion we attempted to classify outcomes according to cognitive, psychomotor, or affective domain, some intended outcomes of clinical learning include elements of all three domains. Two examples are cultural competence and health care quality and patient safety competence.

The U.S. population is becoming increasingly multicultural. Based on the 2014 population projections, by the year 2060, the percentage of non-Hispanic White Americans will fall from 62% to 42%. The percentage of Blacks or African Americans is expected to increase from 13% to 14%, and the percentage of Americans of Asian origin will increase from 5% to 9%. The population of Americans of Hispanic origin is projected to increase from 17% to 29% (Colby & Ortman, 2015). To respond competently to these demographic changes, nursing students must be prepared to deal with diversity in all of its forms (Hines-Martin & Pack, 2009). The AACN Advisory Group on the Competencies for Cultural Competency in Baccalaureate Nursing Education's (2008) rationale for the integration of cultural competence in baccalaureate nursing education is to support the development of patient-centered care that identifies, respects, and addresses differences in patients' values, preferences, and expressed needs. This rationale includes a focus on eliminating health disparities, achieving social justice for vulnerable populations, and functioning in a global environment and in partnership with other health care disciplines.

Cultural competence has no specific end point; it can be understood as an ongoing developmental process by which nurses understand, appreciate, and incorporate cultural expressions and worldviews into the care of patients and interactions with other health care providers. The development of cultural competence begins with awareness of cultural diversity and specific knowledge about cultural values, beliefs, rules, and traditions of the nurse's own culture. A concept related to cultural awareness is that of cultural humility, the belief that one's own culture is not the only or best one. Cultural humility cannot be learned only in the classroom; it requires experience with culturally diverse patients over time and reflection on those experiences (Schuessler, Wilder, & Byrd, 2012).

Promoting culturally competent care is a priority in nursing and in nursing education (Mareno & Hart, 2014). Therefore, clinical teachers should plan learning activities that will challenge learners to explore cultural differences and to develop culturally appropriate responses to patient needs.

Health Care Quality and Patient Safety Competencies

An important set of outcomes of clinical teaching is evidence-based interprofessional practice within a quality improvement (QI) and patient safety framework. Competencies in quality and safety science are an important part of curricula to prepare all health care professionals. In nursing, the QSEN project was initiated in 2005 to transform health care by "addressing the challenge of preparing future nurses with the knowledge, skills, and attitudes necessary to continuously improve the quality and safety of the healthcare systems in which they work" (QSEN, 2014c). The knowledge, skills, and attitudes (KSAs) necessary to deliver safe, quality care are related to six QSEN competencies: patient-centered care, teamwork and collaboration, EBP, QI, safety, and informatics (QSEN, 2014c). These competencies have been integrated into prelicensure and graduate nursing education programs as well as nurse residency programs.

The patient-centered care competency is defined as "Recogniz[ing] the patient or designee as the source of control and full partner in providing compassionate and coordinated care based on respect for patient's preferences, values, and needs" (QSEN, 2014b). QSEN prelicensure KSAs related to this competency include describing cultural, ethnic, and social backgrounds as sources of patient, family, and community values; providing care with respect for the diversity of human experience; and supporting care for patients whose values differ from one's own (QSEN, 2014b). KSAs for graduate students include integrating knowledge of multiple models of pain and suffering; assessing and treating pain and suffering based on patient values, preferences, and expressed needs; and valuing the patient's expertise with his or her own health (QSEN, 2014a). Development of these KSAs can be facilitated through actual and simulated learning activities that allow learners to reflect on their experiences to identify gaps between current practice and practice that is informed by patient needs, values, and preferences.

Teamwork and collaboration is defined as "Function[ing] effectively within nursing and interprofessional teams, fostering open communication, mutual respect, and shared decision-making to achieve quality patient care" (QSEN, 2014b). KSAs related to this competency for prelicensure students include describing scope of practice and roles of health care team members, functioning competently within one's own scope of practice as a team member, and respecting the centrality of the patient as a member of the health care team (QSEN, 2014b). Graduate student KSAs include identifying system barriers and facilitators of team effectiveness, participating in the creation and implementation of systems that support effective teamwork, and valuing the impact of system solutions on team functioning (QSEN, 2014a). Clinical learning activities in settings that offer natural opportunities to function as members of existing interprofessional teams, such as the operating room, promote acquisition of these KSAs.

The definition of EBP is "Integrat[ing] best current evidence with clinical expertise and patient/family preferences and values for delivery of optimal health care" (QSEN, 2014b). For this competency, prelicensure KSAs include describing reliable sources of evidence reports and clinical practice guidelines, consulting with clinical experts before deviating from evidence-based protocols, and valuing the need for continuous practice improvement based on new knowledge (QSEN, 2014b). Graduate student KSAs include determining evidence gaps within specialty practice, using efficient and effective search techniques to answer clinical questions, and valuing the need for ethical performance of research and QI (QSEN, 2014a). Depending on the level of the student, clinical learning activities provide rich opportunities to learn to deliver quality care based on reliable evidence and clinical guidelines for generalist or specialty nursing practice.

QI is defined as "Us[ing] data to monitor the outcomes of care processes and use improvement methods to design and test changes to continuously improve the quality and safety of health care systems" (QSEN, 2014b). KSAs related to this competency for prelicensure students include explaining the merit of measurement and variation in assessing quality of care, contributing to a root cause analysis of a sentinel event; and appreciating the impact of unwanted variation on patient care (QSEN, 2014b). For graduate students, KSAs include describing common quality measures in specialty practice, assuring ethical management of QI projects, and valuing the role of measurement in quality patient care (QSEN, 2014a). Nursing faculty members should create clinical learning opportunities for students to collect data or use existing data to monitor quality of care, and to participate in or conduct QI projects, depending on the level of student.

The safety competency is defined as "Minimiz[ing] risk of harm to patients and providers through both system effectiveness and individual performance" (QSEN, 2014b). Prelicensure KSAs include describing factors that produce a culture of safety, using strategies to reduce reliance on memory, and valuing one's own role in error prevention (QSEN, 2014b). Graduate student KSAs related to this competency include describing best practices for promoting patient and provider safety specialty practice, employing a systems focus rather than individual blame when errors or close calls occur, and valuing the use of organizational error reporting systems (QSEN, 2014a). Nursing faculties should model the safety competency by "appreciat[ing] the cognitive and physical limits of human performance" (QSEN, 2014a), creating a just culture within their nursing education programs, and encouraging students to be forthcoming about and to learn from their errors and close calls. Planning clinical learning opportunities for students to use national patient safety resources in the clinical setting, partner with patients and their families to enhance safe care, and view patient safety through the lens of a total systems approach will facilitate their attainment of the safety KSAs (National Patient Safety Foundation, 2015).

The definition of the informatics competency is "Us[ing] information and technology to communicate, manage knowledge, mitigate error, and support decision making" (QSEN, 2014b). The growing use of electronic health records (EHRs) in various clinical settings requires students to have knowledge of this technology and at least a beginning ability to use EHRs to acquire patient information, use it to plan care, and document assessment findings and care given. The Institute of Medicine's report *The Future of Nursing: Leading Change, Advancing Health* (2011) stated the expectation that nurses "use a variety of technological tools and complex information management systems that require skills in analysis and synthesis to improve the quality and effectiveness of care." This expectation implies that in addition to knowing how to document care electronically, nursing students must understand the concept of meaningful use of health information and value the use of nursing terminologies and classification systems to codify nursing data. Related QSEN KSAs for prelicensure students include giving examples of how technology and information management relate to patient safety and quality of care, using the EHR to document and plan patient care, and appreciating the need to seek lifelong learning of information technology skills (QSEN, 2014b). Graduate student KSAs include critiquing taxonomic and terminology systems used to enhance interoperability of information and knowledge management systems, participating in the creation of clinical decision-making supports and alerts, and appreciating the need for collaboration in developing patient care information systems (QSEN, 2014a). The most effective way to attain these outcomes is to integrate health information technology learning throughout the curriculum instead of offering it in a single course (Skiba, 2010).

UNINTENDED OUTCOMES

Although nurse educators usually have intended outcomes in mind when they design clinical learning activities, those activities may produce positive or negative unintended outcomes as well. Positive unintended outcomes include career choices that students and new graduate nurses make when they have clinical experiences in various settings. Exposure to a wide variety of clinical specialties stimulates learners to evaluate their own desires and competence to practice in those areas and allows them to make realistic career choices. For example, nursing students who do not have clinical learning activities in an operating room are unlikely to choose perioperative nursing as a specialty. However, if students participate in clinical activities in the operating room, some will realize that they are well suited to practice nursing in this area, while others will decide that perioperative nursing is not for them. In either case, students will have a realistic basis for their career choices.

Clinical learning activities can produce negative unintended outcomes as well. Nurse educators often worry that students will learn bad practice habits from observing other nurses in the clinical environment. Often, students are taught to perform skills, document care, or organize their work based on reliable evidence, practice standards or guidelines, the instructor's preferences, or school or agency policy. However, students may observe staff members in the clinical setting who adapt skills, documentation, and organization of work to fit the unique needs of patients or the environment. Students often imitate the behaviors they observe, such as taking shortcuts and using work-arounds while performing skills, including omitting steps that the teacher may believe are important to produce safe, effective outcomes. The power of role models to influence students' behavior and attitudes should not be underestimated. However, the clinical teacher should be careful not to label the teacher's way as correct and all other ways as incorrect. Instead, the teacher should encourage learners to discuss the differences in practice habits that they have observed, evaluate them in terms of evidence for practice, and identify more positive role models.

Another negative unintended outcome of clinical learning may be academic dishonesty. Academic dishonesty is intentional participation in deceptive practices such as lying, cheating, or false representation regarding one's academic work. Clinical teachers often try to instill the traditional health care cultural value that good nurses do not make errors. Even though the Institute of Medicine's report on health care errors (Kohn, Corrigan, & Donaldson, 2000) has caused growing concern about patient safety and the need to prevent errors, a standard of perfection is unrealistic for any practitioner, let alone nursing students and new staff members whose mistakes are an inherent part of learning new knowledge and skills. A teacher's emphasis on perfection in clinical practice may produce the unintended result of student dishonesty to avoid punishment for making mistakes. Punishment for mistakes, in the form of low grades or negative performance evaluations, is not effective in preventing future errors. The unintended result of punishment for mistakes may be that learners conceal errors or lack of knowledge or skill; bluffing their way through tasks or failure to report errors can have dangerous consequences for patients in clinical settings and also creates lost opportunities for learners to learn to correct and then prevent their mistakes (Kohn et al., 2000). If the instructor has established a learning climate of mutual trust and respect, acknowledges the possibility of errors, and assures students of respectful treatment when they admit their inadequacies, students will be less likely to behave dishonestly (Adelman-Mulally et al., 2012). Nursing faculty members and clinical teachers must also be exemplary role models of academic and professional integrity for students (Adelman-Mulally et al., 2012; Tippit et al., 2009).

SUMMARY

Outcomes of clinical teaching include abilities in cognitive, psychomotor, and affective domains that are acquired through clinical teaching and learning. Current nursing education program accreditation criteria focus on evidence that meaningful outcomes of learning have been produced. The effectiveness of clinical teaching can be judged on the extent to which it produces intended learning outcomes.

Clinical learning activities should focus on the development of *knowledge* that cannot be acquired in the classroom or other learning settings. In clinical practice, knowledge is applied to practice. In addition to understanding specific information, higher-level knowledge outcomes include cognitive skill in problem solving, critical thinking, clinical decision making, and clinical reasoning. *Problem solving* ability is an important outcome of clinical teaching. Problems related to patients or the health care environment are typically unique, complex, and ambiguous and often require new methods of reasoning and problem-solving strategies. *Critical thinking* is a process used to determine a course of action after collecting appropriate data, analyzing the validity and utility of the information, evaluating multiple lines of reasoning, and coming to valid conclusions. Critical thinking is facilitated by attitudinal dimensions of self-confidence, maturity, and inquisitiveness. Clinical learning activities help learners to develop discipline-specific critical thinking and *clinical reasoning* skills as they observe, participate in, and evaluate nursing care. *Clinical decision making* involves gathering, analyzing, weighing, and valuing information in order to choose the best course of action from among a number of alternatives. Because nurses rarely know all possible alternatives, benefits, and risks, clinical decision making usually involves some degree of uncertainty. Clinical education should involve learners in realistic situations that require them to make decisions about patients, staff members, and the clinical environment in order to produce this outcome.

Psychomotor skills are another important outcome of clinical learning. Many skills have cognitive and attitudinal dimensions, but clinical teaching typically focuses on the performance component. Psychomotor skill includes the ability to perform proficiently, smoothly, and consistently under varying conditions and within appropriate time limits. *Interpersonal skills* are used to assess client needs, plan and implement patient care, evaluate the outcomes of care, and record and disseminate information. These skills include communication, therapeutic use of self, and teaching patients and others. Interpersonal skills involve knowledge of human behavior and social systems, but there is also a motor component largely comprising verbal and nonverbal behavior. Nurses need *organizational skills* in order to set priorities, manage conflicting expectations, sequence their work to perform efficiently, and delegate nursing tasks to others appropriately. Clinical learning activities provide opportunities for learners to develop leadership and management skills.

Clinical learning also produces important affective outcomes that represent the humanistic and ethical dimensions of nursing. Professional nurses are expected to hold and act on certain values with regard to patient care and to use the processes of moral reasoning, values clarification, and values inquiry. These values are developed and internalized through the process of professional role formation. In an era of rapid knowledge and technological growth, nursing education programs must also produce graduates who are lifelong learners, committed to their own continued professional development.

One example of an outcome that encompasses all three domains is cultural competence. Cultural competence is the ability to provide care that fits the cultural beliefs and practices of patients. This outcome includes understanding and appreciating the similarities and differences between the nurse's and patients' cultures and incorporating cultural expressions and viewpoints into patient care.

Health care quality and patient safety competencies also encompass all three domains. The QSEN competencies are useful for preparing future nurses with the KSAs needed to continuously improve quality of care and safety of health care systems. The QSEN competencies include patient-centered care, teamwork and collaboration, EBP, QI, safety, and informatics. Examples of KSAs for prelicensure and graduate nursing students were provided. The importance of clinical learning activities designed to promote attainment of the competencies was discussed.

Clinical learning activities also produce unintended positive and negative outcomes. Exposure to a wide variety of clinical specialties stimulates learners to evaluate their own desires and competence to practice in those areas and allows them to make realistic career choices. However, observing various role models in the clinical environment may result in students' learning bad practice habits. The unintended result of a teacher's unrealistic emphasis on perfection in clinical practice may be academically dishonest behavior among students, such as concealing lack of knowledge or skill or failing to report errors, both with potentially dangerous consequences.

CNE EXAMINATION TEST BLUEPRINT CORE COMPETENCIES

1. **Facilitate Learning**

   A. Implement a variety of teaching strategies appropriate to
      5. Desired learner outcomes
   G. Model reflective thinking practices, including critical thinking
   H. Create opportunities for learners to develop their own critical thinking skills
   I. Create a positive learning environment that fosters a free exchange of ideas
   J. Show enthusiasm for teaching, learning, and the nursing profession that inspires and motivates students
   K. Demonstrate personal attributes that facilitate learning (e.g., caring, confidence, patience, integrity, respect, and flexibility)
   P. Act as a role model in practice settings

2. **Facilitate Learner Development and Socialization**

   D. Create learning environments that facilitate learners' self-reflection, personal goal setting, and socialization to the role of the nurse
   E. Foster the development of learners in these areas
      1. cognitive domain
      2. psychomotor domain
      3. affective domain
   G. Encourage professional development of learners

REFERENCES

Adelman-Mulally, T., Mulder, C. K., McCarter-Spalding, D. E., Hagler, D. A., Gaberson, K. B., Hanner, M. B., . . . Young, P. K. (2012). The clinical nurse educator as leader. *Nurse Education in Practice, 13*, 29–34. doi:10.1016/j.nepr.2012.07.006

Alfaro-LeFevre, R. (2017). *Critical thinking, clinical reasoning, and clinical judgment: A practical approach* (6th ed.). Philadelphia, PA: Elsevier.

American Association of Colleges of Nursing. (2006). *The essentials of doctoral education for advanced nursing practice.* Washington, DC: Author. Retrieved from http://www.aacn.nche.edu/publications/position/DNPEssentials.pdf

American Association of Colleges of Nursing. (2008). *The essentials of baccalaureate education for professional nursing practice.* Retrieved from http://www.aacn.nche.edu/education-resources/BaccEssentials08.pdf

American Association of Colleges of Nursing. (2011). *The essentials of master's education in nursing.* Washington, DC: Author. Retrieved from http://www.aacn.nche.edu/education-resources/MastersEssentials11.pdf

American Association of Colleges of Nursing Advisory Group on the Competencies for Cultural Competency in Baccalaureate Nursing Education. (2008). Cultural competency in baccalaureate nursing education. Retrieved from http://www.aacn.nche.edu/leading-initiatives/education-resources/competency.pdf

American Association of Colleges of Nursing QSEN Education Consortium. (2012). *Graduate-level QSEN competencies: Knowledge, skills, and attitudes.* Retrieved from http://www.aacn.nche.edu/faculty/qsen/competencies.pdf

American Nurses Association. (2015a). *Code of ethics for nurses with interpretive statements.* Retrieved from http://nursingworld.org/DocumentVault/Ethics-1/Code-of-Ethics-for-Nurses.html

American Nurses Association. (2015b). *Nursing: Scope and standards of practice* (3rd ed.). Silver Spring, MD: Author.

American Nurses Association and National Council of State Boards of Nursing. (n.d.). *Joint statement on delegation.* Retrieved from https://www.ncsbn.org/Delegation_joint_statement_NCSBN-ANA.pdf

Association of periOperative Registered Nurses. (2017). *Guidelines for perioperative practice.* Denver, CO: Author.

Benner, P., Sutphen, M., Leonard, V., & Day, L. (2010). *Educating nurses: A call for radical transformation.* San Francisco, CA: Jossey-Bass.

Colby, S. L., & Ortman, J. M. (2015). *Projections of the size and composition of the U.S. population: 2014 to 2060* (Report No. P25-1143). Retrieved from https://www.census.gov/content/dam/Census/library/publications/2015/demo/p25-1143.pdf

de Menezes, S. S. C., Corrêa, C. G., e Silva, R. de C. G., & da Cruz, D. de A. M. L. (2015). Clinical reasoning in undergraduate nursing education: A scoping review. *Revista da Escola de Enfermagem da USP, 49,* 1032–1039.

Institute of Medicine. (2011). *The future of nursing: Leading change, advancing health.* Washington, DC: National Academies Press.

Iwasiw, C. L., & Goldenberg, D. M. (2014). *Curriculum development in nursing education* (3rd ed.). Burlington, MA: Jones & Bartlett Learning.

Kohn, L., Corrigan, J., & Donaldson, M. (2000). *To err is human: Building a safer health system.* Washington, DC: National Academies Press, Institute of Medicine.

Mareno, N., & Hart, P. L. (2014). Cultural competency among nurses with undergraduate and graduate degrees: Implications for nursing education. *Nursing Education Perspectives, 35,* 83–88.

Nardi, D., & Gyurko, C. C. (2013). The global nursing faculty shortage: Status and solutions for change. *Journal of Nursing Scholarship, 45,* 317–326.

National Council of State Boards of Nursing. (2015). *Test plan for the National Council Licensure Examination for registered nurses.* Retrieved from https://www.ncsbn.org/RN_Test_Plan_2016_Final.pdf

National Council of State Boards of Nursing. (2016). National guidelines for nursing delegation. *Journal of Nursing Regulation, 7,* 5–12. Retrieved from https://www.ncsbn.org/NCSBN_Delegation_Guidelines.pdf

National Patient Safety Foundation. (2015). *Free from harm: Accelerating patient safety improvement fifteen years after "To err is human".* Boston, MA: Author.

Newton, S. E., & Moore, G. (2013). Critical thinking skills of basic baccalaureate and accelerated second-degree nursing students. *Nursing Education Perspectives, 34,* 154–158.

Oermann, M. H., & Gaberson, K. B. (2017). *Evaluation and testing in nursing education* (5th ed.). New York, NY: Springer Publishing.

Quality and Safety Education for Nurses Institute. (2014a). *Graduate QSEN competencies.* Retrieved from http://qsen.org/competencies/graduate-ksas

Quality and Safety Education for Nurses Institute. (2014b). *Pre-licensure KSAs.* Retrieved from http://qsen.org/competencies/pre-licensure-ksas

Quality and Safety Education for Nurses Institute. (2014c). *Project overview: The evolution of the Quality and Safety Education for Nurses initiative.* Retrieved from http://qsen.org/about-qsen/project-overview

Schuessler, J. B., Wilder, B., & Byrd, L. W. (2012). Reflective journaling and development of cultural humility in students. *Nursing Education Perspectives, 33,* 96–99.

Simmons, B. (2010). Clinical reasoning: Concept analysis. *Journal of Advanced Nursing, 66,* 1151–1158.

Skiba, D. (2010). The future of nursing and the informatics agenda. *Nursing Education Perspectives, 31,* 390–391.

Tippit, M. P., Ard, N., Kline, J. R., Tilghman, B. C., Chamberlain, B., & Meagher, P. G. (2009). Creating environments that foster academic integrity. *Nursing Education Perspectives, 30,* 239–244.

Weydt, A. (2010). Developing delegation skills. *The Online Journal of Issues in Nursing, 15*(2), Manuscript 1. Retrieved from http://nursingworld.org/MainMenuCategories/ANAMarketplace/ANAPeriodicals/OJIN/TableofContents/Vol152010/No2May2010/Delegation-Skills.aspx

CHAPTER 3

Developing Clinical Learning Sites

Nursing care occurs in diverse settings where there are patients (individuals, families, groups, and communities) who can benefit from the services of a professional nurse. Professional nurses assume multiple roles as they work with patients of all ages, races, ethnic groups, and cultures. These patients have the full scope of health promotion; health maintenance; and acute, chronic, and rehabilitation care needs.

In an ideal world, all nursing students would have clinical learning activities in all settings, with all patient populations, and in all professional nursing roles, and they would be prepared to adapt to rapid changes with patients, health issues, care locations, and approaches to care. Students would have opportunities to work with people from cultures other than their own and implement care that recognizes the global influences on both health and illness.

Nursing education does not exist in such an ideal world. All students cannot participate in every learning activity, nor can every student provide care for all these diverse groups during their nursing education. Faculty must make difficult choices about clinical education with the hope that the breadth and depth of students' clinical learning activities result in the development of the core competencies and skills needed for safe and effective nursing practice. For students who are already licensed nurses, their clinical experiences must help them grow as professionals as they move to more advanced levels of practice.

The traditional approach to clinical nursing education involves a faculty member working with a group of students (approximately 6–12, although this can vary from program to program), typically on an acute care unit in a hospital, for a portion of a clinical shift. This approach, while frequently used in nursing education, may provide an unpredictable, rapidly changing, and haphazard learning environment (O'Connor, 2015). Factors such as changing patient census, variable diagnoses and acuity of patients, diverse care needs, and staffing issues impact the learning opportunities during clinical practice. Because of the high patient acuity and complexity, many sites do not permit achievement of the full scope of clinical learning objectives. Collaboration with other disciplines, acting as a change agent, being a patient advocate, and the development of many key assessment and psychomotor skills can be difficult in a setting where all patients are critically ill. Because of the increasingly specialized nature of many acute care units (e.g., cardiovascular, orthopedic, and endocrine), it is challenging for students to see a broad scope of patient problems when they have a finite number of clinical hours and a predetermined schedule. Additionally, due to decreasing length of inpatient stays and economic pressures to provide care in outpatient and community settings, limited (and, in some cases, decreased) numbers of clinical learning activities take place on hospital units that provide care for children, individuals with psychiatric illnesses, and women and families during pregnancy and childbirth. Even with these challenges, faculty may still believe that traditional rotations through medical specialty areas with specific numbers of clinical hours in those areas were important. However, they may also include observation experiences and use of a wide variety of alternative settings without clinical teachers directly present to oversee patient care.

Even when traditional acute care placements are appropriate, implementing clinical learning activities in such settings can be challenging. High demand for clinical placements from nursing education programs (often with rapidly increasing enrollments) and other health professional programs have overwhelmed many acute care agencies. Both staff members and patients can be asked to interact with students 24 hours a day, 7 days a week. As a result, acute care agencies often place limitations on the numbers of students per unit or the days and times that students can be present. In some cases, the mandated clinical group size is so limited that some students in a clinical group must be scheduled for observation activities elsewhere so that fewer students are present on the unit. In other cases, the group size has to be kept very small, a remedy that is usually neither economically feasible nor ideal for learning and meeting the educational goals of the course and the program. Engaging in these alternate clinical observation activities may decrease students' opportunity to actively participate in learning the professional nursing role and may also consume the time and resources of staff in these other areas. Faculty members must evaluate the appropriateness of these observation activities, address concerns about student guidance in the absence of a clinical instructor, and support staff members as they encounter different students arriving for observation activities each day.

The rapidly rising cost of health care in acute care settings and the demand for safe, quality care has led to the examination of health care delivery at a national level. The Institute of Medicine's (2011) report, *The Future of Nursing: Leading Change, Advancing Health* encourages the transformation of the health care system from acute care to community settings. Changing health care policies and regulations may overhaul health care access that will ultimately affect nursing and nursing education. Lastly, Benner, Sutphen, Leonard, and Day (2009) reported that more than 50% of nurses work outside the hospital setting, yet a large portion of student learning still takes place in acute care clinical settings. They recommended increasing the variety of clinical settings to allow for a broader scope of experience for students. These widely referenced and respected sources continue to draw national attention to nursing education and should encourage nursing faculty members to continually reexamine clinical nursing education and consider alternate settings for some portion of student clinical learning experiences.

As health care is increasingly delivered in nonacute care settings, clinical learning opportunities in these settings is also increased. Thus, while surgery was once performed almost exclusively in hospitals, many patients now have procedures in freestanding surgical centers. Patients once spent weeks recovering in hospitals after surgery or while recovering from trauma; they now recover at rehabilitation facilities or at home. No longer do patients who need long-term parenteral therapy or antibiotics stay in an inpatient facility. Full management of their care is carried out by nurses working in rehabilitation, long-term care, and home health settings.

Another driving force for the use of diverse settings for clinical learning is a call to increase the global and cultural competencies of graduates of nursing education programs. Major nursing organizations have issued guidelines and suggested competencies for nursing students and programs to develop needed knowledge and development of culturally competent practice (American Association of Colleges of Nursing, 2008; National League for Nursing, 2017). Clinical learning experiences need to support the development of graduates who can provide culturally responsive care and practice from a global perspective. Examples of these experiences include:

- Participation in a cultural immersion experience
- Participation in community projects involving community members—for example, health fairs, community forums and meetings, and the like—to understand concerns, values, and beliefs about health care
- Participation in or attendance at cultural celebrations or religious ceremonies
- Development of partnerships with community organizations such as churches, businesses, schools, or community groups serving vulnerable populations
- Service-learning opportunities working with populations such as immigrants, migrants, underserved, or indigenous groups

Clinical learning activities in diverse settings help to achieve these goals.

REIMAGINING CLINICAL LEARNING SETTINGS

Nursing care can be learned wherever students have contact with patients. Learning objectives do not prescribe a specific setting where the learning activities must take place. The core components of a clinical learning activity can be present in settings other than acute care hospital units and might include patient contact; opportunities for students to have an active role in assessment, goal setting, and then planning, implementing, and evaluating care; clinical reasoning and problem-solving opportunities; competent guidance (from the clinical teacher or someone designated to take on the teaching role in that site); and skill development (intellectual as well as psychomotor).

Benefits

Reimagining and transforming clinical placements for nursing students have multiple benefits. These include preparing students to be a part of a health care system in which the acute care hospital is but one part. Not only will students learn about the varied settings in which health care is provided, but they will also have opportunities to develop skills that these settings are best able to provide. For example, development of a psychomotor skill such as initiation of intravenous therapy, including the clinical assessment and decision-making skills that go with this routine procedure, might be best learned in a perioperative setting. Development of therapeutic communication competencies might be best achieved in rehabilitation settings where it is possible to have sustained patient contact. The best opportunities to learn care planning, evaluation, and revision might be available in a home health setting where multidisciplinary care planning is fully integrated into patient services. The home health setting also lends itself to the development of collaboration skills as well as real-world knowledge about the impact of payer status and insurance reimbursement on the ability of the patient to pay for (and, in many cases, receive) needed care.

Clinical learning activities in community-based settings allow nursing students to work with patients where they live and work. Students see the challenges that patients face as they implement self-care for health promotion and maintenance, as well as see the impact on family members. Collaboration with other members of the health care team is a natural, necessary, and active part of care delivery in community-based settings.

Nursing students can participate in creatively designed, rigorous, high-quality clinical learning activities almost anywhere. This chapter discusses clinical learning opportunities in underused patient care sites, community-based sites, distant sites, and international settings. It also reviews various practical aspects of implementing clinical learning activities in these settings by addressing common agency, faculty, and student problems and suggesting solutions for such problems.

EXAMPLES OF DIVERSE CLINICAL LEARNING SETTINGS

Clinical learning activities in diverse settings include opportunities for students to meet specific learning objectives while caring for patients. Four categories will be used as examples of such activities. The first consists of patient care areas that are not used regularly as clinical learning sites. Some of these patient care sites (e.g., the operating room [OR]) have been virtually eliminated as clinical learning sites by nursing education programs, while others (e.g., outpatient clinics, nursing homes) are underused, despite the rich learning opportunities provided for students in these settings. The second category includes community-based sites where provision of health care may not be the prime focus of the site or agency but provide learning opportunities for clinical nursing students. Examples are schools, camps, senior citizen programs, and housing complexes. An example of learning activities in community-based sites is service learning. Chapter 7 provides more information on planning high-quality service learning activities. With the growth of technology and online nursing education, distance sites provide a third category of diverse clinical learning opportunities. The fourth category is the growing use of international clinical learning activities. Although these learning opportunities may be brief (often 1 week), students gain valuable experiences in diverse international settings while serving as part of a team providing health services.

There are other clinical learning activities not included in this discussion. One is an observation in which students' objectives are best achieved while they maintain a nonparticipant role in the clinical setting. Another is a special event held as part of a clinical rotation (such as a trip to an art gallery or attending a play), designed to help students increase a specific skill, competency, or self-awareness. Also, clinical observations and interactions that are part of a didactic course are not included. Although potentially valuable as learning activities, riding in an ambulance with emergency medical service providers or visiting a hospital, clinic, or patient group as part of a course (whether at home or in another country) is not a clinical learning activity if there is no patient care in which the student participates.

CLINICAL LEARNING IN UNDERUSED PATIENT CARE SITES

With the diversity of clinical practice sites, there are many examples of clinical learning activities in underused patient care sites. Several examples will be used to illustrate how such sites can be optimized.

Outpatient Clinics

Outpatient settings such as primary care practices, specialty clinics, and rehabilitation programs are often difficult to use effectively as clinical learning sites because of the lack of RN role models and the difficulty placing large numbers of students at one site, which can make clinical teaching by the faculty difficult. This can be addressed through placement of students in a single large clinical facility. Major medical centers may have multiple specialty clinics and centers that allow students to participate in a multidisciplinary approach to patient care that may be focused on specific problems. For example, clinics that focus on pain management, wounds, gastroenterology, women's health, behavioral and mental health, diabetes, rehabilitation and sport medicine, and others may be appropriate for student learning. Students will have opportunities to engage in assessment, teaching, and delivery of focused care while interacting with a wide range of health care providers. Nursing staff members provide mentoring of the students while clinical teachers are available onsite and provide regular supervisory visits. Student–teacher conferencing activities allow for an assessment of student learning as well as an opportunity for students to ask questions. Group conferencing with several clinical nursing students can be used to share experiences with other students and enable them to make comparisons and contrasts between the learning settings, the care provided, and the patients seen.

OR and Other Perioperative Settings

Most nursing education programs eliminated an OR clinical rotation from their curricula many years ago, but in doing so, nursing faculties have overlooked many rich clinical learning opportunities. Many hospitalized patients for whom acute care nurses provide care pass though the OR at some time during their hospitalization. Knowledge about patients' surgical experiences can greatly enhance the knowledge and skills of the nurse caring for the patients both before and after surgery. The Association of periOperative Registered Nurses (AORN) reaffirmed their position advocating that all undergraduate professional nursing programs include learning activities in the perioperative setting (AORN, 2015). Perioperative environments are ideal settings for learning application of the nursing process, and perioperative clinical learning activities can contribute to the achievement of a wide variety of program outcomes. In addition to developing expected skills like aseptic technique, students see the use of the latest technology both in the surgical procedures and in the overall care of surgical patients. Possibly most important, students work with a team that demonstrates the interdisciplinary collaboration and communication essential for both safety and high-quality patient care in all settings (AORN, 2015). To help both perioperative staff members and clinical teachers implement such clinical learning activities, the AORN provides learning modules for perioperative experiences.

Nursing students can develop a wide array of psychomotor skills in perioperative settings, such as catheter care, insertion and maintenance of intravenous lines, pain management, skin and wound care, positioning, and care of unconscious patients. They also have opportunities to develop knowledge about legal–ethical issues, collaboration, time and resource management, and safety (Penprase, Monahan, Poly-Drouland, & Prechowski, 2016). Additionally, inclusion of perioperative learning activities in undergraduate nursing curricula will increase nurses' knowledge of patients' surgical experiences. It may also increase the number of nursing students who choose the perioperative specialty after graduation possibly helping to minimize the predicted shortage of nurses in the perioperative setting because "most graduate nurses seek employment in areas where they have had clinical experience" (Doroh & Monahan, 2016; Mott, 2012, Penprase et al., 2016).

Another way to include more perioperative clinical learning activities is with a practicum or capstone experience with preceptor guidance (Penprase et al., 2016). Such capstone courses allow students to apply knowledge and nursing principles learned from various courses throughout the program while being guided by an expert OR clinician. Lastly, ambulatory surgery centers are another related and underused patient care site that may be appropriate for clinical experiences for nursing students (Saunders, Singer, Dugmore, Seaman, & Lake, 2016).

Nursing Homes and Extended Care Facilities

Competency in the care of older adults, including frail elderly individuals, is a desired outcome of all nursing curricula. Given the growing aging population in the United States, almost all graduates will be caring for elderly patients, regardless of their future work setting. An underused clinical learning setting for gaining knowledge and competencies about care for the elderly is the nursing home or extended care facility.

Nursing homes provide an opportunity for students to practice multiple psychomotor skills and learn to provide long-term care to a single patient. In this setting, observation of changes over time is possible while caring for patients with complex needs. With a rich variety of patients, learning needs can be matched with clinical learning assignments as students provide holistic care while developing their health assessment, communication, leadership, and delegation skills with a wide range of residents (Lane & Hirst, 2012). Nursing homes provide many opportunities for students to practice implementing care that has a long-term impact. Bowel and urinary continence programs, programs to improve nutrition, and interventions to increase social interaction are a few examples of such activities.

Another benefit of student clinical learning in nursing homes is the opportunity to learn about the nursing role in improvement of care for the residents of the facility. Clinical teachers can serve as clinical experts and role models, and students have the time needed to implement and support programs that help patients achieve objectives that are hard to meet in today's rapidly changing acute health care environment. These settings also provide rich opportunities to learn and practice delegating nursing tasks to other licensed and unlicensed members of the care team.

There are some barriers to high-quality clinical learning experiences in nursing homes. One barrier is a negative attitude of some students toward elderly people, either preexisting or as a result of a previous nursing home experience. The clinical teacher's attitudes, approach, and active support can help prevent or address students' dislike of the experience (Brynildsen, Bjørk, Berntsen, & Hestetun, 2014). Another barrier facing clinical teachers in this setting is the lack of nursing role models. Clinical teachers can help overcome this concern by being positive role models themselves.

Therefore, it is important to have clinical teachers who are committed to providing quality care for elderly residents, have knowledge about the special needs of aging residents, know regulations impacting nursing homes, and are enthusiastic about caring for this group of patients.

Faculty members need to carefully consider the agency selected for this clinical learning experience. Because there can be wide variability in quality of care provided to residents from facility to facility, it is critical for the faculty to assess indicators of quality in nursing homes and select appropriately. One measure that may provide insight into quality of care is the adequacy of staffing. Evaluating the patterns of staff turnover and retention rates may help determine if the number of RNs and other staff members present during clinical hours is adequate to meet resident needs and to assist students (Mueller, Goering, Talley, & Zaccagnini, 2011). To provide information about other measures of nursing home quality, the Medicare website on nursing homes (www.medicare.gov/nursinghomecompare/search.html) presents reports about nursing home performance on indicators such as quality measures, staffing, and health inspections. This website supplies regular updates and overall ratings for over 15,000 Medicare- and Medicaid-certified nursing homes nationwide.

Once the quality of the nursing home is assessed, the teacher assigned to this clinical site should work on developing a partner relationship with the nursing home staff. This reciprocal relationship will help to build alliances and enable all staff members, teachers, and students to work collaboratively in delivering care, addressing patients' health care needs while providing relevant learning opportunities. Immersion at the clinical facility has been linked to satisfaction, thus Brynildsen et al. (2014) suggest a minimum of a 7-week clinical learning experience to receive maximum learning benefit and ensure student satisfaction. While at the clinical site, faculty need to actively support student learning as they confront care challenges and deal with a variety of social and emotional issues (Algoso, Peters, Ramjan, & East, 2016; Brynildsen et al., 2014). Students can use this experience to improve collaboration skills as they work with a wide variety of staff members, including nursing assistants, licensed practical or vocational nurses, RNs, physical therapists, occupational therapists, dieticians, social workers, and administrators. Lastly, clinical teachers should plan structured orientation programs that provide needed information to adequately prepare students, particularly for the social and clinical aspects they will encounter.

Hospice and Palliative Care

Competency in delivering end-of-life care is an expected student outcome of nursing education, yet many students may not have opportunities to develop skill in caring for these patients. It can be difficult to achieve these competencies in traditional cure-focused clinical settings where students have limited exposure and opportunity to interact with dying patients and their families. Clinical learning in hospice settings is an excellent way to expose students to the issues related to end-of-life care and to provide opportunities to develop many skills needed in all nursing roles and settings. Clinical teachers in community or mental health courses can work with hospice and palliative care providers to arrange for students to partner with hospice nurses and provide care to families receiving hospice services. Clinical teachers can use the End-of-Life Nursing Education Consortium (ELNEC) competencies to guide clinical educational experiences (American Association of Colleges of Nursing, 2013). Given the sensitive issues that arise during end-of-life care, it is important for clinical teachers to consider the emotional needs of students during these experiences and provide opportunities to discuss feelings. This can be accomplished through written reflective journals and conference activities. Faculty can structure clinical conferences to allow students to debrief, reflect, share their experiences, and discuss difficult topics (Bonnel, 2016).

CLINICAL LEARNING IN COMMUNITY-BASED CLINICAL SITES

Almost all patients cared for by nurses in the acute care setting come from and return to the community. In addition, many issues, particularly those related to health promotion and maintenance and management of chronic disease, are best addressed in community settings. Community settings also offer many learning opportunities for development of key skills and competencies that are hard to meet in the acute care environment. For these reasons, inclusion of community-based clinical learning activities in nursing curricula is important. Community-based learning activities are often implemented under the umbrella of service learning. In service learning, students work collaboratively with community partners to meet both course and community objectives. Reflection on the experience and development of a sense of civic engagement are essential components. See Chapter 7 for an in-depth discussion of service learning.

Community-based experiences can occur in a wide variety of settings. These include health departments, schools, home health agencies, camps, shelters, day care centers for children or senior citizens, prisons, clinics, and wellness centers where students complete a wide variety of nursing interventions. The following section provides further details about some of these community-based clinical learning sites.

Childcare Settings

Because childcare-center–based care is provided to about 61% of U.S. children between the ages of 3 and 6 (Federal Interagency Forum on Child and Family Statistics, 2016), this is an opportune site for clinical learning for nursing students. Childcare and early education programs such as Head Start offer many opportunities for nursing students to develop observation, developmental assessment, physical assessment, and teaching skills. Children in these settings have more frequent respiratory illnesses, gastrointestinal illness, and otitis media, thereby providing nursing students with opportunities to learn more about these common childhood conditions and develop health promotion and teaching projects (Crowley, Cianciolo, Krajicek, & Hawkins-Walsh, 2012). Nursing students in these childcare settings can learn to provide a range of health care services that will benefit the children, their families, and even the childcare staff.

Schools

Decreased inpatient pediatric census and improved preventative care have led to the reduction of clinical learning opportunities for nursing students, particularly in smaller community hospitals. When inpatient clinical practice sites are available for clinical experiences, nursing programs report competition with other nursing programs for these sites, resulting in a lack of direct care opportunities (McCarthy & Wyatt, 2014). Nontraditional community-based clinical learning sites such as schools are gaining popularity. School-based clinical learning activities provide excellent alternative opportunities for development of pediatric health assessment and promotion skills. This learning is enhanced if it takes place in the context of an ongoing program that demonstrates the principles of family-centered care and public health nursing rather than being a one-time event when the students drop into a school to provide sporadic care such as taking height and weight measurements or teaching tooth-brushing. Nursing students need to develop skills related to health promotion and well childcare, disease prevention, safety, nutrition, and growth and development. Schools provide ideal opportunities for nursing student development in these areas. Additionally, partnering with a school district for clinical experiences allows students to have learning opportunities involving assessment, teaching, as well as care for children with an array of acute and chronic health conditions. When working with a school, nursing students can also administer medications, practice developmentally appropriate communication, and collaborate with a variety of professionals within the school (Pohl, Jarvill, Adman, & Clark, 2017).

Camps

Another community-based site that can meet many clinical learning objectives, particularly those related to the care of children with acute and chronic illnesses, is a camp. Clinical learning activities in summer camps for children provide a rich learning opportunity for nursing students to learn about growth and development, use physical assessment skills, and manage illnesses and emergencies. Camps that focus on specific health problems or chronic illnesses, such as diabetes, asthma, cancer, or developmental delays, allow nursing students to learn about these health problems during this immersion experience at the camp. Students also develop communication skills, deliver clinical care, engage in interpersonal relationship building, and demonstrate social problem solving (Lau & Wang, 2014). So that they are adequately prepared for the experiences, students may need appropriate clinical clearances (as discussed later in this chapter) and they should also be familiar with the camper's typical health problems and common medications administered. Since camp nurse responsibilities occur around the clock, students need to be prepared to deliver nursing care at all hours of the day and night, and ultimately deal with the camp living conditions and fatigue that may occur. Clinical teachers who guide these learning activities need to provide opportunities for student reflection on their experience and appropriate mentoring during the experience.

Wellness Centers

Wellness centers or interprofessional clinics offer a creative alternative to traditional clinical learning sites. These centers allow nurses, alone or in collaboration with other health care providers, to manage health services that focus on health promotion, disease prevention, health education, and wellness. Typically, these wellness centers or clinics are located in the community in places such as public housing, community or recreation centers, homeless shelters, senior centers, storefronts, or churches where they serve vulnerable and underserved populations. Sometimes, clinical teachers or preceptors serve as clinicians for the site and teach nursing students there as well (Thompson & Bucher, 2013; Wang & Bhakta, 2013). Educators in this dual role as clinical teachers and care providers serve as powerful nursing role models for students, and their first-hand knowledge of the community enriches the students' learning experiences as well as allows them to advocate for the populations served. However, when this clinical model is used, nursing programs face the challenge of providing services during school breaks and holidays, and need to carefully plan programs and activities that are not disrupted by an interruption of services.

At these wellness centers and clinics, students have opportunities to address critical public health problems such as drug, nicotine, and alcohol addictions; stress and anxiety; and violence (National Nurse-Led Care Consortium, 2016). Students gain valuable experience assessing critical community and neighborhood issues and providing needed health services while establishing interprofessional relationships and advocating for those in underserved communities. They can design programs and provide holistic care to vulnerable individuals across the life span.

CLINICAL LEARNING AT DISTANT SITES

Distance education has become a respected and effective method of providing higher education in the United States. Allen and Seaman (2013) reported that 6.7 million students are learning online, with enrollments in online education growing at a substantially faster rate than overall higher education enrollments. Nursing is following this trend. Students choose distance education programs for a variety of reasons, including issues related to distance from, and therefore access to, on-campus programs as well as the convenience of anytime, anyplace learning opportunities. Many distance learning programs operate asynchronously, allowing students to choose what time of the day or week they will participate. This makes distance learning programs especially attractive to adult learners who may be working or raising families or both while furthering their education.

But what about clinical education? Students enrolled in post-licensure undergraduate programs (RN-to-BSN) and graduate-level education may pursue distance education. The content in these programs depends heavily on acquiring not only the didactic knowledge base but also a set of necessary clinical skills. Ultimately, students must be able to demonstrate that they can apply clinical reasoning and function as safe, competent practitioners in a clinical environment. This is the segment of their education that cannot be completely taught or learned using computer technologies. Yet, the literature lacks information that can guide faculty members teaching in these programs, particularly in the clinical education component.

Faculty members in distance education programs need to carefully consider how students will acquire the necessary clinical skills and how these students will be evaluated. Available clinical sites and knowledgeable, skilled preceptors are needed. Typically, those preceptors working with online students are physically located in or near students' own communities, which may be hundreds of miles or more away from the nursing program. Although nurse educators have been able to provide didactic education to students who live almost anywhere using Internet technologies, schools traditionally have had affiliations only with clinical sites located geographically close to their campus, thus requiring development of new clinical sites for distance learners. The process of securing an appropriate clinical placement for students at distant locations involves a series of checks and balances to assure that students receive the education they need. The specific steps involved in selecting, preparing, evaluating, and rewarding preceptors are discussed in more detail in Chapter 12.

Evaluating students in the clinical setting is an ongoing challenge for preceptors and the nursing faculty, but can be particularly challenging with distance education.

Goals of evaluation include identification of student strengths and problem areas as well as documentation of student progress. Faculty members must develop and maintain trusting work relationships with clinical preceptors who are at a distance. Contact between the nursing education program faculty member and the preceptor during a student's clinical experience needs to be timely and consistent. Preceptors need to know how to reach the designated faculty member with questions and concerns. At the same time, teaching and completing student evaluations can be time-consuming for the preceptor, and the nursing education program needs to avoid imposing unnecessary reporting burdens. When working at a distance, electronic communication using email, Skype, or other synchronized audiovisual communication, such as Zoom, can be helpful to busy preceptors and faculty members alike.

Various tools have been developed by faculty members to assist in the evaluation process. Student self-evaluation is essential and includes regular written evaluation, reflection on clinical experiences, and plans for improvement. Involvement of the preceptor in written assessments provides documentation of the preceptor's observations of student performance that are necessary evidence for the faculty member's decision making. Self-identification of areas needing improvement can be stressful for students but is the basis for a mature practitioner's growth and should be fostered by the nursing education program.

Evaluation of clinical competence is more challenging when students are located in a distant setting. Some programs may require students to visit a campus for evaluation sessions and demonstration of essential clinical skills. Sometimes objective structured clinical exams (OSCEs) are used for this evaluation, particularly with nurse practitioner students. These exams assess student clinical competency with standardized patients portraying typical clinical problems. Students rotate through various stations and demonstrate skills such as history taking, assessments, or clinical procedures while a faculty evaluator uses a checklist or other rating tool to evaluate performance (Oranye, Ahmad, Ahmad, & Bakar, 2012). However, this type of evaluation may cause student stress and anxiety by creating a high-stakes testing environment. To ensure valid and reliable assessments of student performance, clinical teachers need to carefully select and train standardized patients and use appropriate data collection tools that are linked to clinical competencies and critical performance elements (Williams & Botwinski, 2012). One promising approach that addresses this concern uses video recordings of student performance with patients in the clinical setting (Strand, Fox-Young, Long, & Bogossian, 2013). Although students in this pilot project had some difficulty with the technical aspect of video recording and uploading files, this method has the potential to provide feedback and assess student performance for distance education students. Other emerging possibilities include telehealth applications, virtual communities, and virtual clinical practicum experiences (Giddens & Walsh, 2010; Grady, 2011; Hawkins, 2012). Regardless of the method used, faculty need to plan for clinical learning at distance sites and carefully consider student guidance and evaluation.

CLINICAL LEARNING IN INTERNATIONAL SITES

Clinical placements in international sites can be rich opportunities to expand students' comfort and competence in the care of diverse patient populations, beyond that which can be gained in coursework focusing on such content. International learning experiences may increase cultural awareness and sensitivity while developing a better understanding of global issues. On a personal level, students may explore values, develop confidence, and learn or refine other skills. Learning activities that take place within the students' own cultures and familiar surroundings do not always help students meet goals related to becoming culturally sensitive, because the patients' world views do not predominate (Saenz & Holcomb, 2009). Nursing students whose clinical activities take place within other cultures, in both developed and developing countries, are challenged intellectually and emotionally to become more culturally aware. Literature reveals that international experiences enhance cultural understanding and increase awareness and respect for cultural differences. These experiences also promote tolerance for different practices and enhance communication. Lastly, students participating in these experiences appreciate different cultural values and beliefs (Asenso, Remier-Kirkham, & Astle, 2013).

Clinical experiences at international sites present unique challenges and require adequate preparation for both the student and the faculty member. Various factors must be considered as part of the planning process. The source institution for the nursing education program may have an international placement office that can assist with arrangements, offer travel suggestions, and facilitate the selection of appropriate sites. Establishing relationships with key personnel at the host location may enhance collaboration and facilitate planning. Once a site has been selected, preliminary and early travel arrangements should be completed because some preparation and planning time may be required. Students and faculty members must ensure that they are protected from developing health problems when traveling abroad. Participants will need to have updated immunizations and maintain current health and travel insurance. Depending upon the location of travel, they may also need to take preventative medications such as antimalarial drugs or get additional vaccinations. Most immunization series must be started well in advance of the planned trip. Students will need passports with an expiration date well beyond the end of the planned learning activity. Some trips, particularly those in developing countries, rural areas, or locations at significantly higher altitudes than students' city of origin, may also require physical conditioning. Students must also be informed of costs, which usually include tuition for the course, transportation, housing and food costs at the site, and cost of day-to-day expenses, including local travel. Completion of necessary paperwork usually includes a waiver of responsibility of the source educational institution and a separate application for the international activity.

Another important part of preparation involves understanding the practice environment, health care system, and nursing regulations at the destination site. Determine what students can legally do at the clinical site. Are there practice boundaries and restrictions on nursing care that they can provide? Students need to be prepared and understand that nursing practice, as well as the settings for that care, will be different. Make sure that students stay within regulated boundaries. Depending on the host location and type of site, verification of licensure of graduate nursing students and accompanying clinical teachers, and protocols to cover any nursing care to be delivered by students may be needed.

An understanding of the overall culture, customs, politics, economics, traditions, communication patterns, and values of the community and country in which they will be placed is also essential. This knowledge will be helpful and will ensure that students demonstrate respect and appreciation for the culture and challenges that the patients face. Practical aspects of life at the distant site must also be addressed. To prevent any misunderstandings while traveling, students need to consider the culture and their roles. Are there predetermined practices, customs, and expectations that they may need to follow? These include appropriate clothing for clinical activities. What does a nurse or volunteer health care provider wear in the host country? What equipment will the student need to provide? In some countries students may need to cover their heads and wear skirts (National League for Nursing, n.d.). Knowing these expectations prior to departing for the trip will facilitate appropriate planning and packing. If students are not fluent in the language spoken in the country, it is helpful to learn some basic language that will be used (e.g., thank you, goodbye) so they have some basic phrases they can use to communicate with others. If technology use is appropriate and available, consider using a mobile application for personal computing devices that assists with language translation. Preparation for day-to-day living conditions, including food and water safety, is essential. Housing should also be considered. Will the students be housed in a hotel, house, dormitory, or tent? Education related to personal safety, including both health and environmental risks, is essential. Lastly, encourage students to investigate common health and illnesses, causes of death, health beliefs, rituals, and practices, as this may facilitate preparation for health promotion and teaching at the clinical site.

Clinical teachers or preceptors must help students to understand that care may be different and that even the most generous care can result in harm. For example, imposing nursing care that cannot be sustained after the team departs is not appropriate, however well-meaning (Gower, Duggan, Dantas, & Boldy, 2016).

Emergency planning also is essential. Make sure that students know what to do if they become separated from the group. Have a frank discussion of what students and clinical teachers should do in case of a natural disaster or act of war or terrorism. Where should they go? When? Whom should they contact and how can that contact be completed? Monitor the U.S. Department of State website (www.travel.state.gov) for travel warnings for U.S. citizens and follow cautions and warnings.

Opportunities for reflection and sharing of experiences are critical because students may encounter emotional issues that need to be addressed. Even with adequate pretrip planning, students may not be prepared for the disparities and complex health issues they encounter, the limited resources available, the stereotypes they may experience, and their ethnocentric thinking (Kokko, 2011). Journaling (traditional or electronic format), development of a photolog, and sharing their experiences with classmates who did not participate provide opportunities for students to explore their feelings and reflect on their learning.

PRACTICAL ASPECTS OF CLINICAL PLACEMENTS IN DIVERSE SITES

When considering practical aspects of clinical placements in diverse sites, there are two major areas of concern. The first reflects the regulatory and accreditation requirements for clinical learning activities; the second involves preparation of the agency, clinical teachers, and students. All clinical learning activities must meet the requirements of state law and regulations (often set by the board of nursing) as well as the policies and requirements of accreditation agencies, the nursing education program (or its parent institution), and the site at which the clinical activities are to take place. Each nursing education program also has procedures in place that describe how contracts and similar formal communication with an agency are to be handled. While often clear from the school's perspective, this is not always the case from the agency's side. This is a very important point for agencies that usually do not negotiate such contracts and for which there is no clearly identified contact person. Some agencies that appear to be freestanding may be part of larger agencies. Where the agency is part of a larger entity (e.g., a hospital system, local government program, state health department, school district, or federal agency such as the Veterans Health Administration), it can be both difficult and time-consuming to get the contract signed by all relevant parties. These agreements can dictate student and faculty requirements needed prior to entering the clinical agency for learning. These agreements are especially important when dealing with smaller agencies that may not have procedures in place related to orientation or placement of students in their facilities. Adhering to the agency guidelines is important to avoid conflicts, especially when multiple programs (nursing and other health professionals) are seeking placements for the same time period. Even if students are at one of the clinical entity's sites, the policy for the overall entity must be followed. Often, smaller and nontraditional sites (e.g., day care settings, church programs, food kitchens) and even some formal agencies that do not have large staffs (e.g., day treatment programs for substance abusers, nursing homes, assisted living facilities) do not require or have a formal orientation program. The clinical teacher should work with the staff to determine what preparation the students need to optimize their learning as well as protect and provide the best care for the patients they will encounter. On the other hand, a larger institution (e.g., a major hospital system) may be the parent organization of smaller community-based programs, and students may need to complete the full agency orientation to be placed in even a small, peripheral program. If these requirements become too onerous, expensive, or time-consuming, the value of clinical learning activities at these sites may be questioned by the nursing education program faculty and administration. Legal aspects of clinical learning experiences are more fully explored in Chapter 6, and a few aspects highly relevant to the use of diverse sites are presented in Exhibit 3.1.

EXHIBIT 3.1

AREAS OF CONSIDERATION WHEN PLACING STUDENTS IN DIVERSE CLINICAL SITES

Legal and Regulatory Issues

- Does the placement meet requirements of relevant state laws and accompanying regulations related to approval, contract, faculty ratios, nature of faculty guidance, and student scope of practice?
- Must the clinical teacher be present for clinical learning activities for students to practice direct patient care?
- Can preceptors be used in the setting and in the manner planned?
- Can the clinical teacher delegate guidance and evaluation of students' learning to a RN on staff at the agency if the clinical teacher is not present but in the building? What if the clinical teacher is not physically present?

Nursing Education Program Issues

- Is a contract required?
- Is travel reimbursement available?

(continued)

- If the planned clinical learning activity will take place over more than the usual hours and day of a traditional clinical activity (e.g., on parts of most days of the week, during school breaks, on weekends), is this reflected in the clinical teacher's workload and compensation?
- Are there specific requirements of the education program's accreditation body that affect the planned clinical learning activity?

Agency Issues

- What are the agency's rules and policies related to nursing student clinical activities?
- Does the agency require a contract with the nursing education program? If so, who handles contracts with education programs?
- How are requests for clinical placements from multiple nursing education and other programs handled?
- What are the agency rules for student clearance (e.g., criminal background, child or elder abuse records, drug screening)?
- If screenings or background checks beyond the requirements of the nursing education program are required, who pays for them?
- Does the nursing education program need to document that students have demonstrated CPR or other competencies?
- What are the health requirements, such as tuberculosis testing or immunizations?
- Are there specific Health Information Portability and Accountability Act or patient privacy statements that must be completed?
- Does the agency need to keep a record of students for legal or regulatory purposes or to obtain future funding based on the value of student service to the organization? If yes, what is needed from the nursing education program?

Student Issues

- What modes of transportation are available? Is there parking?
- What measures will help to ensure safety of students?
- What is the required orientation?

Agency Preparation

As competition for clinical sites continues, clinical teachers seek creative ways to secure effectively and efficiently appropriate student learning opportunities. Clinical agency administrators and educators are also ready to embrace creative approaches that will decrease nursing program competition and rivalry in securing clinical sites while providing an equitable approach that will meet agency, nursing program, and student needs. Educational programs and health care providers must work together to meet common goals. One approach is the formation of a clinical placement consortium. In this model, school representatives, service agency liaisons, and clinical agency representatives meet to find appropriate learning opportunities for all. The use of web-based programs or course management systems is one way to manage and display clinical placement requests and facilitate open communication and negotiation among consortium members (Kline & Hodges, 2006).

Another approach to secure student clinical placements involves development of partnerships between health care organizations and nursing education programs. Academic service partnerships, also known as academic–community partnerships, are formal collaborative relationships between agencies that allow for sharing of knowledge, resources, clinical expertise, and opportunities with the intent of promoting both better patient care and nursing education. Formal partnerships generally allow for better access to clinical placements because the partners have clearly articulated a shared vision and mutually agreed upon goals, and have re-envisioned the roles of teacher and staff members. Partners work together to mobilize talents, leverage resources, and use assets effectively (Baiardi, Brush, & Lapides, 2010; Beal et al., 2012; Broussard, 2011).

Regardless of the type of relationship with the clinical agency or location of the clinical site, there are some basic considerations that will help to ensure a collegial work relationship with agency leaders and nursing staff. Details of the clinical learning activity (when will students be there, what their learning goals are, what they are expected to do, and how they can participate) must be communicated with the staff. Settings that rarely host nursing students, as well as those that often do, can have problems getting this information to the staff members who will have the most contact with the students. Explore if there are methods to electronically share information with staff, such as through email, so that it is disseminated in a convenient and efficient way. Misunderstandings about student activities and objectives do occur and can jeopardize the learning experience. Often course syllabi, clinical objectives, and guides to the clinical learning activity are provided to administrative staff of a clinical agency but may not be shared with the staff members who are directly working with the students and could benefit from access to this information. A meeting with the staff members who will work directly with the students, along with providing multiple copies of these written materials, will facilitate communication and ensure that the right people have the right information.

Including nursing staff in planning clinical learning activities can also prevent potential problems. Seeking input from staff nurses and understanding their workload demands can help clinical teachers plan effectively for student learning activities. Realizing the existing demands on staff members, such as precepting new nurses or supervising other staff members, will help clinical teachers form realistic expectations of the time available to assist students.

Clinical Teacher Preparation

Clinical teachers may need additional education, mentoring, and support as they implement clinical learning activities in new and diverse settings. A highly skilled clinical teacher who is at ease while teaching students to care for acutely ill patients in a critical care unit may not have the knowledge and skills needed to care for those patients in their homes a week after discharge. Like their students, clinical teachers may find that the fine points of adapting care to the home setting while respecting the family in their home and dealing with the virtual loss of the multiple support systems of the acute care setting will be new to them.

The organization and structure of clinical teaching outside of acute care settings will often be new to a faculty member. Some logistical issues will need to be addressed. If the students are not all in the same setting, how will faculty members conduct their clinical teaching activities at multiple sites? How will students and teachers communicate with each other? How will clinical conferences occur? What written assignments will be submitted to the faculty member and how and when will it be returned to students? Electronic technology can provide solutions for some of these issues. Course management platforms can be used to create forums for posting clinical updates and news, submission of course assignments, synchronous discussion boards, or even electronic discussion through Skype. Other electronic communication methods can be used to communicate with students during clinical practice. These methods include cellphones, although they are not always permitted at clinical sites. Short message service (SMS) or text messaging can be used to provide support and instant access between clinical teachers and students during clinical learning experiences activities. Use of this service is inexpensive and easy to use, and it allows for instant connectivity. Some computer applications such as Remind (www.remind.com) are available, which help to schedule automatic announcements and can share messages without revealing the clinical teacher's phone number.

Clinical teachers with nursing students in diverse sites, perhaps at different sites at the same time, have complex teaching obligations. Some sites, particularly those that are community-based or international, work beyond the days, times, or even weeks when traditional clinical learning activities occur, may need to maintain partnerships that work collaboratively to meet student and program needs.

Student Preparation

When students have clinical learning activities in unfamiliar sites or where the learning opportunities are not immediately clear to them, students may feel confused, insecure, isolated, and unprepared for the experience (Leh, 2011). Provision of specific objectives, learning activities, preparation expectations, activity guides, and written expectations will greatly facilitate learning and make the expectations clear. This is especially true if the faculty member will not be present at the site at all times. See Exhibit 3.2 for an example of specific preparation, objectives, activities, and written expectations for a community-based experience. Orientation for the clinical experience is based on agency, site, and student needs. Regardless of the clinical setting, an overall orientation to the course expectations with a review of skills used frequently in the experiences and a discussion about preconceptions and expectations will provide students with essential preparation that will enable them to feel confident and prepared for the experience.

EXHIBIT 3.2

EXAMPLE OF INSTRUCTIONS TO STUDENTS FOR COMMUNITY CLINICAL SITES
Preparation for All Community Clinical Learning Activities

- Review objectives and activities as listed for each assignment and do assigned reading before arriving at the site.
- Review key facts or existing guides (e.g., immunization schedules or classification of hypertension in adults) appropriate for the clinical area.
- Be at the site at the time indicated by your instructor.
- Wear your clean uniform (including identification) and follow the dress code. Dress appropriately for the weather.

(continued)

- Bring a black pen, watch with a second hand, stethoscope, notebook, electronic references, and pocket reference books, as appropriate, for the clinical learning activity.
- Check on transportation and directions to the site.
- Have contact information for your instructor (cell phone number, etc.) with you at all times.
- Share your schedule (where and when you are going) with your class partner.
- Bring a charged cell phone.
- Have the phone number and name of the site contact person.

Specific Preparation Before the Clinical Learning Activity Starts

- Read chapters XX, XX, and XX in the course text.
- Complete and submit the clinical preparation worksheet to your instructor.

General Clinical Activity Guidelines

- Work with the staff for an optimal learning experience.
- Your instructor will visit the site each day and be available by cell phone or text messaging.
- You should complete assessments, documentation, and teaching as described in the following. You may only administer medications under the direct observation of the RN identified by your instructor.
- Review any unfamiliar medical diagnosis, medication, and care needed for patients you are seeing.
- Ask for help if something is unclear.

Clinical Activities

During this clinical learning activity, students will work with staff members to:

1. Follow agency policy for client intake for the visit, including completion of initial assessments and placement of clients and charts with appropriate provider.
2. Review patient's health record for history, diagnoses, medications, and lab test results.
3. Follow patients through the physical exam to the end of the visit, if provider and patient agree.
4. Implement health teaching after review by the instructor.
5. Complete required clinical report.

Student safety during the clinical learning experience will also need to be addressed. This is an issue in all clinical activities, but it is especially important in situations where students may be in an unfamiliar area, making home visits, or going alone or in small groups to clinical sites at various times during the day or evening. Teachers must provide explicit guidelines for student safety during learning activities and document them in the course syllabus. Safety guidelines for home visits and going alone or in small groups to clinical sites should address proper methods of communication with faculty, agency, and patients. Ensure that students have the following information prior to the start of the clinical experience: clinical teacher and emergency contact information, clear travel directions, a reliable vehicle with adequate fuel, availability of a charged cell phone, and guidelines for appropriate dress and behavior while in a patient's home or at an agency or facility without an instructor present. The students must also be prepared for appropriate actions they may need to take if they find themselves in a dangerous situation, be it at an agency, out in the community, or at a patient's home (Leh, 2011).

Regular brief visits by the clinical teacher to each clinical site will help prevent problems and address issues that may arise from staff and students during the experience. Individual and group conferences with students will allow for sharing of experiences and provide additional time to assess learning and growth.

SUMMARY

Nursing care occurs anywhere there are clients who need the services of a professional nurse, and nursing students can learn to provide care wherever they have contact with clients. Traditionally, much of clinical nursing education has occurred in acute care settings because of long-held assumptions about how nurses must be prepared to practice. However, decreasing length of inpatient stays, high patient acuity, economic pressures to provide care in outpatient and community settings, and increasing competition with other educational programs for the same clinical sites have limited clinical learning opportunities located in traditional acute care settings. Using diverse sites for clinical learning activities can prepare nursing students for the challenges of contemporary nursing practice as clients, health needs, care locations, and approaches to care.

This chapter discussed options for planning and providing clinical learning opportunities for undergraduate and graduate nursing students in a wide variety of clinical sites. Examples of clinical learning opportunities in four categories were presented. The first category included patient care areas that are not used regularly as clinical learning sites (e.g., the OR, outpatient clinics, nursing homes, and extended care facilities) despite the rich learning opportunities for students in these settings. The second category included sites where provision of health care is not the prime focus of the site or agency, such as schools, camps, and wellness centers and clinics. The third category is the use of distant clinical sites for online nursing students. The final category is the growing use of international clinical learning opportunities.

Practical aspects of clinical placements in diverse sites were also discussed. Two main areas of concern are the need to meet regulatory and accreditation requirements and the need for adequate preparation of agency staff members, clinical teachers, and students. Examples of methods and tools used for preparation of agency staff members, clinical teachers making the transition from traditional acute care sites, and nursing students were provided.

CNE EXAMINATION TEST BLUEPRINT CORE COMPETENCIES

1. **Facilitate Learning**

   A. Implement a variety of teaching strategies appropriate to
      2. setting
      3. learner needs
      5. desired learner outcomes
   C. Modify teaching strategies and learning experiences based on consideration of learners'

(continued)

      1. cultural background
      2. past clinical experiences
- **D.** Use information technologies to support the teaching–learning process
- **E.** Practice skilled oral and written (including electronic) communication that reflects an awareness of self and relationships with learners (e.g., evaluation, mentorship, and supervision)
- **F.** Communicate effectively orally and in writing with an ability to convey ideas in a variety of contexts
- **H.** Create opportunities for learners to develop their own critical thinking skills
- **M.** Develop collegial working relationships with clinical agency personnel to promote positive learning environments
- **O.** Demonstrate the ability to teach clinical skills
- **P.** Act as a role model in practice settings
- **Q.** Foster a safe learning environment

2. **Facilitate Learner Development and Socialization**

- **D.** Create learning environments that facilitate learners' self-reflection, personal goal setting, and socialization to the role of the nurse
- **E.** Foster the development of learners in these areas:
  1. cognitive domain
  2. psychomotor domain
  3. affective domain
- **F.** Assist learners to engage in thoughtful and constructive self and peer evaluation

3. **Use Assessment and Evaluation Strategies**

- **C.** Use a variety of strategies to assess and evaluate learning in these domains:
  1. cognitive
  2. psychomotor
  3. affective
- **H.** Implement evaluation strategies that are appropriate to the learner and learning outcomes
- **L.** Provide timely, constructive, and thoughtful feedback to learners

4. **Participate in Curriculum Design and Evaluation of Program Outcomes**

- **H.** Collaborate with community and clinical partnerships to support educational goals

6. **Engage in Scholarship, Service, and Leadership**

- **A.** Function as a change agent and leader
  1. Model cultural sensitivity when advocating for change

REFERENCES

Algoso, M., Peters, K., Ramjan, L., & East, L. (2016). Exploring undergraduate nursing students' perceptions of working in aged care settings: A review of the literature. *Nurse Education Today, 36,* 275–28010. doi:1016/j.nedt.2015.08.001

Allen, I. E., & Seaman, J. (2013). *Changing course: Ten years of tracking online education in the United States.* Babson Survey Research Group and Quahog Research Group. Retrieved from http://www.onlinelearningsurvey.com/reports/changingcourse.pdf

American Association of Colleges of Nursing. (2008). Cultural competence in baccalaureate nursing education. Retrieved from http://www.aacn.nche.edu/leading-initiatives/educationresources/competency.pdf

American Association of Colleges of Nursing. (2013). ELNEC fact sheet. Retrieved from http://www.aacn.nche.edu/elnec/about/fact-sheet

Asenso, B. A., Reimber-Kirkham, S., & Astle, B. (2013). In real time: Exploring nursing students' learning during an international experience. *International Journal of Nursing Education Scholarship, 10,* 227–236. doi:10.1515/ijnes.2012.0045

Association of periOperative Registered Nurses. (2015). Value of clinical learning activities in the perioperative setting in undergraduate curricula. Retrieved from http://www.aorn.org/guidelines/clinical-resources/position-statements

Baiardi, J. M., Brush, B. L., & Lapides, S. (2010). Common issues, different approaches: Strategies for community–academic partnership development. *Nursing Inquiry, 17,* 289–296.

Beal, J. A., Alt-White, A., Erickson, J., Everett, L. Q., Fleshner, I., Karshmer, J., … Gale, S. (2012). Academic practice partnerships: A national dialogue. *Journal of Professional Nursing, 28,* 327–332. doi:10.1016/j.profnurs.2012.09.001

Benner, P., Sutphen, M., Leonard, V., & Day, L. (2009). *Educating nurses: A call for radical transformation.* Sudbury, MA: Jossey-Bass.

Bonnel, W. (2016). Clinical performance evaluation. In D. M. Billings & J. A. Halstead (Eds.), *Teaching in nursing: A guide for faculty* (5th ed., pp. 443–462). St. Louis, MO: Elsevier.

Broussard, B. B. (2011). The bucket list: A service-learning approach to community engagement to enhance community health nursing clinical learning. *Journal of Nursing Education, 50,* 40–43. doi:10.3928/01484834-20100930.07

Brynildsen, G., Bjørk, I. T., Berntsen, K., & Hestetun, M. (2014). Improving the quality of nursing students' clinical placements in nursing homes: An evaluation study. *Nurse Education in Practice, 14,* 722–728. doi:10.1016/j.nepr.2014.09.004

Crowley, A. A., Cianciolo, S., Krajicek, M. J., & Hawkins-Walsh, E. (2012). Childcare health and health consultation curriculum: Trends and future directions in nursing education. *Journal for Specialists in Pediatric Nursing, 17,* 129–135.

Doroh, H. M. H., & Monahan, J. C. (2016). Student nurses in the OR: Improving recruitment and retention. *AORN Journal, 103,* 89–94. doi:10.1016/j.aorn.2015.11.003

Federal Interagency Forum on Child and Family Statistics. (2016). *America's children: Key national indicators of well-being.* Washington, DC: U.S. Government Printing Office. Retrieved from https://www.childsttats.gov/americaschildren/glance.asp

Giddens, J. F., & Walsh, M. (2010). Collaborating across the pond: The diffusion of virtual communities for nursing education. *Journal of Nursing Education, 49,* 449–454. doi:10.3928/01484834-20100430-04

Gower, S., Duggan, R., Dantas, J. A. R., & Boldy, D. (2016). Motivations and expectations of undergraduate nursing students undertaking international clinical placements. *Journal of Nursing Education, 55,* 487–494. doi:10.3928/01484834-20160816-02

Grady, J. L. (2011). The virtual clinical practicum: An innovative telehealth model for clinical nursing education. *Nursing Education Perspectives, 32,* 189–194. doi:10.5480/1536-5026-32.3.189

Hawkins, S. Y. (2012). Telehealth nurse practitioner student clinical experiences: An essential educational component for today's health care setting. *Nurse Education Today, 32,* 842–845. doi:10.1016/jnedt.2012.03.008

Institute of Medicine. (2011). *The future of nursing: Leading change, advancing health.* Washington, DC: National Academies Press.

Kline, K. S., & Hodges, J. (2006). A rational approach to solving the problem of competition for undergraduate clinical sites. *Nursing Education Perspectives, 27,* 80–83.

Kokko, R. (2011). Future nurses' cultural competencies: What are their learning experiences during exchange and studies abroad? A systematic literature review. *Journal of Nursing Management, 19,* 673–682. doi:10.1111/j.1365-2834.2011.01221x

Lane, A. M., & Hirst, S. P. (2012). Placement of undergraduate students in nursing homes: Careful considerations versus convenience. *Journal of Nursing Education, 51,* 145–149. doi:10.3928/01484834-20120127-04

Lau, Y., & Wang, W. (2014). Development and evaluation of a learner-centered education summer camp program on soft skills for baccalaureate nursing students. *Nurse Educator, 39,* 246–251. doi:10.1097/NNE0000000000000065

Leh, S. K. (2011). Nursing students' preconceptions of the community health clinical experience: Implications for nursing education. *Journal of Nursing Education, 50,* 620–627. doi:10.3928/01484834-20110729-01

McCarthy, A. M., & Wyatt, J. S. (2014). Undergraduate pediatric nursing education: Issues, challenges, and recommendations. *Journal of Professional Nursing, 30,* 130–138. doi:10.1016/j.profnurs.2013.07.003

Mott, J. (2012). Implementation of an intraoperative clinical experience for senior level baccalaureate nursing students. *AORN Journal, 95,* 445–452. doi:10.1016/j.aorn.2011.05.024

Mueller, C., Goering, M., Talley, K., & Zaccagnini, M. (2011). Taking on the challenge of clinical teaching in nursing homes. *Journal of Gerontological Nursing, 37*(4), 32–38.

National League for Nursing. (n.d.). *Faculty preparation for global experiences toolkit.* Retrieved from http://www.nln.org/docs/default-source/default-document-library/toolkit_facprepglobexp5a3fb25c78366c709642ff00005f0421.pdf

National League for Nursing. (2017). A vision for expanding US nursing education for global health engagement. Retrieved from http://www.nln.org/docs/default-source/about/nln-vision-series-%28position-statements%29/vision-statement-a-vision-for-expanding-us-nursing-education.pdf?sfvrsn=6

National Nurse-Led Care Consortium. (2016). About nurse-managed care. Retrieved from http://www.nncc.us/site/index.php/about-nurse-managed-care

O'Connor, A. B. (2015). *Clinical instruction and evaluation: A teaching resource.* Burlington, MA: Jones & Bartlett.

Oranye, N. O., Ahmad, C., Ahmad, N., & Bakar, R. A. (2012). Assessing nursing clinical skills competence through objective structured clinical examination (OSCE) for open distance learning students in Open University Malaysia. *Contemporary Nurse, 41*, 233–241.

Penprase, B., Monahan, J., Poly-Drouland, L., & Prechowski, S. (2016). Student immersion in perioperative nursing. *AORN Journal, 103*, 189–197. doi:10.1016/j.aorn.2015.12.013

Pohl, C. Jarvill, M., Akman, O., & Clark, S. (2017). Adapting pediatric clinical experiences to a changing health care environment. *Nurse Educator, 42*, 105–108. doi:10.1097/NNE.0000000000000315

Saenz, K., & Holcomb, L. (2009). Essential tools for a study abroad nursing course. *Nurse Educator, 34*, 172–175.

Saunders, R., Singer, R., Dugmore, H., Seaman, K., & Lake, F. (2016). Nursing students' reflections on an interprofessional placement in ambulatory care. *Reflective Practice, 17*, 393–402. doi:110.1080/14623943.2016.1164686

Strand, H., Fox-Young, S., Long, P., & Bogossian, F. (2013). A pilot project in distance education: Nurse practitioner students' experience of personal video capture technology as an assessment method of clinical skills. *Nurse Education Today, 33*, 253–257. doi:10.1016/j.nedt2011.11.014

Thompson, C. W., & Bucher, J. A. (2013). Meeting baccalaureate public/community health nursing education competencies in nurse-managed wellness centers. *Journal of Professional Nursing, 29*, 155–162. doi:10.1016/j.profnurs.2012.04.017

Wang, T., & Bhakta, H. (2013). A new model for interprofessional collaboration at a student-run free clinic. *Journal of Interprofessional Care, 27*, 339–340. doi:10.3109/13561820.2012.761598

Williams, R. L., & Botwinski, C. A. (2012). Identifying strengths and weaknesses in the utilization of objective structured clinical examination (OSCE) in a nursing program. *Nursing Education Perspectives, 33*, 35–39. doi:10.5480/1536-5026-33.1.35

CHAPTER 4

Preparing for Clinical Learning Activities

Nurse educators should consider a number of factors in preparing for clinical learning activities. Equipping students to enter the clinical setting must be balanced with preparing staff members for the presence of learners in a service setting while also respecting the needs of patients. This chapter describes the roles and responsibilities of faculty members, staff members, and others involved in clinical teaching and suggests methods of preparing students and staff members for clinical learning activities. Strategies for crafting clinical learning activities will be discussed in Chapter 7.

UNDERSTANDING THE CONTEXT FOR CLINICAL LEARNING ACTIVITIES

To begin preparations for clinical teaching and learning, nurse educators should reflect on the context in which these activities take place. Teachers and learners use an established health care or community setting for a learning environment, thus becoming guests within that setting. What are the implications for clinical teaching and learning effectiveness under these conditions?

Over the last century, basic preparation for professional nursing has moved from service-based training and apprenticeship to academic educational programs in institutions of higher learning. As a result of this service-education separation, the clinical teacher and students who enter a clinical setting for learning activities are often regarded as guests of the health care agency or community site. They participate in the activities of the established system and attempt to follow the norms of its culture, but they are not a constant presence. They must rely on relationships they develop within the agency to facilitate their sense of belonging to obtain support for student learning (Dahlke & Hannesson, 2016).

Traditionally, clinical teachers and students in an academic nursing education program comprise a temporary system within the permanent culture of the clinical setting. Similarly, a staff development instructor and orientees may represent a temporary system. A temporary system is a set of individuals who work together on a complex task over a limited period of time. Although clinical teachers are professional colleagues to nursing staff members and are viewed as nurses by patients, their primary role is that of educator. Even if they are employed by the agency as a staff member on a casual or part-time basis in addition to their academic positions, faculty members enact a different role in that agency when they are guiding the clinical learning activities of students, and role confusion is often inevitable.

Being a good guest involves knowing and adhering to the established routines, policies, and practices of the clinical setting. Clinical teachers negotiate with staff members for access to learning opportunities and resources while simultaneously protecting students from criticism and preventing errors. Often, students point out discrepancies between nursing staff practice and the standards or procedures that the students were taught. The teacher needs to explain such differences in terms of choice of approach to solving a clinical problem, when appropriate, rather than offering a value judgment. When possible, the clinical teacher should point out staff members who are positive role models of clinical excellence and professionalism. The clinical teacher juggles the complex responsibilities of supporting student learning, developing trusting relationships with staff, and ensuring delivery of safe quality care.

At times, a clinical teacher's desire for positive relationships with staff members, reluctance to delay or slow patient care, and concern for patient and student safety result in minimizing students' risk taking in an effort to prevent errors. For example, teachers may select assignments for students that allow them to demonstrate previously developed competencies rather than choose learning activities that will challenge students to deepen their understanding and develop higher skill levels. If the teacher expects that a student will not be able to complete patient care activities in a timely manner, the instructor may forego a rich opportunity for the student to learn to prioritize, organize, and complete a complex set of tasks for the patient and to work collaboratively with other health care team members to do so efficiently. Excessive gatekeeping actions of this kind do not allow students to exhibit clinical problem solving, organize care activities, and learn to take appropriate, calculated risks.

Although clinical teachers and nursing students are seen as guests in the health care environment, they are also a vital resource to a health care agency. Nursing students represent potential future employees of that organization, and many health care administrators and managers view the presence of nursing students in the facility as a recruitment opportunity (Drake, Pawlowski, & Riley, 2013). Positive clinical learning experiences may encourage nursing students to consider future employment in that agency, and nursing staff members who nurture the development of students can have a powerful influence on such a choice (Brynildsen, Bjørk, Berntsen, & Hestetun, 2014).

Many staff members, however, are unaware of or misinterpret these standards; they expect nursing students to participate fully in all unit activities, assume responsibility for patient care, take the same kinds of patient assignments, and complete the same patient care tasks as do staff members. They may recall their own clinical education as being more rigorous than the contemporary clinical activities that they witness; communicating those perceptions to nursing students can produce self-doubt, discouragement, and dissatisfaction among the novices. The teacher as culture broker must allow students to experience the real world of clinical nursing and, at the same time, communicate to staff members that trends and current issues in nursing education mean that "it's not your mother's nursing school." Keeping clinical agency staff members, managers, and administrators informed about the nature of contemporary nursing education and keeping students updated on current challenges and priorities in the health care environment will help to integrate students more effectively into the real world of clinical nursing.

SELECTING CLINICAL SETTINGS

Clinical teachers may have sole responsibility for selecting the settings in which clinical learning activities occur, or their input may be sought by those who make these decisions. In either case, selection of clinical sites should be based on important criteria such as compatibility of school and agency philosophy, availability of opportunities to meet learning objectives, geographical location, agency licensure or accreditation, availability of positive role models, complexity of patients, level of student, purpose and type of course, and physical resources (Fressola & Patterson, 2017; O'Connor, 2015). In some areas, selection of appropriate clinical settings may be difficult because of competition among several nursing programs, and nursing programs must typically contract with a variety of agencies to provide adequate learning opportunities for students. Additionally, as nursing programs increase enrollments they face the challenge of securing adequate clinical placements, particularly in specialty areas such as pediatrics. Programs may be forced to use numerous clinical sites, which increase the time and energy required for teachers to develop relationships with staff, to obtain necessary information about agencies, and to develop and maintain competence to practice in diverse settings. It also creates an administrative burden to manage clinical agency approval, track student health requirement compliance, and coordinate clinical activities.

Selection Criteria

Nurse educators should conduct a careful assessment of potential clinical sites before selecting those that will be used. Faculty members who are also employed in clinical agencies may provide some of the necessary information, and teachers who have instructed students in an agency can provide ongoing input into its continued suitability as a practice site. State boards of nursing may have specific reporting requirements or forms that need to be completed as part of the selection and approval process for clinical sites. Nursing education programs may need to provide additional information for board of nursing review. For an example of an agency data form see www.portal .state.pa.us/portal/server.pt/community/state_board_of_nursing/12515/licensure_ information/572048#forms. Assessment of potential clinical agencies should address the following criteria:

- *Opportunity to achieve learning outcomes.* Are sufficient opportunities available to allow learners to achieve learning objectives? For example, if planning, implementing, and evaluating preoperative teaching is an important course objective, the average preoperative patient census must be sufficient to permit learners to practice these skills. If the objectives require learners to practice direct patient care, does the agency allow this, or will learners only be permitted to observe? Will learners from other educational programs be present in the clinical environment at the same time? If so, how much competition for the same learning opportunities is anticipated? Will there be adequate patient census to ensure that appropriate learning opportunities are available?
- *Level of the learner.* If the learners are undergraduate students at the beginning level of the curriculum, the agency must provide ample opportunity to practice basic skills. Graduate students need learning activities that will allow them to develop advanced practice skills. Does the clinical agency permit graduate

students to practice independently or under the guidance of a preceptor, without an on-site instructor? Are undergraduate students in a capstone course permitted to participate in clinical learning activities under the guidance of an appropriate staff member as preceptor, without the physical presence of a faculty member?

■ *Degree of control by faculty.* Does the agency staff recognize the authority of the clinical teacher to plan appropriate learning activities for students, or do agency policies limit or prescribe the kinds and timing of student activities? Do staff members restrict the types of learning activities available? Do agency personnel view learners as additions to the staff and expect them to provide service to patients, or do they acknowledge the role of students as learners?

■ *Availability of role models for students.* As previously discussed, students often imitate the behaviors they observe in nursing staff members. Are the agency staff members positive role models for students and new staff nurses? If learners are graduate students who are learning advanced practice roles, are strong, positive role models available to serve as preceptors and mentors? Do they have the educational and experiential qualifications to guide students appropriately? Is staffing adequate to permit staff members to interact with students and participate in their learning, or are they overburdened? Are staff dismissive, exclusionary, and rude, or are they cooperative, inclusive, supportive, and welcoming of students?

■ *Geographical location.* Although geographical location of the clinical agency is not usually the most important selection criterion, it can be a crucial factor when a large number of clinical agencies must be used. Travel time between the campus and clinical settings for faculty and students must be considered, especially if learning activities are scheduled in both settings on the same day. Is travel to the agency via public transportation possible and safe, especially if faculty and students must travel in the evening or at night? Are public transportation schedules convenient; do they allow students and faculty to arrive at the agency in time for the scheduled start of activities, and do they permit a return trip to campus or home without excessive wait times? Does the value of available learning opportunities at the agency outweigh the disadvantages of travel time and cost?

■ *Physical facilities.* Are physical facilities such as conference space, locker rooms, cafeteria or other dining facility, library, and parking available for use by clinical teachers and students?

■ *Staff relationships with teachers and learners.* Do staff members respond positively to the presence of students, engage in effective communications with faculty and students, and welcome appropriate questions from them? Will the staff members cooperate with teachers in selecting appropriate learning activities, participate in orientation activities for faculty and students, and provide useful guidance and feedback about student performance?

■ *Orientation needs.* Some clinical agencies require faculty members to attend scheduled orientation sessions before they take students into the clinical setting. The time required for such orientation must be considered when selecting clinical agencies. If faculty members are also employed in the agency as casual or per diem staff, this orientation requirement may be waived. Can any parts of the orientation be completed without being present in the agency, such as online or via self-study? Is the clinical teacher who is new to a clinical setting permitted to work in the staff nurse role for several days prior to bringing students to the agency, to become familiar with the unit routines and to begin to form collaborative relationships with staff members? Are technology initiatives occurring that require faculty and student orientation, password clearances, and access to computer systems? If so, are there mechanisms in place for training and to allow clinical teachers and students to use these systems as part of the clinical learning activities?

■ *Opportunity for interdisciplinary activities.* As interprofessional skill development emerges as a critical component of nursing education, consider if there are opportunities for learners to practice as members of an interdisciplinary health care team. Will learners have contact with other health care practitioners, such as physical therapists, pharmacists, nutritionists, respiratory therapists, social workers, infection control personnel, and physicians?

■ *Agency requirements.* Unless the educational program and the clinical facility are parts of the same organization, a legal contract or agreement usually must be negotiated to permit students and faculty to use the agency as a clinical teaching site. Such contracts or agreements typically specify requirements such as school and individual liability insurance; competence in cardiopulmonary resuscitation; professional licensure for clinical teachers, graduate students, and RN-to-BSN students; immunization and other health requirements; dress code; use of name tags or identification badges; requirements for student drug testing; and requirements for criminal background checks for students and clinical teachers.

■ *Agency licensure and accreditation.* Accreditation requirements for educational programs may specify that clinical learning activities take place in accredited health care organizations. If the agency must be licensed to provide certain health services, it is appropriate to verify current licensure before selecting that agency as a clinical site.

■ *Costs.* In addition to travel expenses, there may be other costs associated with use of an agency for clinical learning activities. Any fees charged to schools for use of the agency or other anticipated expense to the educational program and to individual clinical teachers and students should be assessed.

■ *Regulatory board approvals.* State boards of nursing often require review and approval of clinical sites before a new site can be used for clinical nursing education. Faculty members or administrators may need to provide information about the health care institution, including bed capacity and average daily patient census, a list of other nursing education programs using the facility, number of students who will use the facility, and specific scheduling information.

Health care agencies are mandating these requirements to ensure patient safety and comply with various regulations. Currently, the Centers for Disease Control and Prevention (CDC; 2017) and the Advisory Committee on Immunization Practices (ACIP) of the CDC recommend that health professions students receive measles, mumps, rubella, hepatitis B, varicella, influenza, tetanus, diphtheria, and pertussis vaccines. The newly revised CDC guidelines also recommend that health care professionals receive human papillomavirus (HPV) and herpes zoster vaccines as appropriate (Kim, Riley, Harriman, Hunter, & Bridges, 2017). Recommendations are regularly updated so teachers need to periodically check these guidelines for new information and consult with health care agencies to align with their requirements. Students may need to demonstrate compliance by showing evidence of immunizations or immunity, or they may require booster immunizations. Additional clinical requirements such as mandatory drug testing may also be specified by health care facilities or the nursing program (Glasgow, Dreher, & Oxholm, 2012). Institutions may require testing for a specific panel of drugs or drug classifications. Typically students have a narrow window of time for completion of the drug testing at the start of a clinical practicum and must follow a specific protocol for this testing. Depending upon state regulations, students may also need to complete a variety of background checks to screen for offenses and criminal arrest records. These background checks may include child abuse, elder abuse, and criminal history checks. Some agencies require that students meet the same requirements that their staff members must meet, which may include financial background checks. As the Fair Credit Reporting Act requires, students should be notified about the purpose of these background checks and must provide written consent (Philipsen et al., 2012). All of these requirements should be communicated to students in print and, for ease of retrieval, in an online electronic format. Clear communication with students about these requirements will help to ensure that students understand them and have sufficient time to gather evidence of completion by the specified deadlines.

The list of clinical requirements may be quite lengthy and may require significant time and financial investment for students to comply; however, they must be completed before a student can begin clinical activities at a clinical site and risk violating the nursing education program's contract with the agency and jeopardize future access to that clinical site. Another concern for the educational institution involves managing these records. When gathering personal information about students, nursing education program personnel need to protect student privacy and prevent inappropriate disclosure of personal information obtained for clinical requirements. Some programs contract with agencies that conduct the background checks and provide reports to the administrator. Student consent is essential when releasing personally identifiable information to such outside agencies to ensure compliance with the Family Education Rights and Privacy Act (FERPA; Shellenbarger & Perez-Stearns, 2010). Thus, nursing education programs should have guidelines for disclosure and a method of keeping this private information separate from students' academic records.

Sufficient time must be allowed before the anticipated start of clinical activities to negotiate a contractual agreement that specifies rights and responsibilities. Legal counsel may be involved in negotiating these legally binding documents that specify roles and responsibilities (Fressola & Patterson, 2017). Clinical teachers must usually have current unencumbered professional nursing licenses for each state in which they instruct in the clinical area, unless the clinical agencies are located in states that have adopted the Nurse Licensure Compact (NLC; National Council of State Boards of Nursing, n.d.). Currently 25 states allow nurses to practice in NLC states as long as they live in a NLC state and hold and meet license requirements in their home state.

PREPARATION OF FACULTY MEMBERS

When selection of the clinical site or sites is complete, the nurse educator must prepare for the teaching and learning activities that will take place there. Areas of preparation that must be addressed include clinical competence, familiarity with the clinical environment, and orientation to the agency or setting.

Clinical Competence

Clinical competence has been documented as an essential characteristic of effective clinical teachers. Clinical competence includes theoretical knowledge, expert clinical skills, and judgment in the practice area in which teaching occurs (Oermann & Gaberson, 2017).

Standards for accreditation and state approval of nursing education programs may require nurse faculty members to have advanced clinical preparation in graduate nursing programs in the clinical specialty area in which they are assigned to teach. In addition, faculty members should have sufficient clinical experience in the specialty area in which they teach. This is particularly important for faculty members who will provide direct, on-site guidance of students in the clinical area; the combination of academic preparation and professional work experience supports the teacher's credibility and confidence. Students often identify the ability to demonstrate nursing care in the clinical setting as an essential skill of an effective clinical instructor (Fressola & Patterson, 2017; Girija, 2012; Huo, Zhu, & Zheng, 2010).

Clinical teachers should maintain current clinical knowledge through participation in continuing education and practice experience. Nurse educators who have a concurrent faculty practice or joint appointment in a clinical agency, or who work part time in a clinical role in addition to their academic assignment, are able to maintain their clinical competence by this means, especially if they practice in the same specialty area and clinical agency in which they teach.

Familiarity With the Clinical Environment

If the clinical teacher is entering a new clinical area, he or she may ask to work with the staff for a few days prior to returning to the site with students. This enables the teacher to practice using equipment and technology that may be unfamiliar and to become familiar with the agency environment, policies, and procedures. If this is not possible, the teacher should at least observe activities or shadow a nursing staff member in the clinical area to discern the characteristics of the patient population, the usual schedule and pace of activities, the types of learning opportunities available to develop desired outcomes, the diversity of health care professionals in the agency, and the presence of other learners (O'Connor, 2015).

As previously mentioned, a clinical agency may require faculty members whose students use the facility to attend an orientation program. Orientation sessions vary in length, from several hours to a day or more, and typically include introductions to administrators, managers, and staff development instructors; clarification of policies such as whether students may administer intravenous medications; review of documentation procedures; and safety procedures. Faculty members may be asked to demonstrate competent operation of equipment, such as infusion pumps, that their students will be using or to submit evidence that they have met the same competency standards that are required of nursing staff members. They may also need computer training so they can access electronic health records.

ADJUNCT AND PART-TIME TEACHERS

As nursing programs face increasing enrollments combined with faculty retirements, fiscal constraints, and changing program needs, adjunct or part-time teachers are often hired for clinical teaching responsibilities. Practicing nurses with their extensive clinical knowledge and expertise in the practice setting may fill the needed teacher vacancies. Drawing upon their knowledge of the clinical setting, they can effectively help students learn nursing care practices; however, these skilled clinicians may lack the necessary education knowledge needed to successfully carry out the clinical teacher role (Johnson, 2016). Specifically, these clinical teachers may need to understand student policies, curriculum, and evaluation practices that are necessary to help students make the connection between theory and practice and provide safe patient care. It is important that all clinical teachers, particularly those newly hired, be oriented to their role, responsibilities, and expectations. Providing opportunities for support and connection with other teachers, integration into the program and faculty development opportunities aimed at addressing clinical teaching and learning needs will enhance retention and success in the clinical teacher role.

PREPARATION OF CLINICAL AGENCY STAFF

Preparation of the clinical agency staff usually begins with the nursing education program's initial contact with the agency when negotiating an agreement or contract between the program and the agency. Establishing an effective working relationship with the nursing staff is an important responsibility of the clinical teacher. Ideally, nursing staff members would be eager to work with the faculty member to help students meet their learning goals. Indeed, in academic health centers and other teaching institutions, participation in education of learners from many health care disciplines is a normal job expectation. Serving as a preceptor or working with students may be used for clinical ladder or magnet status designation evaluation criteria (Pierson, Liggett, & Moore, 2010). Regardless of the reasons for working with students, some staff members will enjoy working with students more than others. Because teachers cannot usually choose which staff members will be involved with students, it is important for the teacher to communicate the following information to all staff members.

Clarification of Roles

Staff members often expect the instructor to be responsible for the care of patients with whom students are assigned to work. Many clinical teachers remark that if they have 10 students and each student is assigned two patients, the instructor is responsible for 30 individuals. These role expectations are both unrealistic and unfair to all involved parties.

Although the clinical teacher is ultimately responsible for student learning, students have much to gain from close working relationships with staff members. Staff members can serve as useful role models of nursing practice in the real world; students can observe how staff members must adapt their practice to fit the demands of a complex, ever-changing clinical environment. At the same time, staff members are often stimulated and motivated by students' questions and the current information that they can share. The presence of students in the clinical environment often reinforces staff members' competence and expertise, and many nurses enjoy sharing their knowledge and skill with novices. Clinical teachers should therefore encourage staff members to participate in the instruction of learners within guidelines that teachers and staff members develop jointly. Students should be encouraged to use selected staff members as resources for their learning, especially when they have questions that relate to specific patients for whom the staff members are responsible.

An important point of role clarification is that the responsibility for patient care remains with staff members of the clinical agency, as mentioned earlier. If a student is assigned learning activities related to care of a specific patient, a staff member, often called the primary nurse, is assigned the overall responsibility for that patient's care. Students are accountable for their own actions, but the primary nurse and student should collaborate to ensure that patient needs are met. Staff members may give reports about patient status and needs to students who are assigned to work with those patients. Students should be encouraged to ask questions of staff members about specific patient care requirements; to share ideas about patient care; and to report changes in patient condition, problems, and tasks that they will not be able to complete, and the need for assistance with tasks (O'Connor, 2015).

Role expectation guidelines such as these should be discussed with staff members and managers. When mutual understanding is achieved, the guidelines may be written and posted or distributed to relevant personnel and students.

Level of Learners

Staff members can have reasonable expectations of learner performance if they are informed of the students' levels of education and experience. Beginning students and novice staff members will need more guidance; staff members working with these learners should expect frequent questions and requests for assistance. More experienced learners may need less assistance with tasks but more guidance on problem solving and clinical decision-making. Sharing this information with staff members allows them to plan their time accordingly and to anticipate student needs.

It is especially important for faculty members to tell agency personnel what specific tasks or activities learners are permitted and not permitted to do. This decision may be guided by educational program or agency policy, the curriculum sequence, or by the specific focus of the learning activities on any given day. For example, during one scheduled clinical session, an instructor may want students to practice communication and active listening skills during health history data collection without relying on physical care tasks. The instructor should share this information with the staff and ask them to avoid involving students in physical care on that day.

Learning Outcomes

The overall purpose and desired outcomes of the clinical learning activities should be communicated to staff members. As demonstrated in the previous example, knowledge of the specific objectives for a clinical session permits staff members to collaborate with the teacher in facilitating learning. If students have the specific learning objective of administering intramuscular injections, staff members can be asked to notify the teacher if any patient needs an injection that day so that the student can take advantage of that learning opportunity.

Knowledge of the learning objectives allows staff members to suggest appropriate learning activities, even if the teacher is unable to anticipate the need. For example, an elderly patient who is confused may be admitted to the nursing unit; the staff nurse who is aware that students are focusing on nursing interventions to achieve patient safety might suggest that a student be assigned to work with this patient.

Need for Positive Role Modeling

The need for staff members to be positive role models for learners is a sensitive but important issue. As previously discussed, teachers often worry that students will learn bad practice habits from experienced nurses who may take shortcuts when giving care. When discussing this issue with staff members, instructors should avoid implying that the only right way to perform skills is the teacher's way. Instead, the teacher might ask staff members to point out when they are omitting steps from procedures and to discuss with learners the rationale for those actions. In this way, staff nurses can model how to think like a nurse, a valuable learning opportunity for nursing students.

Asking staff nurses to be aware of the behaviors that they model for students and seeking their collaboration in fostering students' professional role development is an important aspect of preparing agency staff to work with learners. To accomplish this goal, instructors need to establish mutually respectful, trusting relationships with staff members and to sustain dialogue about role modeling over a period of time.

The Role of Staff Members in Evaluation

Agency staff members have important roles in evaluating learner performance. The clinical performance of learners must be evaluated formatively and summatively. Formative evaluation takes the form of feedback to the student during the learning process; its purpose is to provide information to be used by the learner to improve performance. Summative evaluation occurs at the end of the learning process; its outcome is a judgment about the worth or value of the learning outcomes (Oermann & Gaberson, 2017). Summative evaluations usually result in academic grades or personnel decisions such as promotions or merit pay increases.

Teachers should explain carefully their expectations about the desired involvement of staff members in evaluating student performance. Agency personnel have an important role in formative evaluation by communicating with teachers and learners about student performance. Because staff members are often in close contact with students during clinical activities, their observations of student performance are valuable, but the teacher should keep in mind that staff members may have different expectations for student performance than the instructor does. Staff members should be encouraged to report to the teacher any concerns that they may have about student performance as well as observations of exemplary performance; clinical instructors should accept this input and then validate the report by their own observations. Staff members should also feel free to praise students, point out any errors they may have made, or make suggestions for improving performance. Immediate, descriptive feedback is necessary for learners to improve their performance, and often staff members are better able than teachers to provide this information to students.

However, it is the teacher's responsibility to make summative evaluation decisions. Staff members should know that they are an important source of data on student performance and that their input is valued, but that it is the clinical teacher who ultimately certifies competence or assigns a grade.

PREPARING THE LEARNERS

Students need cognitive, psychomotor, and affective preparation for clinical learning activities. It is the clinical teacher's responsibility to assist students with such preparation as well as to assess its adequacy before students enter the clinical area.

Cognitive Preparation

General prerequisite knowledge for clinical learning includes information about the learning outcomes; the clinical agency; and the roles of teacher, student, and staff member. Additionally, in some nursing education programs, students are able and expected to prepare ahead of time for each clinical learning session (Gubrud, 2016). This preparation may include one or more of the following tasks: gathering information from patient records; interviewing patients and family members; assessing patient needs; performing physical assessment; reviewing relevant pathophysiology, nursing, nutrition, and pharmacology textbooks; and completing written assignments such as a patient assessment, plan of care, concept map, or instructor-designed preparation sheet. In some programs, students complete these types of learning activities during and following their clinical learning activities.

Teachers should ensure that the expected cognitive preparations for clinical learning do not carry more importance than the clinical learning activities themselves. That is, learning should be expected to occur during the clinical learning activities as well as during preclinical preparation. If students receive their learning assignments in advance of the scheduled clinical activity, they can be reasonably expected to review relevant textbook information and to anticipate potential patient problems and needs. If circumstances permit a planning visit to the clinical agency, the student may meet and interview the patient and review the patient's health record. However, requiring extensive written assignments to be completed before the actual clinical activity implies that learning takes place only before the student enters the clinical area. Students cannot be expected to formulate a realistic plan of care before assessing the patient's physical, psychosocial, and cultural needs; this assessment may begin before the actual clinical activity, but it usually comprises a major part of the student's activity in the clinical setting. Thus, preclinical planning should focus on preparations for the learning that will take place in clinical practice. For example, the teacher may require students to formulate a tentative nursing diagnosis from available patient information, formulate a plan for collecting additional data to support or refute this diagnosis, and plan tentative nursing interventions based on the diagnosis. A more extensive written assignment submitted after the clinical activity may require students to evaluate the appropriateness of the diagnosis and the effectiveness of the nursing interventions.

Additionally, because students often copy information from textbooks (or, regrettably, from other students) to complete such requirements, written assignments submitted before the clinical learning activity may not show evidence of clinical reasoning and problem solving, let alone comprehension and retention of the information. For example, some teachers require students to prepare for medication administration during the clinical experience. Students often copy published pharmacologic information without attempting to retain this information and to think critically about why the medication was prescribed or how a particular patient might respond to it. A better approach is to ask students to reflect on the pharmacologic actions of prescribed drugs and to be prepared to discuss relevant nursing care implications, either individually with the instructor or in a group conference. If it is not possible for students to determine in advance which drugs are being used to treat patients whose care they will be participating in, the clinical instructor may ask students to study particular drug classifications and their prototype drugs and to be prepared to seek and use appropriate information resources when the student obtains the drug list. For example, if students are studying nursing care of patients who are at risk of a cerebral vascular accident, they should be familiar with several classifications of antihypertensive drugs and understand the common desired, side, and adverse effects. Students can then formulate a tentative plan of care for these patients and then modify and individualize the plan when they are able to assess specific patients.

Nursing students should learn to use a variety of reference materials both to prepare for clinical practice and as resources during clinical learning activities. Electronic mobile devices are gaining popularity as resources that can be used to access reference materials and save time in the clinical setting (Strandell-Laine, Stolt, Leino-Kilpi, & Saarikoski, 2015). Students can use smartphones, personal digital assistants, tablets, computer applications, and ebooks to support clinical learning (Robb & Shellenbarger, 2014). Faculty members should consider the cost, connectivity issues, training needs, technology support, access, privacy and confidentiality concerns, available software, and student comfort with use if requiring these devices. Teachers may need to plan technology training sessions, collaborate with campus and clinical site technology support personnel, and develop policies and guidelines for appropriate use during clinical learning. Additional information about teaching with technology can be found in Chapter 9.

We recommend that students be expected to complete some cognitive preparation before clinical practice, but extensive, detailed written preparation assignments are unrealistic and often shift focus away from learning *during* clinical activities. Encouraging students' identification and use of appropriate, available information resources during clinical practice facilitates development of clinical reasoning and problem-solving abilities.

Meeting with students during a preclinical conference, either in a group or individually, also allows for assessment of student preparation as well as offer anticipatory guidance. Clinical teachers can use questioning techniques to determine if students have adequate knowledge to care for patients. It also provides an opportunity for clarification about anticipated nursing care and allows for correction of students' misconceptions before patient care is provided. Clinical teachers can assess student preparation and feel assured that students have an appropriate plan for care. Exhibit 4.1 provides sample questions that clinical teachers might use for preclinical conferences with students.

Psychomotor Preparation

Skill learning is an important outcome of clinical teaching. However, the length and number of clinical learning sessions are often limited in nursing education or

---

EXHIBIT 4.1

SAMPLE PRECLINICAL CONFERENCE QUESTIONING

- What are your priority nursing assessments?
- What is your plan of care for the day? What nursing care will you provide first?
- What lab or diagnostic tests were performed recently? What are the results? What are your nursing actions based upon these results?
- What medications are prescribed for your patient that will need to be administered? Why is the patient taking each medication? What are the actions, side effects, and nursing implications of these medications?

new staff orientation programs. In a qualitative study completed by Killam and Heerschap (2013), students reported that lack of practice time and inadequate feedback about psychomotor skill performance were challenges to their learning in the clinical setting. As students develop into competent care providers they need to have adequate time to learn psychomotor skills in a practice setting and be given appropriate and informative feedback to enhance performance. When learning complex skills, it is more efficient for students to practice the parts first in an environment such as a simulation center or skills laboratory, free from the demands of the actual practice setting. In such a setting, students can investigate and discover alternative ways of performing skills, and they can make errors and learn to correct them without fear of harming patients. Thus, students should have ample skill practice time before they enter the clinical area so that they are not expected to perform a skill for the first time in a fast-paced, demanding environment. It is the clinical teacher's responsibility to assure that students have developed the desired level of skill before entering the clinical setting. The use of clinical simulation and technology in a nursing skills lab provides students with realistic learning opportunities to develop psychomotor skills in a controlled environment. Use of clinical simulation activities allows students to practice and refine psychomotor skills and incorporates cognitive and affective learning as well. A literature review of teaching psychomotor skills revealed that teaching methods that provide access to online instruction as part of psychomotor skills teaching was more effective than other approaches (McNett, 2012). Exhibit 4.2 provides additional suggestions for teachers to use for psychomotor skill teaching and learning. Chapter 8 presents a comprehensive discussion of the use of clinical simulation.

EXHIBIT 4.2

STRATEGIES FOR ENHANCING PSYCHOMOTOR SKILL LEARNING

- Focus on commonly used psychomotor skills
- Use a variety of teaching–learning methods (visual, auditory, tactile)
- Physically guide students during early psychomotor skill learning
- Allow students opportunities to test different ways of performing skills but ensure critical elements of the psychomotor skills are performed correctly
- Provide practice opportunities over time, not just a single practice session
- Cluster steps of a psychomotor skill to facilitate memory
- Practice psychomotor skills to become proficient, coordinated, and efficient
- Intersperse psychomotor skill practice with other learning activities
- Design learning activities that allow students to observe skill performance of others
- Alternate psychomotor skill practice and observation of other's skills practice
- Use simulation for psychomotor skill practice and follow this with debriefing
- Provide positive feedback about psychomotor skill performance
- Incorporate prompts or cues to allow students to problem solve during psychomotor skill learning
- Provide formative feedback to correct psychomotor performance errors
- Use summative evaluation to verify skill learning
- Incorporate practice to refresh performance if a psychomotor skill is not used frequently

Source: Adapted from O'Connor (2015) and Oermann, Muckler, and Morgan (2016).

Affective Preparation

Affective preparation of students includes strategies for managing their anxiety and for fostering confidence and positive attitudes about learning. Most students have some anxiety about clinical learning activities. Mild or moderate anxiety often serves to motivate students to learn, but excessive anxiety may impair confidence and interfere with learning (Grobecker, 2016). Students report that their first clinical experience is among the most commonly identified anxiety producing situation for them (Walker & Verklan, 2016). The teacher plays a critical role in mediating that anxiety and stress and may employ strategies to identify students' fears and reduce their anxiety to a manageable level. A preclinical conference session might assess learners' specific concerns and assure students of the teacher's confidence in them, desire for their success, and availability for consultation and guidance during the clinical activities.

For example, during a preclinical conference on the first day of clinical practice in a course, the instructor may state that it is common for students to feel anxious before a clinical activity but that anxiety usually decreases during the experience. The teacher may encourage students to identify and name the specific source and nature of their anxieties; once these are identified, the teacher can help students to use a problem-solving approach to identify helpful responses. For instance, if students express concern that something may happen that they will not know how to handle, the teacher may help students to list all the potential adverse events and then brainstorm possible responses to them. Throughout such a discussion, teachers should reassure students of their availability to answer questions and assist them with clinical reasoning and problem solving during the clinical learning activities. Other strategies, such as orientation, can be used to ensure students are adequately prepared.

Orientation to the Clinical Agency

Like clinical teachers, students also need a thorough orientation to the clinical agency in which learning activities will take place. This orientation may take place before or on the first day of clinical activities. Staff members often assist the teacher in orienting students to the agency and helping them to feel welcome and comfortable in the new environment.

Orientation should include:

- The geographical location of the agency
- The physical setup of the specific unit where students will be placed
- Names, titles, and roles of personnel
- Location of areas such as rest rooms, dining facilities, conference room, locker rooms, public telephones, and library
- Information about transportation and parking
- Agency and unit policies
- Daily schedules and routines
- Emergency protocols (e.g., fire drill, rapid response codes, cardiac arrest procedures, and equipment)
- Patient information documentation systems, including establishment of passwords and acquiring computer access to electronic health records and bedside medication administration systems

In addition, students need to have a telephone number at the clinical setting where they can be contacted in case of family emergency, know what procedures to follow in case of illness or other reason for absence on a clinical day, understand the uniform or dress requirements, and know what equipment to bring (e.g., stethoscope) and what to leave at home (e.g., personal valuables).

Given the growth of informatics in health care settings, faculty need to consider this for student orientation needs. Gone are the days of showing students hard-copy charts and explaining medication administration records and then moving quickly to delivering care. Instead, students need access codes for technology used at the clinical site. They will also need training for computer use, such as bar-coded bedside medication systems and electronic health records, before they can fully deliver care. Preparing students for use of the electronic health record may require a special training session for students. Staff development practitioners or information technology staff may need to schedule designated electronic health record training and arrange access for students. Clinical teachers need to coordinate this technology training with nurse educators and health care information technology personnel. Of course, clinical teachers also need to ensure that they are up to date on this training so that they are prepared to guide student learning in the clinical setting.

Not all of this orientation information needs to be presented on site; some creative clinical teachers have developed electronic resources that provide a virtual tour of the facility. If the agency uses computer software to document patient information, the instructor may be able to acquire a copy of the software application and make it available in the school's computer facility. Or, the nursing program may purchase bar code scanning equipment that can be used to simulate medication administration in clinical practice labs. Learners can be expected to review these resources before coming to the clinical site. Because student and clinical teacher orientation to a clinical facility can be costly and time-intensive for staff development educators, some agencies are now using technology for orientation (Bowers et al., 2011; Brooks & Erickson, 2012; Fura & Symanski, 2014). Self-directed electronic learning modules can be delivered via a website or classroom management system that enables an efficient, flexible, and cost-effective delivery method for training. Mandatory education required by health care facilities, such as fire safety, Health Insurance Portability and Accountability Act (HIPAA) training, infection control, or other topics can be delivered electronically. Clinical teachers and students can review needed training and complete appropriate evaluation materials. Spreadsheets or online systems can efficiently track compliance and completion of learning. Electronic delivery of clinical information can also be used throughout the year to share ongoing updates with clinical teachers and students in an efficient manner.

The First Day

Students almost always perceive the first day of clinical learning activities in a new setting as stressful; this is especially true of learners in their initial clinical nursing course. Students' first exposure to the clinical environment can either promote their independence as learners or foster dependence on the instructor due to fear. Clinical teachers should plan specific activities for the first day that will allow learners to become familiar with and comfortable in the clinical environment and at the same time alleviate their anxiety. These activities may include tours, conferences, games, and special assignments. Another creative option involves having experienced nursing students serve as peer mentors. These experienced students may help reduce anxiety and assist beginning nursing students with a student-led clinical orientation (Knowlton, Hayes, & Jones, 2015).

Even if learners have attended an agency orientation, it is helpful to take them on a tour of the specific areas they will use for learning activities, pointing out locations such as rest rooms, drinking fountains, fire alarms and extinguishers, emergency equipment, elevators, stairwells, and emergency exits. The instructor should introduce learners to staff members by name and title. If students need agency-specific identification badges, parking permits, or passwords for use of the computer system, the teacher may make the necessary arrangements ahead of time or accompany students to the appropriate locations where these items can be acquired. If an empty patient room is available, the instructor may demonstrate the use of equipment such as bed controls, call bell, oxygen delivery systems, and lighting controls.

Special assignments may include review and discussion of patient records, practice of computer documentation, and a scavenger hunt to help learners locate typical items needed for patient care. Exhibit 4.3 is an example of a scavenger hunt activity used in orienting students to a medical–surgical unit of a hospital. Learners may be asked to observe patient care for a specified period of time, interview a patient or family member, shadow a nurse, or complete a short written assignment focused on documenting an observation.

EXHIBIT 4.3

A SCAVENGER HUNT STRATEGY

Anywhere General Hospital
Unit 2C

Work in pairs to search for the location of the items or areas listed in the following. Check them off as you find them.

- Locker room
- Restrooms
- Oxygen tank
- Fire alarms
- Fire extinguishers
- Emergency exits
- Patient health records
- Patient teaching materials
- Nurse manager's office
- Medication dispensing systems
- Linen carts
- Kitchen
- Utility room
- Biohazardous waste containers
- Waterless hand sanitizer dispensers
- Reference materials
- Conference room
- Medical supply carts (intravenous (IV) bags, dressing change materials, gloves)
- Computer work stations
- Pulse oximeter
- Wheelchair

These activities may be followed by a short group conference, during which students are encouraged to discuss their impressions, experiences, and feelings. The teacher should review the roles of student, teacher, and staff members and should emphasize lines of communication. For example, students need to know who to ask for help and under what circumstances—that is, when to ask questions of staff members and when to seek assistance from the teacher. Handouts summarizing these expectations and requirements are useful because students can review them later when their anxiety is lower. If a dining facility is available in the clinical setting, pre- or postclinical conferences may take place in that location to allow students to relax with refreshments away from patient care areas. The conference may conclude by making plans for the next day of clinical practice, including selecting assignments and discussing how learners should prepare for their learning activities. Selection of clinical assignments is discussed in detail in Chapter 7.

SUMMARY

This chapter described the roles and responsibilities of faculty, staff members, and others involved in clinical teaching and suggested strategies for preparing students and staff members for clinical learning.

The teacher and learners comprise a temporary system within the permanent culture of the clinical setting. Negative consequences of this relationship can be avoided by establishing and maintaining regular communication between the instructor and staff members. Clinical teachers function as culture brokers and border spanners to help integrate students more fully into the real world of nursing practice.

Settings for clinical learning should be selected carefully, based on important criteria such as compatibility of school and agency philosophy, licensure and accreditation, availability of opportunities to meet learning objectives, geographical location, availability of positive role models, and physical resources. Selection of appropriate clinical settings may be complicated by competition among several nursing programs for a limited number of agencies. Specific criteria for assessing the suitability of potential clinical settings were discussed.

When clinical sites have been selected, educators must prepare for teaching and learning activities. Areas of preparation include clinical competence, familiarity with the clinical environment, and orientation to the agency. Clinical competence has been documented as an essential characteristic of effective clinical teachers and includes knowledge and expert skill and judgment in the clinical practice area in which teaching occurs. Teachers may maintain clinical competence through faculty practice, joint appointment in clinical agencies, part-time clinical employment, and continuing nursing education activities. The teacher may become familiar with a new clinical setting by working with or observing the staff for a few days prior to returning to the site with students. The clinical agency may require faculty members to attend an orientation program that includes introductions to agency staff, clarification of policies concerning student activities, and review of skills and procedures. Adjunct and part-time clinical teachers need to ensure they are familiar with the curriculum, course, policies, and procedures.

Preparation of the clinical agency staff usually begins with the teacher's initial contact with the agency. Roles of teacher, students, and staff members should be clarified so that staff members have guidelines for their participation in the instruction of learners. An important point of role clarification is that, although students are accountable for their own actions, the responsibility for patient care remains with staff members of the clinical agency. Staff members also need to be aware of specific learning objectives, the level of the learner, the need for positive role modeling, and expectations concerning their role in evaluating student performance. Although staff members' feedback is valuable in formative evaluation, the teacher is always responsible for summative evaluation of learner performance.

Students need cognitive, psychomotor, and affective preparation for clinical learning activities. Cognitive preparation includes information about the learning objectives; the clinical agency; and the roles of teacher, student, and staff member. Students may be expected to prepare for each clinical learning session through reading, interviewing patients, and completing written assignments. However, requirements for extensive written assignments to be completed before the actual clinical activity may imply that learning takes place only before the student enters the clinical area.

The instructor has a responsibility to assess that students have the desired level of skill development before entering the clinical setting. When learning complex skills, it is more efficient for students to practice the parts first in a simulated setting such as a skills laboratory, free from the demands of the actual practice setting. Students should have ample skill practice time before they enter the clinical area so that they are not expected to perform a skill for the first time in a fast-paced, demanding environment.

Affective preparation of students includes strategies for managing their anxiety and for fostering confidence and positive attitudes about learning. Most students have some anxiety about clinical learning activities. Mild or moderate anxiety often serves to motivate students to learn, but excessive anxiety hinders concentration and interferes with learning. In preparation for clinical learning activities, teachers may employ strategies such as a structured preclinical conference to identify students' fears and reduce their anxiety to a manageable level.

Students also need a thorough orientation to the clinical agency in which learning activities will take place. This orientation should include information about the location and physical setup of the agency, relevant agency personnel, agency policies, daily schedules and routines, and procedures for responding to emergencies and for documenting patient information.

Students almost always perceive the first day of clinical learning activities in a new setting as stressful. Clinical teachers should plan specific activities for the first day that will allow learners to become familiar with and comfortable in the clinical environment and at the same time alleviate their anxiety. These activities include tours, conferences, games, and special assignments.

CNE EXAMINATION TEST BLUEPRINT CORE COMPETENCIES

1. **Facilitate Learning**
   - **D.** Use information technologies to support the teaching–learning process
   - **H.** Create opportunities for learners to develop their own critical thinking skills
   - **I.** Create a positive learning environment that fosters a free exchange of ideas
   - **K.** Demonstrate personal attributes that facilitate learning (e.g., caring, confidence, patience, integrity, respect, and flexibility)

(continued)

M. Develop collegial working relationships with clinical agency personnel to promote positive learning environments

O. Demonstrates ability to teach clinical skills

P. Act as a role model in practice settings

Q. Foster a safe learning environment

2. **Facilitate Learner Development and Socialization**

D. Create learning environments that facilitate learners' self-reflection, personal goal setting, and socialization to the role of the nurse

E. Foster the development of learners in these areas
1. cognitive domain
2. psychomotor domain
3. affective domain

4. **Participate in Curriculum Design and Evaluation of Program Outcomes**

A. Demonstrate knowledge of curriculum development including
1. identifying program outcomes
5. selecting appropriate clinical experiences

H. Collaborate with community and clinical partnerships that support the educational goals

5. **Pursue Systematic Self-Evaluation and Improvement in the Academic Nurse Educator Role**

A. Engage in activities that promote one's socialization to the role

E. Participate in professional development opportunities that increase one's effectiveness in the role

6. **Engage in Scholarship, Service, and Leadership**

C. Function effectively within the organizational environment and the academic community
3. Integrate the values of respect, collegiality, professionalism, and caring to build an organizational climate that fosters the development of learners and colleagues.

REFERENCES

Bowers, A. M., Kavanagh, J., Gregorich, T., Shumway, J., Campbell, Y., & Stafford, S. (2011). Student nurses and the electronic medical record. *Computers, Informatics, Nursing, 29,* 692–697. doi:10.1097/NCN.0b013e31822b8a8f

Brooks, C. L., & Erickson, L. K. (2012). What is the solution for clinical nurse educators and the electronic medical record? *Teaching and Learning in Nursing, 7,* 129–132. doi:10.1016/j.teln.2012.06.003

Brynildsen, G., Bjørk, I. T., Berntsen, K., & Hestetun, M. (2014). Improving the quality of nursing students' clinical placements in nursing homes: An evaluation study. *Nurse Education in Practice, 14,* 722–728. doi:10.1016/j.nepr.2014.09.004

Centers for Disease Control and Prevention. (2017). *Recommended immunization schedules for adults.* Retrieved from https://www.cdc.gov.vaccines/schedules/hcp/adult.html

Dahlke, S., & Hannesson, T. (2016). Clinical faculty management of the challenges of being a guest in clinical settings: An exploratory study. *Journal of Nursing Education, 55,* 91–95. doi:10.03928/01484834-20160114-06

Drake, S. H., Pawlowski, U., & Riley, V. (2013). *Developing an effective health care workforce planning model.* Retrieved from https://www.aha.org/content/13/.13wpmwhitepaperfinal.pdf

Fressola, M. C., & Patterson, G. E. (2017). *Transition from clinician to educator: A practical approach.* Burlington, MA: Jones & Bartlett.

Fura, L. A., & Symanski, M. E. (2014). An online approach to orienting clinical nursing faculty in baccalaureate nursing education. *Nursing Education Perspectives, 35,* 324–326. doi:10.5480/12-868.1

Girija, K. M. (2012). Effective clinical instructor: A step toward excellence in clinical teaching. *International Journal of Nursing Education, 4*(1), 25–27.

Glasgow, M. E. S., Dreher, H. M., & Oxholm, C. (2012). *Legal issues confronting today's nursing faculty: A case study approach.* Philadelphia, PA: F. A. Davis.

Grobecker, P. A. (2016). A sense of belonging and perceived stress among baccalaureate nursing students in clinical placements. *Nurse Education Today, 36,* 178–183. doi:10.1016/j.nedt.2015.09.015

Gubrud, P. (2016). Teaching in the clinical setting. In D. M. Billings & J. A. Halstead (Eds.), *Teaching in nursing: A guide for faculty* (5th ed., pp. 282–303). St. Louis, MO: Elsevier.

Huo, X., Zhu, D., & Zheng, M. (2010). Clinical nursing faculty competence inventory—Development and psychometric testing. *Journal of Advanced Nursing, 67,* 1109–1117. doi:10.1111/j.1365-2648.2010.05520.x

Johnson, K. V. (2016). Improving adjunct nursing instructors' knowledge of student assessment in clinical courses. *Nurse Educator, 41,* 108–110. doi:10.1097/NNE.0000000000000205

Killam, L. A., & Heerschap, C. (2013). Challenges to student learning in the clinical setting: A qualitative descriptive study. *Nurse Education Today, 33,* 684–691. doi:10.1016/j.nedt.2012.10.008

Kim, D. K., Riley, L. E., Harriman, K. H., Hunter, P., & Bridges, C. B. (2017). Advisory committee on immunization practices recommended immunization schedule for adults aged 19 years or older—United States. *Morbidity and Mortality Weekly Reports, 66,* 136–138. doi:10.15585/mmwr.mm6605e2

Knowlton, M. C., Hayes, C. A., & Jones, A. M. (2015). Student-led clinical orientation. *Journal of Nursing Education, 54,* 472. doi:10.3928/01484834-20150717-11

McNett, S. (2012). Teaching nursing psychomotor skills in a fundamentals laboratory: A literature review. *Nursing Education Perspectives, 33,* 328–333. doi:10.5480/1536-5026-33.5.328

National Council of State Boards of Nursing. (n.d.). *Nurse licensure compact.* Retrieved from https://www.ncsbn.org/nlc.htm

O'Connor, A. B. (2015). *Clinical instruction and evaluation: A teaching resource* (3rd ed.). Sudbury, MA: Jones & Bartlett.

Oermann, M. H., & Gaberson, K. B. (2017). *Evaluation and testing in nursing education* (5th ed.). New York, NY: Springer Publishing.

Oermann, M. H., Muckler, V. C., Morgan, B. (2016). Framework for teaching psychomotor and procedural skills in nursing. *The Journal of Continuing Education in Nursing, 47,* 278–282. doi:10.3928/00220124-20160518-10

Philipsen, N., Murray, T. L., Belgrave, L., Bell-Hawkins, A., Robinson, V., & Watties-Daniels, D. (2012). Criminal background checks in nursing: Safeguarding the public? *Journal for Nurse Practitioners, 8,* 707–711. doi:10.1016/j.nurpra2012.07.033

Pierson, M. A., Liggett, C., & Moore, K. S. (2010). Twenty years of experience with a clinical ladder: A tool for professional growth, evidence-based practice, recruitment, and retention. *Journal of Continuing Education in Nursing, 41*(1), 33–40. doi:10.3928/00220124-20091222-06

Robb, M., & Shellenbarger, T. (2014). Strategies for searching and managing evidence-based practice resources. *Journal of Continuing Education in Nursing, 45,* 461–466. doi:10.3928/00220124-20140916-01

Shellenbarger, T., & Perez-Stearns, C. (2010). From the classroom to clinical: A Family Educational Rights and Privacy Act primer for the nurse educator. *Teaching and Learning in Nursing, 5,* 164–168.

Strandell-Laine, C., Stolt, M., Leino-Kilpi, H., & Saarikoski, M. (2015). Use of mobile devices in nursing–student teacher cooperation during the clinical practicum: An integrative review. *Nurse Education Today, 35,* 493–499. doi:10.1016/j.nedt.2014.10.007

Walker, D., & Verklan, T. (2016). Peer mentoring during practicum to reduce anxiety in first-semester nursing students. *Journal of Nursing Education, 55,* 651–654. doi:10.3928/01484834-20161011-08

CHAPTER 5

Process of Clinical Teaching

Clinical teaching is a complex interaction between students and teachers. Influencing the clinical teaching process are characteristics of the teacher and learner; the clinical environment and nature of practice within that environment; patients, families, and others for whom students are caring; other health care providers; and the inherent nature of clinical practice with its uncertainties.

The process of clinical teaching is described in this chapter. The chapter provides a framework for the teacher to use in planning clinical activities appropriate for the learning outcomes and students, guiding students in the practice setting, and evaluating clinical performance. A framework assists clinical teachers to create an environment and opportunities for students to learn; the outcomes of those experiences, however, may vary considerably among students because of the many factors that influence the learning process. This chapter also describes characteristics of effective clinical teachers and models of clinical teaching, such as traditional, in which one teacher guides the learning of a small group of students; preceptor; and partnerships, including dedicated education units (DEUs).

TEACHING AND LEARNING

Teaching is a complex process intended to facilitate learning. While the goal of teaching is to lead students in discovering knowledge for themselves, the teacher encourages this discovery through deliberate teaching actions that lead in that direction. Self-discovery does not imply a lack of structure; instead, the teacher provides structure and learning activities for self-discovery by the student.

Clinical teaching is a series of deliberate actions on the part of the teacher to guide students in their learning. It involves a sharing and mutual experience on the part of both teacher and student and is carried out in an environment of support and trust. Teaching is not telling, it is not dispensing information, and it is not merely demonstrating skills. Instead, teaching is *involving* the student as an active participant in this learning. The teacher is a resource person with information to share for the purpose of facilitating learning and acquisition of new knowledge and skills.

Learning is a process through which people change as a result of their experiences. Some of these changes are observable and measurable, for example, the student can explain the evidence base of an intervention or can accurately perform a procedure. In clinical practice, however, new insights, ideas, and perspectives may be as critical to the student's learning and development as overt and measurable behaviors. Learning, therefore, may be a change in observable behavior or performance, or it may reflect a new perception and insight.

The teaching–learning process is a complex interaction of these processes. The teacher is a facilitator of learning, and the student is an active participant. The need for students to be actively involved in their learning is critical in the teaching–learning process, particularly in the clinical setting. When students are actively involved in their learning and perceive a positive teacher–student relationship, they can be honest about their learning needs and how faculty can help them in developing their clinical competencies. Active learning may also foster students' higher level thinking as they reflect on patient problems and possible approaches. Studies on problem-based learning suggest that this method improves students' critical thinking (Gholami et al., 2016; Kong, Qin, Zhou, Mou, & Gao, 2013).

Although teaching and learning are interrelated processes, each may occur without the other. Significant learning may result from the student's clinical activities without any teacher involvement. Similarly, the teacher's carefully planned assignments and learning activities for students may not lead to new learning or development of competencies. The goal of clinical teaching is to create the *environment and activities for learning*, recognizing that each student will gain different insights and outcomes from them.

PROCESS OF CLINICAL TEACHING: FIVE COMPONENTS

The process of clinical teaching includes five steps:

1. Identifying the outcomes for learning
2. Assessing learning needs
3. Planning clinical learning activities
4. Guiding students
5. Evaluating clinical learning and performance

The process of clinical teaching is not linear; instead, each component influences others. For example, clinical evaluation provides data on further learning needs of students that in turn suggest new learning activities. Similarly, as the teacher works with students, observations of performance may alter the assessment and suggest different learning activities.

Identifying Outcomes for Learning

The first step in clinical teaching is to identify the goals and outcomes of clinical practice as discussed in Chapter 2. These intended learning goals and outcomes suggest areas for assessment, provide guidelines for teaching, and are the basis for evaluating learning. Nurse educators identify these outcomes in different ways.

In some nursing programs, the outcomes of learning are stated as objectives to be achieved by students in the clinical course. In other programs, they are expressed in the form of clinical competencies to be demonstrated at the end of the course or for specific clinical activities. Clinical competencies often address 10 areas of learning. These areas are listed in Exhibit 5.1 with examples of competencies in each area.

In some clinical courses, students need to demonstrate learning and performance in all of these areas as well as others specific to the clinical specialty or setting. Other courses may focus on only a few of these areas of learning. Clinical competencies may be stated broadly, similar to most of the examples in Exhibit 5.1, or they can be more specific, such as, "administer intravenous injection of medications." In any clinical course, the competencies should be achievable by students, considering their prior knowledge, skills, and experiences; clinical learning opportunities available in the clinical setting, simulation, and through other learning experiences; and time allotted for clinical practice.

The clinical competencies should be communicated clearly to students, in written form, and understood by them. Similarly, the teacher has an important responsibility in *discussing* these outcomes and related clinical activities with agency personnel, not *telling* them. Agency personnel need input into decisions about the clinical activities

EXHIBIT 5.1

EXAMPLES OF CLINICAL COMPETENCIES

1. Concepts, theories, and other knowledge for clinical practice

   Analyzes the pathophysiological basis for the development of clinical manifestations in common patient conditions.
   Applies multicultural concepts of care to the community.

2. Use of research and other evidence in clinical practice

   Uses evidence on pain management interventions in planning care for patients.
   Evaluates research studies for applicability to long-term care of patients with dementia and their caregivers.

3. Assessment, diagnosis, plan, interventions, and evaluation of outcomes

   Collects data that are developmentally and age appropriate for healthy and ill children.
   Considers multiple nursing interventions for care of patients with complex health problems.

4. Psychomotor and technological skills, other types of interventions, and informatics competencies

   Demonstrates skill in conducting a physical examination.
   Uses health information technology to retrieve critical information for decision making.

5. Values related to care of patients, families, and communities and other dimensions of health care

   Recognizes personal values that might conflict with professional nursing values.
   Accepts cultural, ethnic, and other differences of patients.

   (continued)

6. Communication skills, ability to develop interpersonal relationships, and skill in collaboration with others

   Collaborates with other health providers in care of children with disabilities.
   Communicates effectively with patients, families, staff, and others in the health care setting.

7. Development of knowledge, skills, and values essential for continuously improving the quality and safety of health care

   Identifies issues with quality of care in a clinical setting using relevant measures.
   Participates in analyzing system errors and designing unit-based improvements.

8. Management of care, leadership abilities, and role behaviors

   Manages care effectively for a small group of patients.
   Demonstrates the role and behaviors of a nurse as leader.

9. Accountability and responsibility of the learner

   Accepts responsibility for own actions and decisions.
   Values own role in preventing errors.

10. Self-development and continued learning

    Identifies own learning needs in clinical practice.
    Seeks learning opportunities to develop clinical competencies.

and their match with the goals, philosophy, and care delivery system of the clinical setting. With this input, the teacher may need to alter intended clinical activities and plan simulations and other types of learning opportunities for students.

Students should also have input into the clinical competencies; there may be some already achieved by students and others to be added to meet their individual learning needs and goals. There should be some flexibility in the clinical course as long as students demonstrate the competencies and achieve the essential knowledge and skills for progressing through the nursing program.

It is important for all clinical teachers—full and part time, adjunct, and preceptors—to understand the outcomes of a clinical course and competencies students should develop in it. The course leader is responsible for ensuring that all educators in a course, no matter what their role, use the outcomes and competencies to guide their selection of patients and other learning activities for students and to assess performance.

Assessing Learning Needs

Teaching begins at the level of the learner. The teacher's goal, therefore, is to assess the student's present level of knowledge and skill and other characteristics that may influence achieving the outcomes of the clinical practicum. The first area of assessment involves collecting data on whether the student has the prerequisite knowledge and skills for the clinical situation at hand and for completing the learning activities.

For instance, if the learning activities focus on interventions for health promotion, students first need some understanding of health and behaviors for promoting health. Changing a sterile dressing requires an understanding of principles of asepsis. The teacher's role in assessment of the learner is important so that students engage in learning activities that build on their present knowledge and skills. When students lack the prerequisites, then the instruction can remedy these and more efficiently move students forward in their learning.

Not every student will enter the clinical course with the same prerequisite knowledge and skills, depending on past learning and clinical experiences. The teacher, therefore, should not expect the same entry competencies for all students. Assessment reveals the point at which the instruction should begin and does not imply poor performance for students, only that some learners may need different types of learning activities for the objectives. Assessment may also indicate that some students have already attained certain clinical competencies and can progress to new areas of learning.

The second area of assessment relates to individual characteristics of students that may influence their learning and clinical performance. Students and nurses today represent a diverse group of learners with varied cultural backgrounds, learning styles, ages, and other characteristics. Students bring with them a wealth of life, work, and other experiences. In nursing programs, particularly second-degree programs, there is a wide range of ages of students, reflecting different generations and ways of thinking. Students in a nursing program may be baby boomers (born 1945–1964), Generation Xers (1965–1979), and millennials (1980–2000), with Generation Zers (2001–present) preparing to enter higher education in the next few years. There are different learning styles and expectations across these generations. Students who are Gen Xers and millennials prefer experiential activities and being involved in decisions about their learning activities. Those students, in contrast to older students and most nursing faculty members, are part of the information age and grew up with the Internet. Generational differences may affect how students approach their education. Nurse educators are challenged to design, implement, and evaluate innovative teaching–learning strategies to meet the needs of an increasingly diverse student and patient population (Jeffreys & Dogan, 2013; McLain et al., 2017).

In addition, many students combine their nursing education with other role responsibilities, such as family and work. Information about these characteristics, among others, gives the teacher a better understanding of the students and their responses to different learning situations. Faculty members and clinical nurse educators need to assess individual differences among students and use this knowledge in planning their learning activities.

Planning Clinical Learning Activities

Following assessment of learner needs and characteristics, the teacher plans and then delivers the instruction. In planning the learning activities, the main considerations are the competencies to be developed in the clinical practicum, or outcomes to be met, and individual learner needs. Other factors that influence decisions on clinical activities include evidence of the effectiveness of the clinical teaching method and learning activities being considered, characteristics of the clinical learning environment, and teacher availability to guide learners.

Clinical Competencies/Outcomes of Clinical Course

Clinical learning activities are selected to facilitate students' developing the essential competencies for clinical practice in that course or to meet the outcomes of the clinical practicum, depending on how these are stated by faculty members in the clinical course. The learning activities may include patient care assignments, but care of patients is not the only learning activity in which students engage in the practice setting. The specific competencies to be developed or outcomes to be achieved in that course should guide selection of learning activities. If the competencies focus on communication skills, then the learning activities may involve interviews with patients and families, papers analyzing those interactions, role play, and simulated patient–nurse interactions rather than providing direct care.

Learner Needs

While the clinical outcomes provide the framework for planning the learning activities, the other main consideration is the needs of the student. The activities should build on the student's present knowledge and skills and take into consideration other learner characteristics. Each student does not have to complete the same learning activities; the teacher is responsible for individualizing the clinical activities so that they best meet each student's needs while promoting achievement of the course outcomes.

Learning activities also build on one another. Planning includes organizing the activities to provide for the progressive development of knowledge and skills for each learner.

Evidence on Effectiveness of Clinical Teaching Method and Learner Activities

Decisions about the teaching methods to use and types of activities in which students will participate in the clinical setting should be based on evidence about what works best for promoting student learning. Nurse educators should review the literature to identify evidence to support the teaching methods they are planning and to get ideas about other strategies and activities for students that might be as or more effective. The evidence will also guide how a teaching method is implemented—for example, how to debrief after a simulation and the level of questions to ask to promote higher-level thinking. Evidence-based clinical nursing education involves four phases: (a) asking questions about best practices in teaching students in the clinical setting, (b) searching for research and other evidence to answer those questions, (c) evaluating the quality of the evidence and whether it is ready to be used in clinical teaching, and (d) deciding whether the findings are applicable to one's own clinical course, students, and setting (Oermann, 2009; Oermann & Conklin, 2018).

Characteristics of the Clinical Setting

The size of the agency, the patient population, the educational level and preparation of nurses, their availability and interest in working with students, other types of health care providers in the setting, and other characteristics of the clinical environment should be considered in planning the learning activities. These characteristics are considered in choosing an agency for use in a course, as discussed in Chapter 3, and they also guide the faculty in planning learning activities.

Teacher Availability

The teacher's availability to work with students in the clinical setting is an important consideration in planning the learning activities. Nursing students perceive the teacher's availability to guide their learning as one of the qualities of an effective clinical teacher (Sweet & Broadbent, 2017). The number and level of students in a clinical group, for instance, may influence the type of learning activities planned for a course. Beginning students and nurses new to a clinical practice area may require more time and guidance from the teacher than experienced students and nurses. This principle is also important in distance education and other courses using preceptors; the preceptor should be available to guide students' learning in clinical practice.

Guiding Learners in Clinical Practice

The next step in the process of clinical teaching is guiding learners to acquire the essential knowledge, technological and other skills, and values for practice. Guiding is a facilitative and supportive process that leads the student toward achievement of the outcomes. It is a process of supporting and coaching students in their learning. Guiding is not supervision; supervision is a process of overseeing. Effective clinical teaching requires that teachers guide students in their learning, not oversee their work.

This is the instructional phase in the clinical teaching process—the actual teaching of students in the clinical setting either on site or at a distance. For distance education courses, the instructional phase may be carried out by preceptors, advanced practice nurses (APNs) in the clinical setting, and other providers depending on the course outcomes. With some learning activities, the teacher has a direct instructional role—for instance, demonstrating an intervention to students and questioning them to expand their understanding of a clinical situation. Other teaching activities, though, may be indirect, such as giving feedback on papers and preparing preceptors for their role, among others.

Clinical teaching is more than guiding students in their learning. It also involves assisting them to integrate clinical information and assessment findings, helping them to make clinical judgments, and fostering a spirit of inquiry, among other outcomes (McNelis & Ironside, 2009). In clinical practice, students develop their clinical reasoning skills and learn to think like a nurse.

Clinical education provides the avenue for acquiring the knowledge and behaviors for practice in a particular role, whether it is a beginning professional nurse or new role such as APN. This process requires learning about the role as the initial step and observing and working with nurses in that role as the second step. In clinical instruction, the teacher guides the student in learning about the role and role behaviors of the nurse, and models important values and attributes of the professional in that role. Socialization comes from an integration of clinical and other experiences, not only from the guidance of the teacher. The experiences of students with preceptors, other nurses, and other health care providers contribute to this socialization process.

Skill in Observing Performance

In the process of guiding learners, the teacher needs to be skilled in: (a) observing clinical performance, arriving at sound judgments about that performance, and planning additional learning activities if needed and (b) questioning students to promote their thinking and clinical judgment. Observing students as they learn to care for patients and families and interact with others in the clinical environment allows the teacher to identify continued areas of learning and when assistance is needed from the teacher. This information, in turn, suggests new learning activities for clinical practice.

Observations of students may be influenced by the teacher's values and biases, which may affect *what they see* as they observe a student's performance and their *impressions* of the quality of that performance. All educators should know their own values and biases that might influence their observations of student performance in clinical practice and judgments about student performance of the competencies. Guidelines for observing students are summarized in Exhibit 5.2.

Skill in Questioning Students

The second skill needed by the teacher to effectively guide clinical learning activities is an ability to ask thought-provoking questions without students feeling that they are being interrogated. The ability to think critically is integral to providing safe and quality care, and this skill can be encouraged through the teachers' questions in the clinical setting (Phillips, Duke, & Weerasuriya, 2017). Open-ended questions about students' thinking and the rationale they used for arriving at clinical judgments foster development of higher level cognitive skills. Use of a questioning strategy also helps students begin to think like a nurse (Konradi, 2012).

Faculty members, however, tend to ask low-level questions that focus on recall of information rather than ones that foster critical thinking (Phillips et al., 2017). When questioning students in clinical practice, the teacher should assess understanding of relevant concepts and theories and how they apply to patient care. Other questions can ask students about different approaches and decisions possible in a clinical situation, consequences of each decision, what they would do, and their rationale; possible problems, interventions, and their evidence base; and assumptions underlying their thinking. Questions should encourage learners to think beyond the obvious.

EXHIBIT 5.2

GUIDELINES FOR OBSERVING STUDENTS IN CLINICAL PRACTICE

- Examine your values and biases that may influence observations of students in clinical practice and judgments about clinical performance.
- Do not rely on first impressions for these might change significantly with further observations of the student.
- Make a series of observations before drawing conclusions about clinical performance.
- Share with students on a continual basis observations made of clinical performance and judgments about whether students are meeting the clinical competencies.
- Focus observations on the outcomes of the clinical course or competencies to be achieved.
- When the observations reveal other aspects of performance that need further development, share these with students and use the information as a way of providing feedback on performance.
- Discuss observations with students, obtain their perceptions of performance, and be willing to modify judgments when a different perspective is offered (Oermann & Gaberson, 2017).

The way in which questions are asked is also significant. The purpose of questioning is to encourage students to consider other perspectives and possibilities, not to drill them and create added stress. In the beginning of a clinical course, and particularly in the beginning of the nursing program, the teacher should discuss the purpose of questioning and its relationship to developing thinking and clinical reasoning skills. The teacher can demonstrate the type of questions that will be asked in the course and emphasize that the goal is to help them learn and begin to think like a nurse.

Because questioning is for instructional purposes, students need to be comfortable that their responses will not influence their clinical grades. Instead, the questions asked and answers given are an essential part of the teaching process, to promote learning and development of critical thinking skills, not for grading purposes. Only with this framework will students be comfortable in responding to higher level questions and evaluating alternative perspectives, using the teacher as a resource.

Evaluating Clinical Learning and Performance

The remaining component of the clinical teaching process is evaluation. Clinical evaluation serves two purposes: formative and summative. Through formative evaluation, the teacher monitors student progress toward meeting the outcomes of the clinical course and demonstrating competency in clinical practice. Formative evaluation provides information about further learning needs of students and where additional clinical instruction is needed. Clinical evaluation that is formative is not intended for grading purposes; instead, it is designed to diagnose learning needs as a basis for further instruction.

Summative evaluation, in contrast, takes place at the end of the learning process to ascertain whether the course outcomes have been achieved and competencies developed (Oermann & Gaberson, 2017). Summative evaluation provides the basis for determining grades in clinical practice or certifying competency. It occurs at the completion of a course, an educational program, orientation, and other types of programs. This type of clinical evaluation determines what *has been* learned rather than what *can be* learned.

There are many clinical evaluation strategies that can be used in nursing courses. These are discussed and examples are provided in Chapter 15.

QUALITIES OF EFFECTIVE CLINICAL TEACHERS

Clinical teaching requires an educator who is knowledgeable about the clinical practice area, is clinically competent, knows how to teach, relates effectively to students, and is enthusiastic about clinical teaching. The teacher also serves as a role model for students or selects clinicians who will model important professional behaviors.

There has been much research in nursing education on characteristics and qualities of an effective clinical teacher. Every clinical teacher should be aware of behaviors that promote learning in the practice setting and ones that impede student learning.

Knowledge

Teachers in nursing, as in any field, need to have expertise in the subject they are teaching. In clinical teaching, this means that educators are knowledgeable about the types of patient problems in the clinical setting, nursing care measures, new treatments and technologies in patient care, and related research. Teachers must be up-to-date in the area of clinical practice in which they are working with students. This is particularly true in the traditional model of clinical teaching, in which the teacher is responsible for planning and guiding student learning in practice.

Clinical Competence

Teachers cannot guide student learning in clinical practice without being competent themselves. Clinical competence is an important characteristic of effective clinical teaching in nursing (Lovric, Prlic, Zec, Puselijic, & Zvanut, 2015). Teachers need to be experts in the area of clinical practice in which they are teaching, maintain their clinical skills, be able to explain and demonstrate nursing care in a real situation, and guide students in developing essential clinical competencies. This quality of teaching may be problematic for faculty members who teach predominantly in the classroom or change practice settings frequently and do not keep current in an area of clinical practice. It is up to the teacher to maintain clinical expertise and skills.

Skill in Clinical Teaching

Skill in clinical teaching includes the ability of the teacher to assess learning needs, plan instruction that meets those needs and fosters achievement of the outcomes of the clinical course, guide students in developing their clinical competencies, and evaluate learning fairly. These teaching skills are described more specifically in Exhibit 5.3.

The clinical teacher needs to know *how to teach*. While this seems obvious, in some settings, clinical teachers, preceptors, and others working with students are not prepared educationally for their roles. They have limited knowledge about how to guide students' learning in the clinical setting and assess their performance. Being an expert clinician is not enough. In a study by Lovric et al. (2015), students rated teaching ability among the most important competencies of a clinical nurse educator.

Skills in evaluating clinical performance both formatively, for feedback, and summatively, at the end of a period of time in the clinical course, are critical for effective teaching. Research has shown that effective teachers are fair in their evaluations of students, correct student errors without belittling students and diminishing their self-confidence, and give prompt feedback that promotes further learning and development.

Interpersonal Relationships With Students

The ability of the clinical teacher to interact with students, both on a one-to-one basis and as a clinical group, is another important teacher behavior. Qualities of an effective teacher in this area are showing confidence in students, respecting students, being honest and direct, supporting students and demonstrating caring behaviors, being approachable, and encouraging students to ask questions and seek guidance when needed. Considering the demands on students as they learn to care for patients, students need to view the teacher as someone who supports them in their learning. In a study by Hanson and Stenvig (2008), students identified three attributes of a good clinical nursing educator. These were knowledge, interpersonal relationships with students, and use of appropriate teaching strategies.

EXHIBIT 5.3

CLINICAL TEACHING SKILLS

- Assesses learning needs of students, recognizing and accepting individual differences
- Plans assignments that help in transfer of learning to clinical practice, meet learning needs, and promote acquisition of knowledge and development of competencies
- Communicates clearly to students outcomes of learning and expectations of students in clinical practice
- Considers student goals and needs in planning the clinical activities
- Structures clinical assignments and activities in clinical practice so they build on one another
- Explains clearly concepts and theories applicable to patient care
- Demonstrates effectively clinical skills, procedures, and use of technology
- Provides opportunities for practice of clinical skills, procedures, and technology and recognizes differences among students in the amount of practice needed
- Is well prepared for clinical teaching
- Develops clinical teaching strategies that encourage students to problem solve, arrive at clinical decisions, and think critically in a clinical situation
- Asks higher level questions that assist students in thinking through complex clinical situations and cases requiring critical thinking
- Encourages students through teaching and assessment to think independently and beyond accepted practices and to try out new interventions
- Varies clinical teaching strategies and learning activities to stimulate student interest and meet individual needs of students
- Guides learning and students' use of resources for learning
- Is available to students in clinical practice when they need assistance
- Serves as a role model for students
- Provides specific, timely, and useful feedback on student progress
- Shares observations of clinical performance with students
- Encourages students to evaluate their own performance
- Corrects mistakes without belittling students
- Exhibits fairness in evaluation

Personal Characteristics of the Clinical Teacher

Personal attributes of the teacher also influence teaching effectiveness. These attributes include enthusiasm, a sense of humor, willingness to admit limitations and mistakes honestly, patience, and flexibility when working with students in the clinical setting. Students often describe effective teachers as ones who are friendly and provide an opportunity for them to share feelings and concerns about patients. An effective clinical teacher is approachable (Sweet & Broadbent, 2017). Three other personal qualities important in teaching in any setting are integrity, perseverance, and courage (Glassick, Huber, & Maeroff, 1997). While these characteristics were originally used to describe the teacher as a scholar, they are just as important in carrying out the clinical teaching role. Integrity implies truthfulness with students and fairness in dealing with them in the process of learning and in clinical evaluation. The teacher develops an atmosphere of trust for students to engage in open discussions, examine alternatives, and discuss conflicting opinions with the faculty member. Fairness "involves the presentation of one's own interpretations and conclusions in ways that keep open an examination of alternatives" (Glassick et al., 1997, p. 64).

In clinical teaching, faculty members and other educators need to self-assess and recognize areas of teaching to be improved. They should be willing to reflect on their teaching and evaluation practices and consider better ways of designing clinical activities and guiding students in their learning. Good teachers, like good scholars, strive to perfect their teaching skills over time and avoid stagnation in their teaching approaches.

STRESSES OF STUDENTS IN CLINICAL PRACTICE

Clinical practice is inherently stressful. In the clinical setting, students face uncertainties and unique situations that they may not have encountered in their prior learning. For some students, clinical practice is stressful because they are unsure about approaches and interventions to use. Interacting with the teacher, other health care providers, the patient, and family members may also contribute to the stress that students experience in clinical practice.

Other stresses, from the students' perspective, relate to the changing nature of patient conditions, a lack of knowledge and skill to provide care to patients, excessive workload, unfamiliarity in the clinical setting, working with difficult patients, developing technological skills, and being observed and evaluated by the teacher (Blomberg et al., 2014; Li, Wang, Lin, & Lee, 2011; Moscaritolo, 2009; Suresh, Matthews, & Coyne, 2013). In a study by Li et al. (2011), stress from lack of knowledge and skills for practice was ranked highest by students. Studies also document student stress in academic and personal situations, but students perceive clinical stresses more intensely (Jimenez, Navia-Osorio, & Diaz, 2010).

In many of these studies, the clinical teacher and behaviors of the teacher created the most stress for students. This finding reinforces the need for the faculty to develop supportive and trusting relationships with students in the clinical setting and be aware of the stressful nature of clinical learning activities. A climate that supports the process of learning in clinical practice is dependent on a caring relationship between teacher and student rather than an adversarial one.

Learning in clinical practice occurs in public under the watchful eye of the teacher, the patient, and others in the setting. By keeping the nature of clinical learning in mind and using supportive behaviors when interacting with students, the teacher can reduce some of the stress that students naturally feel in clinical practice.

STRESSFUL NATURE OF CLINICAL TEACHING

Clinical teaching can be stressful for the teacher. First, it is time consuming. A three-credit theory or online course usually requires 3 hours per week of instruction, one clock hour for each credit hour, not including preparation time. However, a three-credit clinical course may require 6 to 9 hours of clinical teaching a week, two to three clinical practice hours per credit hour, and even more in some nursing education programs. This time commitment for clinical teaching may create stress for faculty members who are also involved in research, scholarship, professional service, and their own clinical practice. In many nursing education programs, faculty members do academic advisement of students and are responsible for writing grant proposals, conducting research, writing for publication, serving on committees, providing community service, and maintaining a clinical practice. These multiple roles are demanding for clinical educators.

In addition to demands associated with the multiple roles of a nursing faculty member, other aspects of clinical teaching may be stressful. These include:

- Coping with the many expectations associated with clinical teaching
- Feeling exhausted at the end of a clinical teaching experience with students
- Too heavy a workload
- Pressure to maintain clinical competence or a clinical practice without time to do so
- Feeling unable to satisfy the demands of students, clinical agency personnel, patients, and others
- Teaching inadequately prepared students

For some new clinical teachers, their stress relates to a lack of preparation for their role. While clinicians have expert knowledge and skills in their specialty area, they may have limited knowledge of how to teach. Reid, Hinderer, Jarosinski, Mister, and Seldomridge (2013) emphasized that preparation for the role of clinical teacher was essential to promote job satisfaction and reduce attrition. They prepared experienced clinicians as part-time clinical teachers using multiple teaching strategies (face-to-face and online instruction, simulations, and group mentoring sessions). As part of the preparation they also explored challenges faced by clinical teachers and provided mentoring for new faculty members.

The aim of the Eastern Shore Faculty Academy and Mentorship Initiative, a collaboration among three nursing programs, was to facilitate the transition of expert clinicians to part-time clinical educators to meet the needs for faculty in the region. The initiative addressed the nursing faculty shortage by developing a pool of highly qualified and diverse part-time clinical nurse educators who are shared across programs (Hinderer, Jarosinski, Seldomridge, & Reid, 2016).

Novice faculty members and teachers new to a nursing education program should find a mentor in the school who can support them as they learn the educator role in that setting. Mentors can be good sources of guidance on how to balance clinical teaching with other roles. Adjunct and part-time clinical educators also need a mentor to help them develop as effective clinical teachers. The mentor can be a resource for the clinical teacher and provide a link to the nursing program.

MODELS OF CLINICAL TEACHING

There are different models of clinical teaching: traditional, in which the teacher is directly responsible for guiding students in the clinical setting; preceptor; and clinical teaching partnership, including DEUs. In the preceptor and partnership models, preceptors and others in the clinical setting provide the clinical instruction, with the faculty member responsible for overall planning, coordinating the experience, grading clinical practice, and assuming other course-related responsibilities.

Traditional Model

In the traditional model of clinical teaching, the educator provides the instruction and evaluation for a small group of nursing students and is on site during the clinical experience. A benefit of this model is the opportunity to assist students in using the concepts and theories learned in class, through online instruction, in readings, and through other learning activities in patient care. The teacher can select clinical activities that best meet the students' needs and are consistent with course goals and objectives. Because the clinical teacher is involved to varying degrees with the nursing curriculum overall, the clinical activities may be more carefully selected to reflect the concepts that students are learning in the course than when preceptors or partners provide the instruction. In addition, the faculty member may be more committed to student learning and development and meeting course goals than preceptors or clinicians hired only for clinical teaching, often on a short-term basis.

Disadvantages, though, are the large number of students for whom faculty members may be responsible; not being accessible to students when needed because of demands of other students in the group; teaching procedures, clinical skills, and use of technologies for which the faculty member may lack expertise; the time commitment of providing on-site clinical instruction for faculty members with multiple other roles; and high costs for the nursing program. Clinical nurse educators who are part time or adjunct may not be sufficiently familiar with the philosophy and goals of the program, overall curriculum, clinical competencies developed prior to and following the course in which they are teaching, and other program characteristics, which may affect their planning of clinical activities for students and their expectations of students in the course. It is critical for the full-time faculty to prepare and orient part-time and adjunct faculty members involved in clinical teaching so they are not only aware of their role and responsibilities but also understand how their course relates to the overall nursing curriculum.

In the traditional model, the clinical learning experiences are dependent on patients in the setting at the time when students are present. As patients' conditions change, students may lack the requisite knowledge and skills to care for them. Nielsen (2009) identified another disadvantage in that students in acute care settings may prepare for particular assignments, but when they arrive on the unit, the patient is discharged. In courses in which students provide total patient care, they have limited time for contact with other patients in the setting. Nielsen proposed a concept-based approach in which students focus their learning on concepts—for example, oxygenation—and clinical practice provides experiences in those concepts across different patients. Nielsen, Noone, Voss, and Mathews (2013) described their model of clinical teaching, which is based on the intentional planning of clinical learning activities based on course competencies rather than a focus on total patient care experiences.

Another disadvantage of the traditional model of clinical teaching is that the educator and students may not be part of the health care system in which students have clinical practice. They are outsiders to the clinical setting and may not understand the system of care in that setting and its culture. As such, faculty members must work closely with the managers and clinical nursing staff to ensure an effective clinical experience for students. It is up to the faculty member to develop a working relationship with the staff, which is essential to create an environment for learning and take advantage of experiences available in the setting. In the traditional model of clinical teaching, faculty members who are not also practicing in the clinical setting often invest extensive time in developing and maintaining these relationships.

The relationships that nursing faculty members develop in the clinical setting are not only with nursing staff but also involve other health care providers. With the emphasis on interprofessional care, nursing students need clinical learning activities in which they examine their own role in relationship to other providers, collaborate with other health professionals, and learn to work as a team. This learning can occur with simulations. Simulations that involve nursing, medical, pharmacy, and other students provide a way for students to learn to collaborate and gain an understanding of different perspectives to patient care. Interprofessional education with simulation is an effective strategy to teach students about collaborative models of care delivery and prepare future health professionals to work effectively within teams (Buhse & Della Ratta, 2017; Horsley et al., 2016; Reed et al., 2016; Rossler, Buelow, Thompson, & Knofczynski, 2017).

Preceptor Model

In the preceptor model of clinical teaching, an expert nurse in the clinical setting works with the student on a one-to-one basis in the clinical setting. Preceptors are staff nurses and other nurses employed by the clinical agency who, in addition to their ongoing patient care responsibilities, provide on-site clinical instruction for students and new graduate nurses. In addition to one-to-one teaching, the preceptor guides and supports learners and serves as a role model.

In the preceptor model of clinical instruction, the faculty member from the nursing program serves as the coordinator, liaison between the nursing education program and clinical setting, and resource person for the preceptor. The faculty member, however, is typically not on site during the clinical practicum. The preceptor model involves sharing clinical teaching responsibilities between nursing program faculty members and expert clinicians from the practice setting.

One strength of the preceptor model is the consistent one-to-one relationship of the student and preceptor, providing an opportunity for the student to work closely with a role model. This close relationship promotes professional socialization and enables students to gain an understanding of how to function in the role for which they are being prepared. Other advantages of preceptorships are that students are able to work closely with a clinical expert in the field, improve their critical thinking and decision-making skills, and learn new clinical skills under the guidance of the preceptor. Through these experiences with the preceptor, students develop their self-confidence (Lewis & McGowan, 2015).

Potential disadvantages of the preceptor model are lack of integration of didactic learning and clinical practice; lack of flexibility in reassigning students to other preceptors if needed; and time and other demands made on the preceptors. Preceptors must be well prepared for their roles. This preparation should include instruction on methods to facilitate adult learning, teaching methods, communication, evaluation, and conflict resolution consistent with the specific goals of the nursing program (McClure & Black, 2013). To meet individual needs of preceptors, in one agency the preceptor preparation program was redesigned to include two levels: an introductory workshop for new preceptors and an advanced workshop for experienced preceptors. Preceptor competencies were developed specific to the organization and used to guide program development (Gueorguieva et al., 2016). Although preceptors should be prepared educationally for this role, some preceptors may lack clinical teaching skills. For effective teaching, the preceptor must be skilled as a teacher with the same qualities as other clinical educators described earlier in this chapter. In distance education courses, students typically have clinical experiences, guided by preceptors, in sites close to their home.

Partnership Model

There are varied types of partnerships in nursing education. Some of these are the result of nursing program faculties and administrators searching for ways to increase student enrollment and cope with budgetary constraints, a nursing faculty shortage, and not enough clinical sites, and others are intended to address the gap in preparation for practice readiness (American Association of Colleges of Nursing, 2008; Gorton & Foss, 2018; Wyte-Lake, Tran, Bowman, Needleman, & Dobalian, 2013). Didion, Kozy, Koffel, and Oneail (2013) described an academic–clinical partnership to better prepare students for improving the quality and safety of health care. In this partnership, students practice in a stable clinical setting rather than rotating across clinical sites to enable them to learn about system issues and gain experience in working with a health care team.

Partnerships vary widely. In some programs, the partnership model is a collaborative relationship between a clinical agency and nursing program that involves sharing a clinician and academic faculty member. The clinician teaches students in the clinical setting, with the faculty member serving as course coordinator, and the faculty member in turn contributes to the clinical agency—for example, by conducting research and serving as a consultant, or practicing as an APN in the agency. Expertise and services are shared between the partners. In this type of partnership, the clinician may work with a graduate or prelicensure nursing student on an individualized basis or may teach a small group of prelicensure students, as in the traditional clinical teaching model. At both the undergraduate and graduate levels, the faculty member works closely with the clinicians and agency to ensure the selection of relevant clinical activities for students.

Another example of a partnership for clinical teaching is the clinical scholar model, which originated in 1984 as a joint initiative between the University of Colorado College of Nursing and University of Colorado Hospital. In this model, clinical nurse experts coordinate student placements and learning experiences, provide consistent instruction for nursing students, and contribute to the evaluation of students' clinical competencies. These clinical experts are master's prepared in nursing and have a minimum of 5 years of experience in a nursing specialty practice and 2 years of employment in the health care agency (Gorton & Foss, 2018). This model gives students an opportunity to be taught by expert clinicians practicing in the setting. Other partnerships are community based, linking education, practice, and research.

Another type of partnership is the DEU, which is a unit within a clinical setting or a setting that is dedicated to teaching nursing students. A DEU is a triad of students, faculty members, and clinical nursing staff who collaborate to create a learning environment for students. While there are varied DEU models in the United States and other countries, a common element is the active engagement of nursing and other staff in the education of students. In these models, nurse clinicians serve as clinical teachers with academic faculty members in the role as liaison, guiding the clinician to ensure a quality clinical experience and that course outcomes are met. The goal of this model is to better prepare nursing students for clinical practice and with fewer faculty members from the school of nursing (Dapremont & Lee, 2013; Moscato, Nishioka, & Coe, 2013). The key to sustaining DEUs depends on the interest of clinicians to teach students and provide support for their learning (Mulready-Shick & Flanagan, 2014).

DEUs have been found to increase agency capacity, allowing schools to place more students in the setting than with a traditional clinical course or preceptorship (Hill, Foster, & Oermann, 2015; Moscato et al., 2013). Both students and staff report satisfaction with this model of clinical teaching. Another benefit of a DEU is that the agency partner can often reduce orientation time for new graduate nurses who had DEU clinical experiences in the setting (Sharpnack, Koppelman, & Fellows, 2014). While DEUs are used typically in acute care for prelicensure students, the model is also found in diverse patient care settings such as long-term care (Melillo et al., 2014), maternal–newborn units (Raines, 2016), and intensive care (Koharchik et al., 2016).

Selecting a Clinical Teaching Model

There is no one model that meets the needs of every nursing education program, clinical course, or group of students. The teacher should select a model considering these factors:

- Educational philosophy of the nursing program
- Philosophy of the faculty about clinical teaching
- Goals and intended outcomes of the clinical course and activities
- Level of nursing student
- Type of clinical setting
- Availability of preceptors, expert nurses, and other people in the practice setting who provide clinical instruction
- Willingness of clinical agency personnel and partners to participate in teaching students and other educational activities

SUMMARY

The process of clinical teaching begins with identification of the goals and outcomes for clinical learning and proceeds through assessing the learner, planning clinical learning activities, guiding students, and evaluating clinical learning and performance. The goals and outcomes suggest areas for assessment, provide guidelines for teaching, and are the basis for evaluating learning. They may be expressed in the form of clinical objectives, outcomes, or competencies and may be established for an entire course or for specific clinical activities. The outcomes of clinical practice should be communicated clearly to students, in written form, and understood by them. Similarly, the teacher has an important responsibility in discussing these outcomes and related clinical activities with agency personnel.

Teaching begins at the level of the learner. The teacher's goal, therefore, is to assess the student's present level of knowledge and skill and other characteristics that may influence developing the clinical competencies. This assessment is important so that students engage in learning activities that build on their present knowledge and skills. When students lack the prerequisites, then the instruction can remedy these deficiencies and more efficiently move students forward in their learning. The second area of assessment relates to individual characteristics of students that may influence their learning and clinical performance, such as age, learning style, and cultural background.

Following assessment of learner needs and characteristics, the teacher plans and then delivers the instruction. In planning the learning activities, the main considerations are the objectives and individual learner needs. The next step in the process of clinical teaching is that of guiding learners to acquire essential knowledge, skills, and values for practice. In this process of guiding learners, the teacher needs to be skilled in (a) observing clinical performance, arriving at sound judgments about that performance, and planning additional learning activities if needed and (b) questioning learners to encourage critical thinking but without interrogating them.

The last component of the clinical teaching process is evaluation. Clinical evaluation can be formative or summative. Through formative evaluation, the teacher monitors student progress in meeting the clinical outcomes and demonstrating competency in clinical practice. Summative evaluation, in contrast, takes place at the end of the learning period to ascertain whether the outcomes have been achieved and competencies developed. It occurs at the completion of a course, an educational program, orientation, and other types of programs. This type of clinical evaluation determines what *has been* learned rather than what *can be* learned.

Teaching in the clinical setting requires an educator who is knowledgeable, is clinically competent, knows how to teach, relates effectively to students, and is enthusiastic about clinical teaching. The research in nursing education over the years has substantiated that these qualities are important in clinical teaching.

Clinical practice is stressful for students. Students have identified dimensions of clinical learning that often produce anxiety, such as fear of making a mistake that would harm the patient; interacting with the patient, the teacher, and other health care providers; the changing nature of patient conditions; a lack of knowledge and skill for giving care to patients; and working with difficult patients, among others. In some research studies, students have reported that the teacher is a source of added stress for them. These findings highlight the need for the teacher to develop supportive and trusting relationships with students in the clinical setting and to be aware of the stressful nature of this learning experience. A climate that supports the process of learning in clinical practice is dependent on a caring relationship between teacher and student rather than an adversarial one.

The teacher chooses a model for clinical teaching: traditional, preceptor, or partnership, including the DEU model. In the traditional model of clinical teaching, the instruction and evaluation of a group of students are carried out by a faculty member. In the preceptor model of clinical teaching, an expert nurse in the clinical setting works with the student typically on a one-to-one basis. The preceptor also guides and supports the learner and serves as a role model. The faculty member is typically not on site during the clinical experience but has important responsibilities for the course, such as serving as course coordinator, providing the classroom instruction, serving as a liaison between the nursing education program and clinical setting, and being a resource person for the preceptor.

Partnerships were also described in this chapter. The partnership model varies with the academic institution but is generally a collaborative relationship between the nursing education program and a clinical agency or with the community. Partnerships emphasize collaboration among partners to meet the needs of the partners and community as a whole. Another type of partnership is the DEU, in which agency nursing staff teach prelicensure nursing students with the unit assuming responsibility for creating a supportive learning environment. In these models, nurse clinicians serve as clinical teachers with academic faculty members in the role of liaison, guiding the clinician to ensure a quality clinical experience and that course outcomes are met.

CNE EXAMINATION TEST BLUEPRINT CORE COMPETENCIES

1. **Facilitate Learning**
   A. Implement a variety of teaching strategies appropriate to
      1. content
      2. setting (clinical)
      3. learner needs
      4. learning style
      5. desired learner outcomes
      6. method of delivery
   B. Use teaching strategies based on
      1. educational theory
      2. evidence-based practices related to education
   C. Modify teaching strategies and learning experiences based on consideration of
      1. cultural background
      2. past clinical experiences
      3. past educational and life experiences
   F. Communicate effectively orally and in writing with an ability to convey ideas in a variety of contexts
   G. Model reflective thinking practices, including critical thinking
   H. Create opportunities for learners to develop their own critical thinking skills
   I. Create a positive learning environment that fosters a free exchange of ideas
   J. Show enthusiasm for teaching, learning, and the nursing profession that inspires and motivates students
   K. Demonstrate personal attributes that facilitate learning (e.g., caring, confidence, patience, integrity, respect, and flexibility)
   L. Respond effectively to unexpected events that affect instruction
   M. Develop collegial working relationships with clinical agency personnel to promote positive learning environments
   N. Use knowledge of evidence-based practice to instruct learners
   O. Demonstrate ability to teach clinical skills
   P. Act as a role model in practice settings
   Q. Foster a safe learning environment

2. **Facilitate Learner Development and Socialization**
   A. Identify individual learning styles and unique learning needs of learners
   B. Provide resources for diverse learners to meet their individual learning needs
   C. Advise learners in ways that help them meet their professional goals
   D. Create learning environments that facilitate learners' self-reflection, personal goal setting, and socialization to the role of the nurse
   E. Foster the development of learners in these areas
      1. cognitive domain
      2. psychomotor domain
      3. affective domain
   F. Assist learners to engage in thoughtful and constructive self and peer evaluation
   H. Encourage professional development of learners

5. **Pursue Systematic Self-Evaluation and Improvement in the Academic Nurse Educator Role**
   A. Engage in activities that promote one's socialization to the role
   D. Demonstrate a commitment to lifelong learning
   E. Participate in professional development opportunities that increase one's effectiveness in the role
   F. Manage the teaching, scholarship, and service demands as influenced by the requirements of the institutional setting

(continued)

6. **Engage in Scholarship, Service, and Leadership**

    B. Engage in scholarship of teaching
        1. Exhibit a spirit of inquiry about teaching and learning, student development, and evaluation methods
        2. Use evidence-based resources to improve and support teaching
    C. Function effectively within the organizational environment and academic community
        3. Integrate the values of respect, collegiality, professionalism, and caring to build an organizational climate that fosters the development of learners and colleagues

REFERENCES

American Association of Colleges of Nursing. (2008). *Essentials of baccalaureate education for professional nursing.* Retrieved from http://www.aacn.nche.edu/education-resources/BaccEssentials08.pdf

Blomberg, K., Bisholt, B., Kullen Engstrom, A., Ohlsson, U., Sundler Johansson, A., & Gustafsson, M. (2014). Swedish nursing students' experience of stress during clinical practice in relation to clinical setting characteristics and the organisation of the clinical education. *Journal of Clinical Nursing, 23,* 2264–2271. doi:10.1111/jocn.12506

Buhse, M., & Della Ratta, C. (2017). Enhancing interprofessional education with team-based learning. *Nurse Educator, 42.* [E-pub ahead of print]. doi:10.1097/nne.0000000000000370

Dapremont, J., & Lee, S. (2013). Partnering to educate: Dedicated education units. *Nurse Education in Practice, 13,* 335–337. doi:10.1016/j.nepr.2013.02.015

Didion, J., Kozy, M. A., Koffel, C., & Oneail, K. (2013). Academic/clinical partnership and collaboration in Quality and Safety Education for Nurses education. *Journal of Professonional Nursing, 29,* 88–94. doi:10.1016/j.profnurs.2012.12.004

Gholami, M., Moghadam, P. K., Mohammadipoor, F., Tarahi, M. J., Sak, M., Toulabi, T., & Pour, A. H. (2016). Comparing the effects of problem-based learning and the traditional lecture method on critical thinking skills and metacognitive awareness in nursing students in a critical care nursing course. *Nurse Education Today, 45,* 16–21. doi:10.1016/j.nedt.2016.06.007

Glassick, C. E., Huber, M. T., & Maeroff, G. I. (1997). *Scholarship assessed.* San Francisco, CA: Jossey-Bass.

Gorton, K., & Foss, K. (2018). Partnerships with clinical settings: Roles and responsibilities of nurse educators. In M. H. Oermann, J. C. De Gagne, & B. C. Phillips (Eds.), *Teaching in nursing and role of the educator: The complete guide to best practice in teaching, evaluation, and curriculum development* (2nd ed., pp. 203–230). New York, NY: Springer Publishing.

Gueorguieva, V., Chang, A., Fleming-Carroll, B., Breen-Reid, K. M., Douglas, M., & Parekh, S. (2016). Working toward a competency-based preceptor development program. *Journal of Continuing Education Nursing, 47,* 427–432. doi:10.3928/00220124-20160817-10

Hanson, K. J., & Stenvig, T. E. (2008). The good clinical nursing educator and the baccalaureate nursing clinical experience: Attributes and praxis. *Journal of Nursing Education, 47,* 38–42.

Hill, R. Y., Foster, B., & Oermann, M. (2015). Dedicated education unit model for a transition into practice course. *Journal of Continuing Education in Nursing, 46,* 403–408. doi:10.3928/00220124-20150821-02

Hinderer, K. A., Jarosinski, J. M., Seldomridge, L. A., & Reid, T. P. (2016). From expert clinician to nurse educator: Outcomes of a faculty academy initiative. *Nurse Educator, 41,* 194–198. doi:10.1097/nne.0000000000000243

Horsley, T. L., Reed, T., Muccino, K., Quinones, D., Siddall, V. J., & McCarthy, J. (2016). Developing a foundation for interprofessional education within nursing and medical curricula. *Nurse Educator, 41*(5), 234–238. doi:10.1097/nne.0000000000000255

Jeffreys, M. R., & Dogan, E. (2013). Evaluating cultural competence in the clinical practicum. *Nursing Education Perspectives, 34,* 88–94.

Jimenez, C., Navia-Osorio, P. M., & Diaz, C. V. (2010). Stress and health in novice and experienced nursing students. *Journal of Advanced Nursing, 66,* 442–455. doi:10.1111/j.1365–2648.2009.05183.x

Koharchik, L., Jakub, K., Witsberger, C., Brooks, K., Petras, D., Weideman, Y., & Antonich, M. G. (2016). Staff nurse's perception of their role in a dedicated education unit within the intensive care unit. *Teaching and Learning in Nursing, 12,* 17–20. doi:10.1016/j.teln.2016.11.001

Kong, L. N., Qin, B., Zhou, Y. Q., Mou, S. Y., & Gao, H. M. (2013). The effectiveness of problem-based learning on development of nursing students' critical thinking: A systematic review and meta-analysis. *International Journal of Nursing Studies.* doi:10.1016/j.ijnurstu.2013.06.009

Konradi, D. B. (2012). Learning to think like a professional nurse: A critical questions strategy. *Journal of Nursing Education, 51,* 359–360. doi:10.3928/01484834-20120522-03

Lewis, S., & McGowan, B. (2015). Newly qualified nurses' experiences of a preceptorship. *British Journal of Nursing, 24*(1), 40–43. doi:10.12968/bjon.2015.24.1.40

Li, H.-C., Wang, L. S., Lin, Y.-H., & Lee, I. (2011). The effect of a peer-mentoring strategy on student nurse stress reduction in clinical practice. *International Nursing Review, 58,* 203–210. doi:10.1111/j.1466-7657.2010.00839.x

Lovric, R., Prlic, N., Zec, D., Puseljic, S., & Zvanut, B. (2015). Students' assessment and self-assessment of nursing clinical faculty competencies: Important feedback in clinical education? *Nurse Educator, 40,* E1–E5. doi:10.1097/nne.0000000000000137

McClure, E., & Black, L. (2013). The role of the clinical preceptor: An integrative literature review. *Journal of Nursing Education, 52,* 335–341. doi:10.3928/01484834-20130430-02

McLain, R. M., Fifolt, M., Dawson, M. A., Su, W., Milligan, G., Davis, S., & Hites, L. (2017). Student success survey: Supporting academic success for at-risk nursing students through early intervention. *Nurse Educator, 42,* 33–37. doi:10.1097/nne.0000000000000322

McNelis, A., & Ironside, P. (2009). National survey on clinical education in prelicensure nursing education programs. In N. Ard & T. M. Valiga (Eds.), *Clinical nursing education: Current reflections* (pp. 29–38). New York, NY: National League for Nursing.

Melillo, K. D., Abdallah, L., Dodge, L. Dowling, J. S., Prendergast, N., Rathbone, A., . . . Thorton, C. (2014). Developing a dedicated education unit in long-term care: A pilot project. *Geriatric Nursing, 35*(2014), 264–271. doi:10.1016/j.gerinurse.2014.02.022

Moscaritolo, L. (2009). Interventional strategies to decrease nursing student anxiety in the clinical learning environment. *Journal of Nursing Education, 48,* 17–23.

Moscato, S. R., Nishioka, V. M., & Coe, M. T. (2013). Dedicated education unit: Implementing an innovation in replication sites. *Journal of Nursing Education, 52,* 259–267. doi:10.3928/01484834-20130328-01

Mulready-Shick, J., & Flanagan, K. (2014). Building the evidence for dedicated education unit sustainability and partnership success. *Nursing Education Perspectives, 35,* 287–293. doi:10.5480/14-1379

Nielsen, A. E. (2009). Educational innovations. Concept-based learning activities using the clinical judgment model as a foundation for clinical learning. *Journal of Nursing Education, 48,* 350–354.

Nielsen, A. E., Noone, J., Voss, H., & Mathews, L. (2013). Preparing nursing students for the future: An innovative approach to clinical education. *Nurse Education In Practice, 13,* 301–309. doi:10.1016/j.nepr.2013.03.015

Oermann, M. H. (2009). Evidence-based programs and teaching/evaluation methods: Needed to achieve excellence in nursing education. In M. Adams & T. Valiga (Eds.), *Achieving excellence in nursing education* (pp. 63–76). New York, NY: National League for Nursing.

Oermann, M. H., & Conklin, J. L. (2018). Evidence-based teaching in nursing. In M. H. Oermann, J. C. De Gagne, & B. C. Phillips (Eds.), *Teaching in nursing and role of the educator: The complete guide to best practice in teaching, evaluation, and curriculum development* (2nd ed., pp. 363–378). New York, NY: Springer Publishing.

Oermann, M. H., & Gaberson, K. B. (2017). *Evaluation and testing in nursing education* (5th ed.). New York, NY: Springer Publishing.

Phillips, N. M., Duke, M. M., & Weerasuriya, R. (2017). Questioning skills of clinical facilitators supporting undergraduate nursing students. *Journal of Clinical Nursing.* Advance online publication. doi:10.1111/jocn.137611

Raines, D. A. (2016). A dedicated education unit for maternal-newborn nursing clinical education. *Nursing for Women's Health, 20*(1), 21–27. doi:10.1016/j.nwh.2015.12.005

Reed, T., Horsley, T. L., Muccino, K., Quinones, D., Siddall, V. J., McCarthy, J., & Adams, W. (2016). Simulation using TeamSTEPPS to promote interprofessional education and collaborative practice. *Nurse Educator, 42*(3), E1–E5. doi:10.1097/nne.0000000000000350

Reid, T. P., Hinderer, K. A., Jarosinski, J. M., Mister, B. J., & Seldomridge, L. A. (2013). Expert clinician to clinical teacher: Developing a faculty academy and mentoring initiative. *Nurse Education in Practice, 13,* 288–293. doi:10.1016/j.nepr.2013.03.022

Rossler, K. L., Buelow, J. R., Thompson, A. W., & Knofczynski, G. (2017). Effective learning of interprofessional teamwork. *Nurse Educator, 42,* 67–71. doi:10.1097/nne.0000000000000313

Sharpnack, P. A., Koppelman, C., & Fellows, B. (2014). Using a dedication education unit clinical education model with second-degree accelerated nursing program students. *Journal of Nursing Education, 53,* 685–691. doi:10.3928/01484834-20141120-01

Suresh, P., Matthews, A., & Coyne, I. (2013). Stress and stressors in the clinical environment: A comparative study of fourth-year student nurses and newly qualified general nurses in Ireland. *Journal of Clinical Nursing, 22,* 770–779. doi:10.1111/j.1365-2702.2012.04145.x

Sweet, L., & Broadbent, J. (2017). Nursing students' perceptions of the qualities of a clinical facilitator that enhance learning. *Nurse Education in Practice, 22,* 30–36. doi:10.1016/j.nepr.2016.11.007

Wyte-Lake, T., Tran, K., Bowman, C. C., Needleman, J., & Dobalian, A. (2013). A systematic review of strategies to address the clinical nursing faculty shortage. *Journal of Nursing Education, 52,* 245–252. doi:10.3928/01484834-20130213-02

CHAPTER 6

Ethical and Legal Issues in Clinical Teaching

Clinical teaching and learning take place in a social context. Teachers, students, staff members, and patients have roles, rights, and responsibilities that are sometimes in conflict. These conflicts create legal and ethical dilemmas for clinical teachers. This chapter discusses some ethical and legal issues related to clinical teaching and offers suggestions for preventing, minimizing, and managing these difficult situations.

USE OF SOCIAL MEDIA

Online social networking is a useful and popular means of communication and collaboration. Social media forms include Facebook, Twitter, LinkedIn, Instagram, Myspace, YouTube, and Pinterest, among others. Many nursing students at every educational level are active users of social media, especially members of the millennial generation who are "digital natives." Health care professionals' conduct both on and off the job is held to ethical and legal standards and guidelines; personal and professional identities overlap and are difficult to separate. Nursing students may be unaware of their responsibilities with regard to social media use in the context of nurse–patient relationships and as members of the profession of nursing. Therefore, nursing faculty members and students may encounter ethical and legal consequences of social media misuse (Stephens & Gunther, 2016; Westrick, 2016).

Misuse of social media becomes a source of regulatory concern when role boundary violations occur (Spector & Kappel, 2012). The American Nurses Association (ANA) *Code of Ethics for Nurses with Interpretative Statements* (2015) emphasizes the obligation of nurses to act within the professional role and to maintain role boundaries in relationships with patients. Boundary violations can occur when students "friend" or "follow" patients or former patients on social media, resulting in harm to patients (Westrick, 2016).

The *Code of Ethics* (ANA, 2015) also specifically mentions social media in emphasizing the nurse's obligation to maintain patient privacy. Confidentiality can be breached when information about patients is posted on social media sites, even without revealing a patient's name. Patients have a right to privacy, and sometimes information can be pieced together from various postings (possibly by different people) resulting in identification of a specific patient. Such disclosures often are unintentional, but they can have serious consequences for patients (Westrick, 2016).

In addition to potential harm to patients, social media misuse can have serious consequences for nursing students, nursing education programs, and health care facilities. While nursing students cannot be disciplined by state boards of nursing, they may face disciplinary action, including course failure or dismissal, by the nursing education program. Additionally, nursing education programs' working relationships with clinical agencies could be damaged by students' boundary violations and breaches of confidentiality, and future nursing students could lose valuable clinical learning opportunities in those settings. Health care facilities can face fines for student violations of the U.S. Health Insurance Portability and Accountability Act (HIPAA) of 1996 (discussed later in this chapter), and students could be subject to private legal actions by patients or consequences for violating laws (Westrick, 2016).

Nursing education programs should develop and enforce explicit policies regarding the use of electronic communication and social media, including specific consequences for policy violations. Professional guidelines such as the ANA's *Code of Ethics* (2015), ANA's *Principles for Social Networking and the Nurse* (2011a) and *Social Networking Principles Toolkit* (2011b), and the National Council of State Boards of Nursing's (NCSBN) *A Nurse's Guide to the Use of Social Media* (2011) can be referenced in these policies. Students may be required to sign documents affirming that they have reviewed and agree to adhere to the nursing education program social media use policies (Westrick, 2016).

Nursing faculty members should discuss guidelines for nurses' appropriate use of social media with students. These guidelines include:

- *Conduct standards.* Nursing students are held to the same professional, legal, and ethical behavior as licensed nurses. While engaged in clinical learning activities, they are subject to agency policies and requirements. Conduct outside of class and clinical practica may be evaluated according to the same professional standards.
- *Protecting patient privacy.* Do not post or transmit individually identifiable patient information, including names, images, or any information that can reasonably be used to identify patients. Do not transmit patient information to anyone who does not have a legitimate care-based or legal need to know.
- *Maintaining nurse-patient boundaries.* Establish, communicate, and enforce professional boundaries with patients in social media. Nurses should not participate in online social relationships with patients or former patients.
- *Viewing by others.* Evaluate all online communication and behavior with the understanding that it could be viewed by patients, educators, colleagues, and employers or potential employers. Even if later deleted, the data remain on a server and could be retrieved by others or discovered by a court of law.
- *Separate online personal and professional information.* Use the privacy settings on social media sites to keep personal and professional online activities separate. However, these precautions do not guarantee that information will not be disseminated by others in less protected formats.
- *Response to questionable content.* Take appropriate action regarding posting of social media content that reflects incompetent, unethical, illegal, or impaired practice. Bring questionable content to the attention of colleagues who posted

it so that they may take appropriate action. If the posted content poses a risk to patient safety or privacy, report it to a supervisor or teacher and, if action is not taken, to the appropriate external authorities.

■ *Development of policy.* Participate in the development of institutional policy concerning online conduct that raises legal and ethical concerns. Such policies should address remedial action for patients and nonpunitive correction and training for nurses whose questionable online conduct is unintentional.

■ *Respect for colleagues and employers.* Avoid discussing school- or work-related issues online, including complaints about classmates, teachers, clinical agencies, or the educational institution. Do not make disparaging, threatening, harassing, derogatory, or other offensive comments about others. These activities may constitute cyber-bullying. Such behavior also may be detrimental to effective health care team functioning, with patient safety ramifications, and may result in sanctions against the nurse. (ANA, 2011a; NCSBN, 2011; Westrick, 2016)

Faculty members should review the ethical and legal standards and guidelines for social media use with students on a regular basis (e.g., yearly or every semester) and may reinforce these concepts using case studies or simulations.

ETHICAL ISSUES

Ethics are standards of conduct based on beliefs about what is good and bad, obligations related to good and bad acts, and principles underlying decisions to conform to these standards. Ethical standards make it possible for nurses, patients, teachers, and students to understand and respect each other. Contemporary bioethical standards are related to respect for human dignity, autonomy, and freedom; beneficence; justice; veracity; privacy; and fidelity (Oermann & Gaberson, 2017). These standards are important considerations for all parties involved in clinical teaching and learning.

Learners in a Service Setting

If the word *clinical* means "involving direct observation of the patient," clinical activities must take place where patients are. Traditionally, learners encounter patients in health care service settings, such as acute care, extended care, and rehabilitation facilities. With the increasing focus on controlling health care costs and primary prevention, however, patients increasingly receive health care in the home, community, and school environments. Whatever the setting, patients are there to receive health care, staff members have the responsibility to provide care, and students are present to learn. Are these purposes always compatible?

Although it has been more than three decades since Corcoran (1977) raised ethical questions about the use of service settings for learning activities, those concerns still are valid. In the clinical setting, nursing students or new staff members are learners who are somewhat less skilled than experienced practitioners. Although their activities are observed and guided by clinical teachers, learners are not expected to provide cost-effective, efficient patient care services. On the other hand, patients expect quality service when they seek health care; providing learning opportunities for students is not usually their priority. The ethical standard of *beneficence* refers to the duty to help, to produce beneficial outcomes, or at least to do no harm. Is this standard violated when the learners' chief purpose for being in the clinical environment is to learn, not to give care?

Patients who encounter learners in clinical settings may feel exploited or fear invasion of their privacy; they may receive care that takes more time and creates more discomfort than if provided by expert practitioners. The presence of learners in a clinical setting also requires more time and energy of staff members, who are usually expected to give and receive reports from students, answer their questions, and demonstrate or help with patient care. These activities may divert staff members' attention from their primary responsibility for patient care, interfere with their efficient performance, and affect their satisfaction with their work.

Because achieving the desired outcomes of clinical teaching requires learning activities in real service settings, teachers must consider the rights and needs of learners, patients, and staff members when planning clinical learning activities. The clinical teacher is responsible for making the learning objectives clear to all involved persons and for ensuring that learning activities do not prevent achievement of service goals. Patients should receive adequate information about the presence of learners in the settings where they are receiving care before giving their informed consent to participate in clinical learning activities. The teacher should ensure the learners' preparation and readiness for clinical learning as well as his or her own presence and competence as an instructor, as discussed in Chapter 4.

Student–Faculty Relationships

Respect for Persons

As discussed in Chapter 1, an effective and beneficial relationship between clinical teacher and student is built on a base of mutual trust and respect. Although both parties are responsible for maintaining this relationship, the clinical teacher must initiate it by demonstrating trust and respect for students. A trusting, respectful relationship with students demonstrates the teacher's commitment to ethical values of respect for human dignity and autonomy. Because civil behavior is learned, teachers must model discretion, attentiveness, respectful communication, and professional behavior in all encounters with students, colleagues, patients, and staff members in the clinical setting (Altmiller, 2012).

Incivility is a form of disrespect for persons. Both nursing faculty members and nursing students perceive incivility to be a growing concern in nursing education (Luparell, 2011). Academic incivility is behavior in the form of words, actions, or gestures that is intended to be rude or disrespectful, that interferes with the teaching–learning process, and that leads to mental and physical distress among those in that environment. It can span a broad continuum of behaviors including lack of preparation for learning activities, unwillingness to engage in the learning process, tardiness, unauthorized use of cell phones or other devices, distracting side conversations, insulting the instructor, intimidation, physical aggression against other students or teachers, and making direct threats of violence (Altmiller, 2012; Rad & Moonaghi, 2016; Robertson, 2012). In clinical practice, uncivil behavior can negatively affect patient safety by disrupting interdisciplinary team functioning and hampering clear, timely communication of patient information (Clark & Springer, 2010). If nursing students do not learn civil interaction with patients, team members, and those in authority, they are likely to become uncivil employees in the health care system (Rad & Moonaghi, 2016).

Student factors that may contribute to academic incivility include anxiety "derived from a perpetual fear of failure" (Robertson, 2012, p. 26) as well as competing demands of occupational workload and family responsibilities, financial stress, time management challenges, and mental health and personal issues (Clark & Springer, 2010). These stressors exhaust students' adaptive coping mechanisms, resulting in fear, desperation, and intense frustration manifested in the form of anger, impulsivity, impaired judgment, and incivility.

Faculty conduct may exacerbate academic incivility, including teaching behaviors that perpetuate or amplify student anxiety, such as arrogance, superiority, and abuse of authority; gossip about students; expression of anger; threats regarding grades; publicly embarrassing or ridiculing students in clinical settings; lack of clarity in the course syllabus about expectations for student performance, evaluation, and conduct; perceived favoritism toward some students, and inability to manage or overlooking uncivil student behavior (Altmiller, 2012; Clark & Springer, 2010; Rad & Moonaghi, 2016; Robertson, 2012). Thus, student anxiety is magnified by teachers whose teaching practices gravitate toward opposite ends of the spectrum. Some teachers fail to clearly communicate their expectations, while others use rigid and oppressive pedagogies that lack caring and respect. Students and teachers become preoccupied with self-preservation rather than the educational task at hand, and each group assigns blame to the other (Robertson, 2012).

The most effective approach to managing incivility in clinical teaching focuses on prevention while simultaneously specifying and implementing progressive disciplinary measures if the proactive methods fail. The faculty must establish clear policies about the administration of each course (e.g., attendance, unsafe clinical practice) and expectations for student performance, evaluation, and behavior, including the repercussions of uncivil behavior. These expectations should be included in course syllabi and discussed with students at the beginning of the academic term. A set of behavioral standards to which students and faculty must adhere minimizes misunderstandings and misalignment of expectations. These standards may be developed collaboratively by teachers and students, regularly reviewed with students, and referenced in course syllabi (Robertson, 2012). As previously mentioned, teachers must consistently adhere to such behavioral standards and model the civil behavior they wish to see in students.

Unfortunately, neither detailed course syllabi nor a widely communicated set of conduct standards will prevent all acts of incivility. "In such instances, a well-written protocol not only affords clarity and guidance, but it also promotes the consistent handling of classroom incivility" (Robertson, 2012, p. 25). This protocol should also be shared with students so that they are aware that a standardized approach to conduct violations will be used by faculty members and administrators. The protocol should clearly specify progressive discipline for infractions, which may include an oral or written warning or reprimand, removal from the clinical environment for a specified period of time, a disciplinary hearing, or dismissal from the nursing education program, depending on the severity of the infraction. As is the case for all such policy development, the faculty is advised to seek guidance from the institution's legal counsel to make sure that student rights are protected and that the policy and procedures are consistent with those of the governing institution. Additionally, a carefully crafted and publicized protocol has no power unless it is consistently applied by all faculty members with support from program administrators.

Fairness and Justice

The ethical standard of justice refers to fair treatment—judging each person's behavior by the same standards. Clinical teachers must evaluate each student's performance by the same standard. Students may perceive a clinical teacher's behavior as unfair when the teacher appears to favor some students by praising, supporting, and offering better learning opportunities to them more than others. In a study of student perceptions of incivility, Altmiller (2012) found that students identified the power gradient between students and teachers as a source of potential and actual unequal treatment. They cited experiences of gender, ethnic, and racial bias and discrimination, and feared that the teacher's authority and power would discourage teachers from restraining those biases. Developing social relationships with some students could be perceived as favoritism by other students. Teachers often find it challenging to set appropriate role boundaries for teacher–student relationships. While their primary role is that of teacher, they also want to model caring behavior to students, be supportive to students who are struggling, and be approachable and student-friendly (Poorman, Mastorovich, & Webb, 2011). However, in their desire to "make visible [their] concern for students" (Poorman et al., 2011, p. 373), teachers may cross the line into inequitable treatment based on personal feelings. The teacher's relationships with students can be friendly and warm but should be collegial without being personal and social.

As previously discussed, nurse educators should be prudent about their use of social networking sites such as Facebook and Twitter. Faculty members have used Twitter to communicate with students, build relationships with them, and enhance their learning. However, these uses of social networking sites should be separate from the teacher's personal use of these technologies. Befriending students on their Facebook page and following them on Twitter raises faculty–student boundary issues and implies an egalitarian relationship that does not acknowledge the power advantage that faculty members hold (Oermann & Gaberson, 2017; Westrick, 2016). Inviting students to sign up as friends or followers to a Facebook or Twitter account that the teacher uses for social interaction with peers invites their discovery of information that the teacher might prefer to be private.

Students' Privacy Rights

When students have a succession of clinical instructors, it is common for the instructors to communicate information about student performance. Learning about the students' levels of performance in their previous clinical assignment helps the next instructor to anticipate their needs and to plan appropriate learning activities for them. Although students usually benefit when teachers share such information about their learning needs, personal information that students reveal in confidence should not be shared with other teachers. The U.S. Family Educational Rights and Privacy Act of 1974, as amended, restricts disclosure of students' academic information to individuals who have a legitimate need to know; written permission from students is necessary to discuss their performance with anyone else. Evaluative statements about student performance should not be shared with other faculty members, but information about a student's need for a particular learning activity or more practice with a specific skill is necessary for a teacher to provide the appropriate guidance.

Additionally, when sharing information about students, teachers should focus on factual statements about performance without adding personal judgments.

Characterizing or labeling students is rarely helpful to the next instructor, and such behavior violates ethical standards of privacy as well as respect for persons.

Because clinical teachers in nursing education programs are professional nurses, they sometimes experience conflict regarding their knowledge of students' health problems. As nurses, they might tend to respond in a therapeutic way if a student revealed personal information about a health concern, but as teachers, their primary obligation is to a teacher–student relationship. Absent any existing institutional policy or compelling evidence that the personal information should be disclosed to protect the safety of the student or other person, educators should follow the principle of what action would best promote student learning.

Clinical teachers who are aware of a student's health problem should also avoid making special exceptions for this student that would not be available to other students. Students who need special accommodations because of a health problem should request them from the institution's disability services officer. If accommodations are granted, the clinical teacher should discuss with the student how they will be made available. See the discussion on students with disabilities later in this chapter.

Competent Teaching

Applying the ethical standard of beneficence to teaching, students have a right to expect that their clinical teachers are competent, responsible, and knowledgeable. As discussed in Chapter 5, clinical competence, including expert knowledge and clinical skill, is an essential characteristic of effective clinical teachers. In addition, clinical teachers must be competent in facilitating students' learning activities, including planning appropriate assignments and giving specific, timely feedback on individual student performance. Examples of unethical behavior related to clinical teacher competence include not being available for guidance in the clinical setting and not planning sufficiently for a clinical learning activity that maximizes student learning.

Academic Dishonesty

Although cheating and other forms of dishonest behavior are believed to be common in the classroom environment, academic dishonesty can occur in clinical settings as well. Academic dishonesty is defined as intentional participation in deceptive practices regarding the academic work of self or others. Dishonest acts include lying, cheating, plagiarizing, altering or forging records, falsely representing oneself, and knowingly assisting another person to commit a dishonest act (Tippett et al., 2009). While we discuss academic dishonesty as an ethical violation, it can also be classified as a legal issue when it serves as the basis of a disciplinary action.

Examples of academic dishonesty in the clinical setting include:

- *Cheating:* A student copies portions of a classmate's case study analysis and presents the assignment as her own work. Similarly, a student who asks for a staff member's assistance to calculate a medication dose but tells the instructor that he did the work alone is also cheating.
- *Lying:* A student tells the instructor that she attempted a home visit to a patient but the patient was not at home. In fact, the student overslept and missed the scheduled time of the visit.

- *Plagiarism:* While preparing materials for a patient teaching project, a student paraphrases portions of a published teaching pamphlet without citing the source.
- *Altering a document:* A staff nurse orientee appends information to the documentation of nursing care for a patient on the previous day without noting it as a late addition.
- *False representation:* As a family nurse practitioner student begins a physical examination, the patient addresses the student as "doctor." The student continues with the examination and does not tell the patient that he is a nurse.
- *Assisting another in a dishonest act:* Student A asks Student B to cover for her while she leaves the clinical agency to run a personal errand. The teacher asks Student B if he has seen Student A; Student B says that he thinks she has accompanied a patient to the physical therapy department.

Although some of the previous examples may appear to be harmless or minor infractions, dishonest acts should be taken seriously because they can have harmful effects on patients, learners, faculty–student relationships, and the educational program. Clinical dishonesty can jeopardize patient safety if learners fail to report errors or do not receive adequate guidance because their competence is assumed (Bavier, 2009). Mutual trust and respect form the basis for effective teacher–learner relationships, and academic dishonesty can damage a teacher's trust in students. Dishonest acts that are ignored by teachers contribute to an environment that supports academic dishonesty, conveying the impression to students that this behavior is acceptable or at least excusable (Tippett et al., 2009). Additionally, honest students resent teachers who fail to deal effectively with cheating.

Students who are dishonest in school are more likely to conceal or deny errors in the workplace or violate professional conduct standards (Smith, 2012). For this reason, most nurse faculty members are conscientious about holding students accountable to standards of integrity and imposing severe consequences as permitted by policy. However, student appeals of these decisions are often overturned or modified by grade appeal panels comprising faculty members from nonclinical disciplines who may not understand the serious implications for patient safety (Bavier, 2009).

Clinical academic dishonesty usually results from one or more of the following factors:

- *Competition, desire for good grades, and heavy workload.* Competition for good grades in clinical nursing courses may result from student misunderstanding of the evaluation framework. If students believe that a limited number of good grades are available, they may compete fiercely with their classmates, sometimes leading to deceptive acts in an attempt to earn the highest grades. Additionally, many nursing students have additional pressures related to employment and family responsibilities; they may feel overloaded and unable to meet all of the demands of a rigorous nursing education program without resorting to cheating. "Higher education is increasingly a high stakes environment where a student's retention in or progression through a program, [retention of a] scholarship or loan, parental approval, or other significant factor is dependent on academic success" (Tippitt et al., 2009, p. 239).
- *Emphasis on perfection.* As discussed in Chapter 2, clinical teachers often communicate the expectation that good nurses do not make mistakes.

Although nurse educators attempt to prepare practitioners who will perform carefully and skillfully, a standard of perfection is unrealistic. Students naturally make mistakes in the process of learning new knowledge and skills, and punishment for mistakes, in the form of low grades or a negative performance evaluation, will not prevent these errors. In fact, it is the fear of punishment that often motivates students to conceal errors, and errors that are not reported are often harmful to patient safety (Kohn, Corrigan, & Donaldson, 2000).

■ *Poor role modeling.* The influence of role models on behavior is strong. Nursing students and novice staff nurses who observe dishonest behavior of teachers and experienced staff members may emulate these examples, especially when the dishonest acts have gone unnoticed, unreported, or unpunished (Tippitt et al., 2009).

Clinical teachers can use a variety of approaches to discourage academic dishonesty. They should be exemplary role models of honest behavior for learners to emulate (Tippitt et al., 2009). They should acknowledge that mistakes occur in the learning process and create a learning climate that allows students to make mistakes in a safe environment with guidance and feedback for problem solving.

In a study of how nurse educators determine passing or failing nursing student clinical behaviors, Tanicala, Scheffer, and Roberts (2011) concluded that:

> With the growing focus in health care on creating a culture of safety, versus the current approach of blame and punishment in both practice and education, . . . nursing clinical education must engage in a culture shift . . . from individual student error to analyzing errors from an educational perspective. (p. 160)

However, students need reassurance that, if humanly possible, teachers will not allow them to make errors that would harm patients. Finally, each nursing education program should develop a policy that defines academic dishonesty and specifies appropriate penalties for violations. This policy should be communicated to all students, reviewed with them at regular intervals, and applied consistently and fairly to every violation (Tippitt et al., 2009).

When enforcing the academic integrity policy, it is important to apply ethical standards to protect the dignity and privacy of students. A public accusation of dishonesty that is found later to be ungrounded can damage a student's reputation. The teacher should speak with the student privately and calmly, describe the student's behavior and the teacher's interpretation of it, and provide the student with an opportunity to respond to the charge. It is essential to keep an open mind until all available evidence is evaluated, because the student may be able to supply a reasonable explanation for the behavior that the teacher interpreted as cheating.

LEGAL ISSUES

It is beyond the scope of this book to discuss and interpret all federal, state, and local laws that have implications for clinical teaching and evaluation, and the authors are not qualified to give legal advice to clinical teachers regarding their practice. We recommend that clinical teachers refer questions about the legal implications of policies and procedures to the legal counsel for the institution in which they are employed; concerns about a teacher's legal rights in a specific situation are best referred to the individual's attorney. However, this section discusses common legal issues that often arise in the practice of clinical teaching.

Students With Disabilities

Two federal laws have implications for the education of learners with disabilities. The Rehabilitation Act of 1973, Section 504, prohibits public postsecondary institutions that receive federal funding from denying access or participation to individuals with disabilities. The Americans with Disabilities Act (ADA) of 1990 and the ADA Amendment Act of 2008 guarantee persons with disabilities equal access to educational opportunities if they are otherwise qualified for admission. A qualified individual with a disability is one who has a physical or mental impairment that substantially limits one or more of that individual's major life activities, or that the individual has a record of or is regarded as having such impairment.

In the ADA amendments, the definition of disability did not change, but the interpretation of disability is more expansive, providing protection to a wider range of individuals with disabilities. In determining whether an individual is disabled, the following three conditions apply:

1. The effects of ameliorating agents cannot be considered. For example, a person with epilepsy whose seizures are controlled by medications or one who uses a hearing aid to correct hearing loss is still considered to have a qualifying condition if one or more life activities are affected.
2. Conditions that are in remission or episodic are considered to be disabilities if, when they are active, they have a similar effect on one or more life activities.
3. The term "life activities" is now more broadly defined to include "seeing, hearing, eating, smelling, sleeping, breathing, walking, speaking, bowel and bladder control, learning, reading, writing, spelling, concentrating, thinking, communicating, perceiving and other neurologic functions, working, performing self care and other manual tasks" (Southern Regional Education Board [SREB], n.d.).

In nursing education programs, qualified individuals with disabilities are those who meet the essential eligibility requirements for participation, with or without modifications (SREB, n.d.). A common goal of nursing education programs is to produce graduates who can function safely and competently in the roles for which they were prepared. For this reason, it is appropriate for those who make admission decisions to determine whether applicants could be reasonably expected to develop the necessary competence. The first step in this decision process is to define the core performance standards necessary for participation in the program. Because nursing is a practice discipline, core performance standards include cognitive, sensory, affective, and psychomotor competencies. The SREB recommended that core performance standards be published in catalogs, on websites, in application materials, and in program descriptions for the state board of nursing and accrediting bodies. They should also be made available to students, faculty members, staff members, and agencies in which students have clinical learning activities. All applicants to nursing education programs should be informed of the core performance standards to allow them to make initial judgments about their qualifications. Under the ADA as amended, nursing education programs cannot base admission or progression decisions on the core performance standards. Instead, the standards should be used to assist applicants and students to determine their need for accommodations (SREB, n.d.).

Persons with disabilities who are admitted to nursing education programs are responsible for informing the institution of the disability and requesting reasonable accommodations. Each nursing education program must determine on an individual basis whether the necessary modifications can be reasonably made. The nursing faculty, administration, and staff should cooperate with other institutional units to identify auxiliary aids and services, such as building accessibility and assistive devices, that students with identified disabilities may need. Reasonable accommodations for participating in clinical learning activities might include (SREB, n.d.):

- Allowing additional time for a student with a qualified learning disability to complete an assignment
- Allowing additional time to complete the program
- Scheduling clinical learning activities in facilities that are readily accessible to and usable by individuals with disabilities
- Providing the use of an amplified stethoscope for a student with a hearing impairment
- Providing qualified readers or interpreters

Reasonable accommodations do not include lowering academic standards or eliminating essential technical performance requirements (Smith, 2012). However, nurse educators need to distinguish essential from traditional functions by discussing such philosophical issues as whether individuals who will never practice bedside nursing in the conventional manner should be admitted to nursing education programs.

Disabilities may be visible (e.g., limited mobility, visual or hearing deficit, physical or functional loss of a limb) or invisible (e.g., learning disability, behavioral health problem, chronic illness). As previously discussed, clinical teachers should not attempt to determine whether accommodation is indicated, nor should they decide on the specific type of accommodation necessary. The disabilities services officer of the educational institution determines whether the student is a qualified individual with a disability and, if so, whether the disability requires accommodations. This officer then issues a formal, written description of the required clinical accommodations, usually to the student, who decides whom to share it with. Accommodation statements should not be shared with others without the student's written permission. The purpose of accommodation is to provide the student with a disability the means to compensate for it so that full participation in the clinical learning activity is possible.

Many nursing faculty members voice concerns about the capacity of students with physical disabilities to perform physical tasks associated with nursing practice. A clinical teacher of a student with a physical disability should carefully analyze a planned learning activity to identify the essential elements necessary to produce desired outcomes, keeping in mind that much of the professional nurse's work is intellectual. Is it more important for a nursing student to demonstrate the ability to reposition a patient or to demonstrate the ability to assess the patient's skin integrity and pulmonary and circulatory function, recognize the need for repositioning, delegate the task to a licensed or unlicensed staff member and supervise that person as necessary, and evaluate the patient outcomes? Students with disabilities are the best sources of information about their disabilities and the limitations that they present, adaptations they have learned to compensate for them, and what accommodations have worked in the past. After appropriate accommodations are provided, however, students with disabilities must be evaluated according to the same criteria as other students.

In cases where a student with a disability is at risk of clinical failure, it is important that faculty members and administrators have clearly and consistently documented any offer and provision of accommodations and the student's subsequent use or non-use of them. Evaluations should be based on a genuine substantive assessment of the student's performance with any appropriate accommodations. The student must have been notified, orally and in writing, about her or his clinical practice deficiencies and the related consequences well before a grading decision was made. The clinical teacher must have provided constructive feedback about the student's performance, suggested specific improvements, and provided a time frame within which those improvements must be made.

Due Process

Another legal issue related to clinical teaching is that of student rights to due process. The 14th Amendment of the U.S. Constitution specifies that the state cannot deprive a person of life, liberty, or property without due process of law. With regard to the rights of students to due process, however, this constitutional protection extends only to those enrolled in public institutions. Students at private institutions may base a claim against the school on discrimination or contract law (Smith, 2012). For example, if a private school publishes a code of student rights and procedures for student grievances in its student handbook, those documents may be regarded as part of a contract between the school and the student. In paying and accepting tuition, the student and the school jointly agree to abide by this code of rights and set of procedures. A student may sue on the basis of breach of contract if the school does not follow the stated due process procedures.

Courts hold different standards for due process based on whether it applies to academic or disciplinary decisions. Academic decisions pertain to issues related to performance and academic standing, such as assigning a failing grade in a course, delaying progress, and dismissal from a program because of failure to maintain acceptable academic standing. Academic due process concerns both the *process* used to inform students of their academic standing and the *basis* for a decision regarding academic standing. Thus, *procedural due process* relates to the fairness of the process used to make academic decisions, and *substantive due process* relates to the basis for those decisions. A student appeal of an academic decision may allege a violation of either type of due process rights, but courts do not usually intervene in faculty members' evaluation of student academic or clinical performance. "Applying the principle of judicial deference, courts examining cases pertaining to faculty's evaluation of students usually uphold the faculty's decision, if there was an adherence to standard academic norms and the procedures used were fair and reasonable" (Smith, 2012, p. 5). The following legal principles apply to substantive due process (Smith, 2012):

- Students must be informed in advance about the academic standards that will be used to judge their performance.
- Student performance should be evaluated using the stated standards or criteria and grades assigned according to the stated policy. A teacher's

academic decision should be based on a genuine substantive evaluation of the student's performance. All students should be evaluated according to the same standards; academic decisions should not be arbitrary or capricious.

If a student believes that a grade or other academic decision is unfair, the stated appeal or grievance process should be followed. Usually, the first level of appeal is to the teacher or group of teachers who assigned the grade. If the conflict is not resolved at that level, the student usually has the right of appeal to the administrator to whom the teacher reports. The next level of appeal is usually to a student standing committee or appeal panel of nursing faculty members. Finally, the student should have the right to appeal the decision to the highest level administrator in the nursing education program and then to the appropriate academic administrators at the parent institution.

Procedural due process concerns the fairness of the process by which academic decisions are made. Students should be notified about their academic deficiencies and the related consequences well before grading decisions are made. Ideally, notification occurs orally and in writing. To further protect students' procedural due process rights, the teacher should provide constructive feedback about their performance, suggest specific improvements, and provide a timeframe within which those improvements must be made. Evaluation of clinical performance is as much an academic decision as is assessment of classroom work, and the same procedural due process protections should be followed.

Of course, if students exhaust every level of appeal and are still not satisfied with the outcome, they have the right to seek relief in the court system. It is important to note that the courts will allow such a lawsuit to go forward only if there is evidence that the student has first exhausted all internal school remedies. However, if the educational program faculty and administrators have followed substantive due process procedures as described above, it is unlikely that the academic decision will be reversed. In particular, the courts will likely exercise judicial deference to the educational program if the student's complaint concerns a requirement of passing an exit examination to graduate because of the potential consequence to the program of a low National Council Licensure Exam (NCLEX®) pass rate (Smith, 2012). In due process appeals to a court of law, the burden of proof that academic due process was denied rests with the student. With regard to due process for academic decisions, the key to resolving conflict and minimizing faculty liability is in maintaining communication with students whose performance is not meeting standards.

Disciplinary decisions such as dismissal on the basis of misconduct or dishonesty require a higher level of due process than is required for academic actions. Unlike academic decisions that require professional judgments and are therefore beyond the scope of judicial review, disciplinary actions can be reviewed by the courts' traditional fact-finding procedures (Smith, 2012).

Disciplinary decisions are made when a student violates the law or regulation by engaging in prohibited activity. All colleges and universities have rules, standards, conduct codes, and policies that students are expected to meet, usually published in the institutional catalog and student handbook. Nursing education programs often have specific expectations regarding adherence to professional codes of conduct that are consistent with but go above and beyond the rules and standards of the parent institution. These publications must also explicate the procedures that will be followed if these rules are violated (Smith, 2012).

Disciplinary due process includes the following components:

- The student is provided with adequate written notice, including specific details concerning the misconduct. For example, a notice may inform the student that she failed to attend a required clinical activity; that neither the faculty member nor nursing unit secretary was informed of the anticipated absence, in violation of school policy on professional conduct; and that, because this incident represented the third violation of professional conduct standards, the student would be dismissed from the program according to the sanctions provided in the policy.
- The student is provided the opportunity for a fair, impartial hearing on the charges. Students have the right to speak on their own behalf, to present witnesses and evidence, and to question the other participants in the case (usually teachers and administrators). Using the example above, the student might present evidence that she did attempt to call the faculty member to report her absence; this evidence could include the date and time of the call, the name of the person with whom she spoke, and a copy of a telephone bill verifying the date, time, and number called. Although the student and the faculty member are entitled to the advice of legal counsel, neither attorney may question or cross examine witnesses.
- The student has the right to appeal an unfavorable decision by the hearing panel to an appeals panel or a designated administrator. Usually, this administrator or, ultimately, the university or college president has the authority to make the final decision (Smith, 2012).

If the final decision is to uphold the dismissal, students have the right to seek remedy from the court system if they believe that due process was not followed. However, in disciplinary cases, the burden of proof that due process was denied rests with the student.

Negligence, Liability, and Unsafe Clinical Practice

When determining whether a given action meets the criteria for professional negligence, the overall standard of care is what an ordinary, reasonable, and prudent person would have done in the same context. The standard of care for a nursing student is not what another nursing student would have done; students are held to the same standards of care as RNs. The NCSBN Model Nurse Practice Act (2014a), Article V, Section 10 includes the statement that the nurse practice act does not prohibit the practice of nursing by a student in an approved nursing education program as long as the student "is under the auspices of the program [and] . . . acts under the supervision of an RN serving for the program as a faculty member or teaching assistant" (p. 7). Another section of the Model Act (Article VII, Section 2) states that each nurse is required to know and adhere to the requirements of the nurse practice act, that nurses are accountable for their decisions based on their education and experience, and that nurses must practice with reasonable skill and safety. The concept of personal liability also applies to cases of professional negligence. Each person is responsible for his or her own behavior, including negligent acts. Students are liable for their own actions as long as they are performing according to the usual standard of care for their education and experience, and they seek guidance when they are uncertain what to do. Therefore, it is not true that students practice under the faculty member's license.

Teachers are not liable for negligent acts performed by their students as long as the teacher has (a) selected appropriate learning activities based on objectives;

(b) determined that students have prerequisite knowledge, skills, and attitudes necessary to complete their assignments; and (c) provided competent guidance. However, teachers are liable for their negligent actions if they make assignments that require more knowledge and skill than the learner has developed or if they fail to guide student activities appropriately. The NCSBN Model Rules (2014b) include statements about the grounds for disciplining an RN. These include failure to competently guide student clinical learning activities as a clinical teacher. Even if the clinical teacher was not negligent in making assignments or guiding student learning, he or she is likely to be named as a defendant in any lawsuit arising from a nursing student's alleged negligence or malpractice. For this reason, clinical teachers should carry sufficient individual professional liability insurance to cover the costs of defending themselves, even if their employers provide insurance coverage for faculty members.

If a student demonstrates clinical performance that is potentially unsafe, the student and the teacher who made the assignment may be liable for any subsequent injury to the patient. However, because time for learning must precede time for evaluation, is it fair for the teacher to assign a failing grade in clinical practice before the end of the course, when to do so would prevent the student's access to learning opportunities for which he or she has paid tuition? In this case, denying access to clinical learning activities because of unsafe practice or inadequate clinical reasoning should not be considered an academic grading decision. Instead, it is an appropriate response to protecting the rights of patients to safe, competent care—a disciplinary decision.

The teacher's failure to take such protective action potentially places the teacher and the educational program at risk for liability. Instead of denying the student access to all learning opportunities, removal from the clinical setting should be followed by a substitute assignment that would help the student to remove the deficiency in knowledge, skill, or attitude. For example, the student might be given a library assignment to acquire the information necessary to guide safe patient care, or an extra skills laboratory session could be arranged to allow more practice of psychomotor skills. A set of standards of safe clinical practice and a program policy that enforces the standards are helpful guides to faculty decision making and action while protecting student and faculty rights. Exhibit 6.1 is an example of safe clinical practice standards, and Exhibit 6.2 is an example of a policy that enforces these standards.

EXHIBIT 6.1

STANDARDS OF SAFE CLINICAL PRACTICE

XXXXXX UNIVERSITY
SCHOOL OF NURSING
BSN PROGRAM

STANDARDS OF SAFE CLINICAL PRACTICE

In clinical practice, students are expected to demonstrate responsibility and accountability as professional nurses with the goal of health promotion and prevention of harm to self and others. The School of Nursing faculty believes that this goal will be attained if each student's clinical practice adheres to the Standards of Safe Clinical Practice. Safe clinical performance always includes, but is not limited to, the following behaviors:

1. Practice within boundaries of the nursing student role and the scope of practice of the RN.

(continued)

2. Comply with instructional policies and procedures for implementing nursing care.
3. Prepare for clinical learning assignments according to course requirements and as determined for the specific clinical setting.
4. Demonstrate the application of previously learned skills and principles in providing nursing care.
5. Promptly report significant client information in a clear, accurate, and complete oral or written manner to the appropriate person or persons.

ACKNOWLEDGMENT

I have read the XXXXXX University School of Nursing Standards of Safe Clinical Practice and I agree to adhere to them. I understand that these standards are expectations for my clinical practice and will be incorporated into the evaluation of my clinical performance in all clinical courses. Failure to meet these standards may result in my removal from the clinical area, which may result in clinical failure due to inability to achieve the required learning outcomes.

Signature and Date

EXHIBIT 6.2

POLICY ON SAFE CLINICAL PRACTICE

XXXXXX UNIVERSITY
SCHOOL OF NURSING
BSN PROGRAM

SAFE CLINICAL PRACTICE POLICY

POLICY

During enrollment in the XXXXXX University School of Nursing BSN Program, all students, in all clinical activities, are expected to adhere to the Standards of Safe Clinical Practice. Failure to abide by these standards will result in disciplinary action, which may include dismissal from the nursing program.

PROCEDURES

1. Students will receive a copy of the Standards of Safe Clinical Practice, and they will be reviewed during the Annual Nursing Assembly at the beginning of each academic year. At that time, students will be required to sign an agreement to adhere to the standards. Each student will retain one copy of the agreement, and one copy will be retained in the student's file.
2. Violation of these standards will result in the following disciplinary action:
   a. First Violation
      1. Student will be given an immediate oral warning by the faculty member. The incident will be documented by the faculty member on the *Violation of Standards of Safe Clinical Practice* form. One copy of this form will be given to the student, and one copy will be kept in the student's record.
      2. At the discretion of the faculty member, the student may be required to leave the clinical unit for the remainder of that day. The student may be given an alternative assignment.
      3. If this violation is of a serious nature, it may be referred to the associate dean and the dean of nursing for further disciplinary action as in b and c below.

(continued)

  b. Second Violation
   1. The faculty member will document the incident on the *Violation of Safe Clinical Practice* form. Following discussion of the incident with the student, the faculty member will forward a copy of the form to the associate dean for review and recommendation regarding further action.
   2. The recommendation of the associate dean will be forwarded to the dean of nursing for review and decision regarding reprimand or dismissal. This disciplinary action process will be documented and placed in the student's record.
  c. If the student has not been dismissed and remains in the program following the above disciplinary action, any additional violation will be documented and referred as above to the associate dean and the dean of nursing for disciplinary action, which may include dismissal from the program.
  d. The rights of students will be safeguarded as set forth in the XXXXXX University *Code of Student Rights, Responsibilities, and Conduct* published in the current *XXXXXX University Student Handbook.*

Documentation and Record Keeping

Teachers should keep records of their evaluations of student clinical performance. These records may include anecdotal notes, summaries of faculty–student conferences, progress reports, and summative clinical evaluations. These records are helpful in documenting that students received feedback about their performance, areas of teacher concern, and information about student progress toward correcting deficiencies.

An anecdotal note is a narrative description of the observed behavior of the student in relation to a specific learning objective. The note may also include the teacher's interpretation of the behavior, recorded separately from the description. Limiting the description and optional interpretation to a specified clinical objective avoids recording extraneous information, which is an ineffective use of the teacher's time. Anecdotal notes should record both positive and negative behaviors so as not to give the impression that the teacher is biased against the student. Students should review these notes and have an opportunity to comment on them; used in this way, anecdotal notes are an effective means of communicating formative evaluation information to students (Oermann & Gaberson, 2017). Some sources recommend that both teacher and student sign the notes.

Writing anecdotal notes for every student, every day, is unnecessarily time consuming. An effective, efficient approach might be to specify a minimum number of notes to be written for each student in relation to specified objectives. A student whose performance is either meritorious or cause for concern might prompt the instructor to write more notes.

Records of student–teacher conferences are likewise summaries of discussions that focused on areas of concern, plans to address deficiencies, and progress toward correcting weaknesses. These conferences should take place in private and should address the teacher's responsibility to protect patient safety, concern about the student's clinical deficiencies, and a sincere desire to assist the student to improve. During the conference, the student has opportunities to clarify and respond to the teacher's feedback. At times, an objective third party such as a department chairperson or program director may be asked to participate in the conference to witness and clarify the comments of both teacher and student. The conference note should record the date, time, and place of the conference; the names and roles of participants; and a summary of the discussion, recommendations, and plans. The note may be signed only by the teacher or by all participants, according to institutional policy or guidelines.

Because they contain essentially formative evaluation information, anecdotal notes and conference notes should not be kept in the student's permanent record. Teachers should keep these documents in their private files, taking appropriate precautions to ensure their security, until there is no reasonable expectation that they will be needed. In most cases, when the learner successfully completes the program or withdraws in good academic standing, these records can be discarded (again, taking appropriate security precautions). It is unlikely that successful learners will appeal favorable academic decisions. However, it is recommended that anecdotal records and conference notes be kept for longer periods when there is a chance that the learner may appeal the grade or other decision. The statute of limitations for such an appeal is a useful guide to deciding how long to keep those materials. It is recommended that teachers consult with legal counsel if there is a question about institutional policy on retention of records.

Patient Privacy Laws

HIPAA, created in 1996, affirms patients' fundamental right to privacy for their personal health information. HIPAA privacy rules apply to "covered entities" such as hospitals, clinics, and rehabilitation centers. Nursing education programs that place students at these sites for clinical learning activities usually are not considered covered entities but "business associates" that are bound by the same privacy standards. Nursing students thus are subject to HIPAA rules while engaged in clinical learning activities at these facilities. Additionally, they should understand that HIPAA rules apply to their private conduct outside of their clinical practice (Westrick, 2016).

The 2009 Health Information Technology for Economic and Clinical Health (HITECH) Act is another federal law that protects patient information. It includes a requirement for patient notification of any breach of confidentiality and a tiered structure of civil penalties for violations (Melnik, 2013).

Additionally, there may be state laws protecting patient information, enabling patients to file civil lawsuits for breach of confidentiality. According to common law doctrine, patients also have a right to sue for "invasion of privacy" on the basis of harm resulting from disclosure of personal information.

Patient privacy laws, while protecting patient rights, have created new challenges for clinical nurse educators. Because of privacy concerns regarding disclosure of individually identifiable health information, many health care facilities have adopted policies and procedures that may pose barriers to clinical teaching and learning.

Most health care organizations require nursing education programs to provide documentation that their students have been oriented to the requirements of HIPAA. If numerous clinical sites are used by a program, this requirement can be onerous if each agency requires students to attend or complete its own HIPAA orientation. Nursing education administrators may be able to negotiate with all clinical agencies to agree on the basic content of the required orientation, recognizing that the requirement could be met in various ways. Students are typically asked to sign a verification that they have been oriented to HIPAA requirements and that they agree to abide by those requirements. This orientation and verification should be repeated at regular intervals (e.g., yearly or each semester).

Because health care agencies also usually require nursing education programs to provide verification that nursing students have met specified health requirements, this verification process may create HIPAA concerns. If the nursing education program collects, receives, or transmits students' individually identifiable health information, it could be deemed responsible for maintaining reasonable and appropriate administrative, technical, and physical safeguards to ensure the integrity and confidentiality of the information and to protect against any reasonably anticipated threats to the security of the information and unauthorized uses or disclosures of it. Some clinical agencies request specific health data as evidence that students have met clinical health requirements, such as a rubella titer result. However, if the nursing education program complies with this request and the agency misuses the information in any way, both the education program and the clinical agency risk claims of unauthorized release or use of protected information about individual students.

Many nursing education programs avoid these potential complications by requiring a licensed health care provider to verify that a student has met all specified clinical health requirements. This verification, including dates for immunizations and a signed statement that the student's general health is adequate to allow full participation in the nursing program, is kept in the nursing education program files, but the raw data remain the property of the student and his health care provider. Another approach to resolving these concerns is to have all nursing students examined and tested by the student health service of the parent institution, with the raw data stored in that office and notification to the nursing education program that the clinical health requirements have or have not been met. It is wise to seek the advice of the school, college, or university counsel about how requirements for verification of students' health status by clinical agencies should be handled so that an appropriate policy can be developed and implemented.

As previously discussed, social media use can result in HIPAA violations, sometimes inadvertently. Students should adhere to professional guidelines for social media use, including not posting or transmitting information that might be used to identify patients to anyone who does not have a legitimate right to know. Students may be required to sign documents affirming that they have been informed of HIPAA requirements and that they agree to adhere to them.

SUMMARY

Because clinical teaching and learning take place in a social context, the rights of teachers, students, staff members, and patients are sometimes in conflict. These conflicts create legal and ethical dilemmas for clinical teachers. This chapter discussed selected ethical and legal issues related to clinical teaching.

Online social networking is a useful and popular means of communication and collaboration, but nursing faculty members and students may encounter ethical and legal consequences of social media misuse. The ANA *Code of Ethics for Nurses with Interpretative Statements* emphasizes the obligation of nurses to act within the professional role and to maintain role boundaries in relationships with patients. Boundary violations can occur when students "friend" or "follow" patients or former patients on social media. Nurses also have an obligation to maintain patient privacy; confidentiality can be breached when information about patients is posted on social media sites, sometimes inadvertently. Social media misuse can have serious consequences for patients, nursing students, nursing education programs, and health care facilities. Nursing education programs should develop and enforce explicit policies regarding the use of electronic communication and social media, including specific consequences for policy violations; professional guidelines for use of social media can be used to inform policy development. Guidelines for appropriate use of social media should be reviewed regularly with students; examples of these guidelines were provided in the chapter.

Ethical standards such as respect for human dignity, autonomy, and freedom; beneficence; justice; veracity; privacy; and fidelity are important considerations for all parties involved in clinical teaching and learning. Students must learn to apply these standards to nursing practice, and teachers must apply them in their relationships with students as well as their teaching and evaluation responsibilities. Incivility in nursing education was discussed, with suggestions for how to prevent it and manage it.

Specific ethical issues related to clinical teaching and learning include the presence of learners in a service setting, the need for faculty–student relationships to be based on justice and respect for persons, students' privacy rights, teaching competence, and academic dishonesty. Legal issues that have implications for clinical teaching and learning include educating students with disabilities, student rights to due process for academic and disciplinary decisions, standards of safe clinical practice, student and teacher negligence and liability, documentation and record keeping regarding students' clinical performance, and potential violations of HIPAA requirements with regard to student health information.

Suggestions were offered for preventing, minimizing, and managing these difficult ethical and legal situations. Laws and institutional policies often provide guidelines for action in specific cases. However, these suggestions should not be construed as legal advice, and teachers are advised to seek legal counsel in regard to specific questions or problems.

CNE EXAMINATION TEST BLUEPRINT CORE COMPETENCIES

1. **Facilitate Learning**

   E. Practice skilled oral and written (including electronic) communication that reflects an awareness of self and relationships with learners (e.g., evaluation, mentorship, and supervision)
   K. Demonstrate personal attributes that facilitate learning (e.g., caring, confidence, patience, integrity, respect, and flexibility)
   P. Act as a role model in practice settings

2. **Facilitate Learner Development and Socialization**

   A. Identify individual learning styles and unique learning needs of learners with these characteristics:
      4. at-risk (e.g., educationally disadvantaged, learning and/or physically challenged, social, and economic issues)
   B. Provide resources for diverse learners to meet their individual learning needs
   D. Create learning environments that facilitate learners' self-reflection, personal goal setting, and socialization to the role of the nurse

(continued)

E. Foster the development of learners in these areas:
  3. affective domain

3. Use Assessment and Evaluation Strategies

  B. Enforce nursing program standards related to
   1. admission
   2. progression
   3. graduation
  K. Advise learners regarding assessment and evaluation criteria
  L. Provide timely, constructive, and thoughtful feedback to learners

5. Pursue Systematic Self-Evaluation and Improvement in the Academic Nurse Educator Role

  H. Practice according to legal and ethical standards relevant to higher education and nursing education

6. Engage in Scholarship, Service, and Leadership

  C. Function effectively within the organizational environment and the academic community
   3. Integrate the values of respect, collegiality, professionalism, and caring to build an organizational climate that fosters the development of learners and colleagues

REFERENCES

Altmiller, G. (2012). Student perceptions of incivility in nursing education: Implications for educators. *Nursing Education Perspectives, 33,* 15–20.

American Nurses Association. (2011a). ANA's principles for social networking and the nurse: Guidance for registered nurses. Retrieved from http://www.nursingworld.org/MainMenuCategories/ThePracticeofProfessionalNursing/NursingStandards/ANAPrinciples/Principles-for-Social-Networking.pdf

American Nurses Association. (2011b). Social networking principles toolkit. Retrieved from www.nursingworld.org/socialnetworkingtoolkit

American Nurses Association. (2015). Code of ethics for nurses with interpretive statements. Retrieved from http://nursingworld.org/DocumentVault/Ethics-1/Code-of-Ethics-for-Nurses.html

Bavier, A. R. (2009). Holding students accountable when integrity is challenged. *Nursing Education Perspectives, 30,* 5.

Clark, C. M., & Springer, P. J. (2010). Academic nurse leaders' role in fostering a culture of civility in nursing education. *Journal of Nursing Education, 49,* 319–325.

Corcoran, S. (1977). Should a service setting be used as a learning laboratory? An ethical question. *Nursing Outlook, 25,* 771–774.

Family Educational Rights and Privacy Act, 20 U.S.C. § 1232g; 34 CFR Part 99 (1974).

Health Insurance Portability and Accountability Act (HIPAA) of 1996. Public Law 104–191.

Kohn, L., Corrigan, J., & Donaldson, M. (2000). *To err is human: Building a safer health system.* Washington, DC: National Academies Press, Institute of Medicine.

Luparell, S. (2011). Incivility in nursing: The connection between academic and clinical settings. *Critical Care Nurse, 31,* 92–95.

Melnik, T. (2013). Avoiding violations of patient privacy with social media. *Journal of Nursing Regulation, 3*(4), 39–44.

National Council of State Boards of Nursing. (2011). *A nurse's guide to the use of social media.* [Brochure]. Retrieved from https://www.ncsbn.org/NCSBN_SocialMedia.pdf

National Council of State Boards of Nursing. (2014a). Model nurse practice act. Retrieved from https://www.ncsbn.org/12_Model_Act_090512.pdf

National Council of State Boards of Nursing. (2014b). Model rules. Retrieved from https://www.ncsbn.org/14_Model_Rules_0914.pdf

Oermann, M. H., & Gaberson, K. B. (2017). *Evaluation and testing in nursing education* (5th ed.). New York, NY: Springer Publishing.

Poorman, S. G., Mastorovich, M. L., & Webb, C. A. (2011). Helping students who struggle academically: Finding the right level of involvement and living with our judgments. *Nursing Education Perspectives, 32,* 369–374.

Rad, M., & Moonaghi, H. K. (2016). Strategies for managing nursing students' incivility as experienced by nursing educators: A qualitative study. *Journal of Caring Sciences, 5,* 23–32.

Robertson, J. E. (2012). Can't we all just get along? A primer on student incivility in nursing education. *Nursing Education Perspectives, 33,* 21–26.

Smith, M. (2012). The legal, professional, and ethical dimensions of higher education in nursing (2nd ed.). New York, NY: Springer Publishing.

Southern Regional Education Board. (n.d.). The Americans with Disabilities Act: Implications for nursing education. Retrieved from http://www.sreb.org/publication/americans-disabilities-act

Spector, N., & Kappel, D. (2012). Guidelines for using electronic and social media: The regulatory perspective. *Online Journal of Issues in Nursing, 17*(3), Manuscript 1. Retrieved from http://www.nursingworld.org/MainMenuCategories/ANAMarketplace/ANAPeriodicals/OJIN/TableofContents/Vol-17-2012/No3-Sept-2012/Guidelines-for-Electronic-and-Social-Media.html

Stephens, T. M., & Gunther, M. E. (2016). Twitter, millenials, and nursing education research. *Nursing Education Perspectives, 37,* 23–27.

Tanicala, M. L., Scheffer, B. K., & Roberts, M. S. (2011). Pass/fail nursing student behaviors Phase I: Moving toward a culture of safety. *Nursing Education Perspectives, 32,* 155–161.

Tippitt, M. P., Ard, N., Kline, J. R., Tilghman, J., Chamberlain, B., & Meagher, P. G. (2009). Creating environments that foster academic integrity. *Nursing Education Perspectives, 30,* 239–244.

Westrick, S. J. (2016). Nursing students' use of electronic and social media: Law, ethics, and e-professionalism. *Nursing Education Perspectives, 37,* 16–22.

SECTION II

Strategies for Effective Clinical Teaching

CHAPTER 7

Crafting Clinical Learning Assignments

One of the most important responsibilities of a clinical teacher is crafting clinical assignments that are related to desired learning outcomes, appropriate to students' levels of knowledge and skill, and challenging enough to motivate learning. Although directing a learner to provide comprehensive nursing care to one or more patients is a typical clinical assignment, it is only one of many possible assignments, and not always the most appropriate choice. This chapter presents a framework for selecting clinical learning assignments and discusses several alternatives to the traditional total patient care assignment.

PATIENT CARE VERSUS LEARNING ACTIVITY

When planning assignments, clinical teachers typically speak of selecting patients for whom students will provide care. However, as discussed in Chapter 1, the primary role of the nursing student in the clinical area is that of learner, not nurse. Although it is true that nursing students need contact with patients in order to apply classroom learning to clinical practice, caring for patients is not synonymous with learning. In a classic study of the use of the clinical laboratory in nursing education, Infante (1985) took the position that nursing students are *learning to care* for patients; they are not nurses with *responsibility for patient care*. Providing patient care does not guarantee transfer of knowledge from the classroom to clinical practice; instead, it often reflects work requirements of the clinical agency.

Many faculty members assume that caring for patients always constitutes a clinical assignment for students on every level of the nursing education program. Even in their earliest clinical courses, nursing students typically have responsibility for patient care while learning basic psychomotor and communication skills. However, given the high patient acuity level in most acute care settings, beginning-level nursing students are not ready to provide total care for the typical patient in such environments, and this early responsibility for patient care often creates anxiety that interferes with learning.

As discussed in Chapter 2, changes in health care, technology, society, and education influence the competencies needed for professional nursing practice.

Learning outcomes necessary for safe, competent nursing practice today include cognitive skills of problem solving, clinical decision making, critical thinking, and clinical reasoning, in addition to technical proficiency. If nurse educators are to produce creative, independent, assertive, and decisive practitioners, they cannot assume that students will acquire these competencies through patient care assignments. To produce these outcomes, clinical teachers should choose clinical assignments from a variety of learning activities, including participation in patient care.

FACTORS AFFECTING SELECTION OF CLINICAL ASSIGNMENTS

The selection of learning activities within the context of the clinical teaching process was discussed earlier. Clinical activities help learners to apply knowledge to practice, develop skills, cultivate professional values, and form the role of professional nurse. Clinical assignments should be selected according to criteria such as the learning objectives of the clinical activity; needs of patients; availability and variety of learning opportunities in the clinical environment; and the needs, interests, and abilities of learners.

Learning Outcomes

The most important criterion for selection of clinical assignments is usually the desired learning outcome. The teacher should structure each clinical activity carefully in terms of the learning objectives, and each clinical activity should be an integral part of the course or educational program. In some nursing education programs, one set of course objectives applies to both the classroom and clinical learning outcomes; in others, separate but related sets of objectives are created to reflect the different emphases of "knowing that" (classroom learning outcome) and "knowing how" (clinical learning outcome).

Whatever method of specifying desired outcomes is used, it is essential that the clinical teacher, students, and staff members understand the purpose and goals of each clinical activity (Woodley, 2018). Depending on the level of the learner, students may have difficulty envisioning how broad program or course outcomes can be achieved in the context of a specific clinical environment. It is the clinical teacher's role to translate these outcomes into specific clinical objectives and to select and structure learning activities so that they relate logically and sequentially to the goals. The clinical teacher should share with each student the rationale for his or her specific clinical assignment to help students to focus on the learning opportunities presented by each unique assignment.

Learner Characteristics

As previously discussed, the learner's educational level or previous experience; aptitude for learning; learning style; and specific needs, interests, and abilities should also influence the selection of clinical assignments. The teacher must consider these individual differences; all learners do not have the same needs (Woodley, 2018), so it is unreasonable to expect them to have the same learning assignments on any given day.

For example, Student A learns skills at a slower pace than other students at the same level. The instructor should plan assignments so that this student has many opportunities for repetition of skills with feedback. If the objective is to learn the skills of medication administration, most students might be able to learn those skills in a reasonable amount of time in the context of providing care to one or more patients. Student A might learn more effectively with an assignment to administer all medications to a larger group of patients over the period of a day or more, without other patient care responsibilities. When the student has acquired the necessary level of skill, the next clinical assignment might be to administer medications while learning other aspects of care for one or more patients.

Students who are able to achieve the objectives of the essential curriculum (see Chapter 1) rather quickly might receive assignments from the enrichment curriculum that allow them to focus on their individual needs. For example, a student who is interested in exploring perioperative nursing might be assigned to follow a patient through a surgical procedure, providing preoperative care, observing or participating in the surgery, assisting in immediate postoperative care in the postanesthesia care unit, and presenting a plan for home care in a postclinical conference. Taking learners' interests and professional development goals into account when planning enrichment activities will motivate students and individualize their learning experiences.

Needs of Patients

Patient needs and care requirements should also be considered when planning clinical assignments for students. In relation to the learning objective, will the nursing care activities present enough of a challenge to the learner? Are they too complex for the learner to manage?

Even if patients signed consents for admission to the health care facility that included an agreement to the participation of learners in their care, their wishes regarding student assignment and those of their family members should be respected. At times of crisis, patients and family members may not wish to initiate a new nurse–patient relationship with a nursing student. Nursing staff members who have provided care to these patients can often help the clinical teacher determine whether student learning needs and specific patient and family needs can both be met through a particular clinical assignment.

As mentioned previously, the patient acuity level in a given clinical setting affects the selection of learning opportunities for nursing students. When the acuity level is high, it may not be possible for a clinical teacher to assign every student to learn to care for patients with many complex needs. In this case, some students may be assigned to apply their knowledge to the care of two or more relatively stable patients to develop their prioritization and time management skills, or two or more students may be assigned to plan, organize, deliver, evaluate, and document care for one patient with complex needs. Variations in student–patient ratio assignment options are described in more detail later in this chapter.

Timing of Activities and Availability of Learning Opportunities

Because the purpose of clinical learning is to foster application of theory to practice, clinical learning activities should be related to what is being taught in the classroom.

Ideally, clinical activities are scheduled concurrently with relevant classroom content so that learners can make immediate transfer and application of knowledge to nursing practice. However, there is little evidence of a relationship between clinical learning outcomes and the structure, timing, and organization of clinical learning activities.

The availability of learning opportunities to allow students to meet objectives often affects clinical assignments. The usual schedule of activities in the clinical facility may determine the optimum timing of learning activities. For example, if the learning objective for a new nursing student is "Identify sources of information about patient needs from the electronic health record," it might be difficult for students to gain access to patient records at change of shift when many health care team members are using the available computers to document care. Thus, scheduling learners to arrive at the clinical site at midmorning may allow better access to the resources necessary for learning.

Some clinical settings, such as outpatient clinics and operating rooms, may be available to both patients and students only on a daytime, Monday through Friday, schedule. In other settings, however, scheduling clinical learning activities during evening or nighttime hours or on weekend days may offer students better opportunities to meet certain objectives. If the learning objective is "Implement health teaching for the parents of a premature or ill neonate," the best time for students to encounter parents may be during evening visiting hours or on weekends. Using these time periods for clinical activities may also prevent two or more groups of learners from different educational programs being in the same clinical area simultaneously, affecting the availability of learning opportunities.

Of course, learning activities at such times may conflict with family, work, and other academic schedules and commitments for both teachers and students. In some cases (e.g., with the use of preceptors), it is not necessary for the teacher to be present in the clinical setting with learners, thereby allowing more flexible scheduling of clinical activities. However, flexibility is necessary to take advantage of learning opportunities when they are available.

The clinical teacher should broadly interpret the objectives for a clinical course to take full advantage of the learning opportunities in each clinical setting. If the instructor knows what concepts the students are learning in the classroom, he or she can find various clinical learning opportunities in different settings. For example, if the focus is wound healing, students could have learning activities involving patients with postoperative wounds, pressure ulcers, traumatic wounds, or arterial or venous chronic leg ulcers. It is not necessary for every student to have a similar learning opportunity if all learning activities enable students to apply the same concept in practice. In postclinical conference, students can be guided to discuss the various ways in which they applied a particular concept or principle; this debriefing activity will broaden their clinical knowledge and help them to identify similarities and differences among the various patient responses to a common alteration in health status.

OPTIONS FOR LEARNING ASSIGNMENTS

The creative teacher may craft clinical assignments from a wide variety of learning activities. Several options for making assignments are discussed.

Teacher-Selected or Learner-Selected Assignments

Although it is the teacher's responsibility to specify the learning objective, learners should have choices of learning activities that will help them achieve the objective. Having a choice of assignment or at least a choice between options selected by the teacher motivates students to be responsible for their own learning and fully engage in the learning activity. Allowing learners to participate in selecting their own assignments may also reduce student anxiety.

Of course, the teacher should offer guidance in selecting appropriate learning activities through questions or comments that require students to evaluate their own needs, interests, and abilities. Sometimes teachers need to be more directive; a student may choose an assignment that clearly requires more knowledge or skill than the student has developed. In this case, the teacher must intervene to protect patient safety as well as to help the student make realistic plans to acquire the necessary knowledge and skill. Other students may choose assignments that do not challenge their abilities; the teacher's role is to support and encourage such students to take advantage of opportunities to achieve higher levels of knowledge and skill.

Skill Focus Versus Total Care Focus

As previously discussed, the traditional clinical assignment for nursing students is to give total care to one or more patients. However, not all learning objectives require students to practice total patient care. For example, if the objective is, "Assess patient and family preparation for postoperative recovery at home," the student does not have to provide total care to the postoperative patient in order to meet the objective. The student could meet the objective by interviewing the patient and family, observing a case manager's assessment of the patient and family's readiness for discharge or a physical therapist's assessment of the patient's ability to perform physical activities, and reviewing the patient's electronic health record. Additionally, total patient care is an integrative activity that can be accomplished effectively only when students are competent in performing the component skills.

As previously discussed, all students do not need to be engaged in the same learning activities at the same time. Depending on their individual learning needs, some students might be engaged in activities that focus on developing a particular skill, while others could be practicing more integrative activities such as providing total patient care.

For example, if students are learning physical assessment skills, some students could be assigned to practice auscultation by listening to breath, heart, and abdominal sounds of a variety of patients without having the responsibility of performing other patient care activities. In postclinical conference, these students should share their insights about the commonalities and differences among their assessment findings and relate them to the patients' histories and pathophysiologies. A different group of students could perform assessment rounds during the next clinical practice day.

One advantage to assigning some students to learning activities that do not involve total patient care is that the clinical teacher is more available for closer guidance of students when they are learning to care for patients with complex needs. Staggering assignments in this way helps the clinical teacher better meet the learning needs of all students.

Student–Patient Ratio Options

Although the traditional clinical assignment takes the form of one student to one patient, there are other assignment options. These options include:

- *One student/one patient or multiple patients.* One student is responsible for certain aspects of care or for comprehensive care for one or more patients. The student works alone to plan, implement, and evaluate nursing care. This type of assignment is advantageous when the objective is to integrate many aspects of care after the student has learned the individual activities.
- *Multiple students/one patient.* Two or more students are assigned to plan, implement, and evaluate care for one patient. Each learner has a defined role, and all collaborate to meet the learning objective. Various models of dual or multiple assignment exist. For example, three students would read the patient record, review the relevant pathophysiology, and collaborate on an assessment and plan of care. Student A reviews information concerning the patient's medications, administers and documents all scheduled and prn (when-needed) medications, and manages the intravenous infusions. Student B focuses on providing and documenting all other aspects of patient care. Student C evaluates the effectiveness of the plan of care, assists with physical care when needed, interacts with the patient's family, and provides reports to appropriate staff members. Members of the learning team can switch roles on subsequent days. This assignment strategy is particularly useful when patients have complex needs that are beyond the capability of one student, although it can be used in any setting with a large number of students and a low patient census. Other advantages include reducing student anxiety and teaching teamwork and collaborative learning.
- *Multiple students–patient aggregate.* A group of students is assigned to complete activities related to a community or population subgroup at risk for certain health problems. For example, a small group of students might be assigned to conduct a community assessment to identify an actual or potential health problem in the aggregate served by the clinical agency. Clinical activities would include interviewing community residents and agency staff members, identifying environmental and occupational health hazards, documenting the availability of social and health services, and performing selected physical assessments on a sample of the aggregate. The student group would then analyze the data and present a report to the agency staff and community members. Advantages of this assignment strategy include promoting a focus on the community as client, teaching collaboration with other health care providers and community members, and reinforcement of group process.

Management Activities

Some clinical assignments are chosen to enable learners to meet outcomes related to nursing leadership, management and improvement of patient care, and health care organizational goals. Undergraduate nursing students are usually introduced to concepts and skills of leadership and management in preparation for their future roles in complex health care systems. These students often benefit from clinical assignments that allow them to develop skill in planning and managing care for a group of patients. For example, a senior baccalaureate student may enact the role of team leader for other nursing students who are assigned to provide total care for individual patients.

The student team leader may receive reports about the group of patients from agency staff, plan assignments for the other students, give reports to those students, supervise and coordinate work, and communicate patient information to staff members.

Master's and doctoral students may be preparing for management and administrative roles in health care organizations; their clinical activities might focus on enacting the roles of first-level or middle manager, patient care services administrator, clinical nurse leader, or case manager. Often, such clinical assignments involve the participation of a preceptor (see Chapter 12).

Guided Observation

Observation is an important skill in nursing practice, and teachers should provide opportunities for learners to develop this skill systematically. Observing patients in order to collect data is a prerequisite to problem solving, clinical reasoning, and clinical decision making. To make accurate and useful observations, the student must have knowledge of the phenomenon and the intellectual skill to observe it: the what and how of observation. As a clinical learning assignment, observation should not be combined with an assignment to provide care. If students do not have concurrent care responsibilities, they are free to choose the times and sometimes the locations of their observations. The focus should be on observing purposefully in order to meet a learning objective.

Observation also provides opportunities for students to learn through modeling. By observing another person performing a skill, the learner forms an image of how the task or behavior is to be performed, which serves as a guide to learning. For this reason, it is helpful to schedule learners to observe in a clinical setting before they are assigned to practice activities. However, scheduling an observation before the learner has acquired the prerequisite knowledge is unproductive; the student may not be able to make meaning out of what is observed.

Written observation guidelines can be used effectively to prepare learners for the activity and to guide their attention to important data during the observation. Exhibit 7.1 is an example of an observation guide to prepare students for a group observation activity in an operating room. Note the explicit expectations that, before the observation, students will read, think critically, and anticipate what they will see. The presence of a clinical teacher or other resource person to answer questions and direct students' attention to pertinent items or activities is also helpful. Students may be asked to evaluate the observation activity by identifying learning outcomes, what they did and did not like about the activity, and the extent to which their preparation and the participation of the instructor was helpful. Exhibit 7.2 is a sample evaluation tool for an observation activity.

EXHIBIT 7.1

EXAMPLE OF AN OBSERVATION GUIDE

Operating Room Observation Guide

Purposes of the Observation Activity

1. To gain an overview of perioperative nursing care in the intraoperative phase.
2. To observe application of principles of surgical asepsis in the operating room.
3. To distinguish among roles of various members of the surgical team.

(continued)

General Information

You are expected to prepare for this observation and to complete an observation guide while you are observing the surgical procedure. Please read your medical–surgical nursing textbook, pp. 195 to 200, for a general understanding of nursing roles in the intraoperative phase.

Bring this observation guide and a pen or pencil on the day of your observation. The guide will be collected and reviewed by the instructor at the end of the observation activity.

Most likely, you will observe either a coronary artery bypass graft or an aortic valve replacement. Please review the anatomy of the heart, specifically the coronary vessels and valves. In addition, read the following pages in your medical–surgical nursing textbook: coronary artery disease, pp. 1058 to 1059 and 1069 to 1085; valvular heart disease (aortic stenosis), pp. 1131 to 1132 and 1135 to 1139.

After you have completed your reading assignment, attempt to answer the questions in the first section of the observation guide (Preparation of the Patient) related to preparations that take place before the patient comes to the operating room. Don't be afraid to make some educated guesses about the answers; we will discuss them and supply any missing information on the day of your observation.

Complete the remaining sections of the observation guide during your observation. The instructor will be available to guide the observation and to answer questions.

Preparation of the Patient

1. Who is responsible for obtaining the consent for the surgical procedure? Why?
2. Who identifies the patient when he or she is brought into the operating room? Why?
3. What other patient data should be reviewed by a nurse when the patient is brought to the operating room (sign-in protocol)? Why?
4. Who transfers the patient from transport bed to the operating room bed? What safety precautions are taken during this procedure?
5. What is the nurse's role during anesthesia induction?
6. What team members participate in the time-out protocol? Identify elements of the protocol that protect the safety of this patient.
7. When is the patient positioned for the surgical procedure? Who does this? What safety precautions are taken? What special equipment may be used?
8. What is the purpose of the preoperative skin preparation of the operative site? When is it done? What safety precautions are taken?
9. What is the purpose of draping the patient and equipment? What factors determine the type of drape material used? What safety precautions are taken? Who does the draping? Why?
10. What nursing diagnoses are commonly identified for patients in the immediate preoperative and early intraoperative phases?

Preparation of Personnel

1. Apparel: Who is wearing what? What factors determine the selection of apparel? How and when do personnel don and remove apparel items? What personal protective equipment is used and why?
2. Hand antisepsis: Which personnel use hand antisepsis techniques to prepare for the procedure? When? Which method is used?
3. Gowning and gloving: What roles do the scrub person and the circulator play?

Roles of Surgical Team Members

1. Surgeons and assistants (surgical residents, interns, medical students)
2. Nurses and surgical technologists
3. Anesthesia personnel
4. Others (perfusion technologist, radiologic technologist, pathologist, laser operator, etc.)

(*continued*)

Maintenance of Aseptic Technique

1. Movement of personnel
2. Sterile areas and items
3. Nonsterile areas and items
4. Handling of sterile items

Equipment

1. Lighting: Who positions it? How? When?
2. Monitoring: What monitors are used? Who is responsible for setting up and watching this equipment?
3. Blood/other fluid infusion: Who is responsible for setting up and monitoring this equipment?
4. Electrosurgical device: What is this equipment used for? Who is responsible for it? What safety precautions are taken?
5. Suction: What is this equipment used for? Who is responsible for setting up and monitoring it?
6. Smoke evacuator: What is this equipment used for? Who is responsible for setting up and using it?
7. Patient heating/cooling equipment: What is this equipment used for? Who is responsible for setting up and monitoring it?
8. Other equipment

Intraoperative Nursing Diagnoses

1. What nursing diagnoses are likely to be identified for this patient in the intraoperative period?

Conclusion of Procedure

1. What elements of the sign-out protocol are implemented at this time?
2. How is the patient hand-over communication conducted? What personnel are involved? Were the essential elements included?
3. What nursing diagnoses are likely to be identified for this patient in the early postoperative period?

EXHIBIT 7.2

EXAMPLE OF STUDENT EVALUATION OF A GUIDED OBSERVATION ACTIVITY

Student Evaluation of Operating Room Observation

1. To what extent did you prepare for this learning activity?
   ___ I completed all assigned readings and attempted answers to all questions on the first section of the observation guide.
   ___ I completed all assigned readings and attempted to answer some of the observation guide questions.
   ___ I completed some of the assigned readings and attempted to answer some of the observation guide questions.
   ___ I didn't do any reading, but I tried to answer some of the observation guide questions before I came to the operating room.
   ___ I didn't do any reading, and I didn't answer any observation guide questions before I came to the operating room.
2. How would you rate the overall value of this learning activity?
   ___ It was excellent; I learned a great deal.
   ___ It was very good; I learned more than I expected to.

(continued)

____ It was good; I learned about as much as I expected to.
____ It was fair; I didn't learn as much as I expected to.
____ It was poor; I didn't learn anything of value.
3. How would you rate the value of the observation guide in helping you to prepare for and participate in the observation?
____ Extremely helpful in focusing my attention on significant aspects of perioperative nursing care.
____ Very helpful in guiding me to observe activities in the operating room.
____ Helpful in guiding my observations but at times distracted my attention from what I wanted to watch.
____ Only a little helpful; it seemed like a lot of work for little benefit.
____ Not at all helpful; it distracted me more than it helped me to observe what was going on in the operating room.
4. How would you rate the helpfulness of the instructor who guided your operating room observation?
____ Excellent; helped me to analyze, synthesize, and evaluate the activities I observed.
____ Very good; answered my questions and focused my attention on important activities.
____ Good; was able to answer some questions, attempted to make the activity meaningful to me.
____ Fair; I probably could have learned as much without an instructor present.
____ Poor; distracted me or interfered with my learning; I could have learned more without an instructor present.
5. What was the most meaningful part of this learning activity for you? What was the most important or surprising thing you learned?
6. What was the least meaningful part of this observation activity? If there is something that you would change, suggest a specific change to make it better.

Service Learning

Another option for clinical learning assignments is service learning. Service learning differs from volunteer work, community service, fieldwork, and internships. Volunteer and community service focus primarily on the service that is provided to the recipients, and fieldwork and internships primarily focus on benefits to student learning. Service learning benefits the community and students, and allows students to see the value of service to vulnerable populations (Beauvais, Foito, Pearlin, & Yost, 2015). Service learning is an academic credit-earning learning activity in which students:

■ Participate in an organized service activity that meets identified community needs
■ Reinforce course content
■ Reflect on the service activity to gain a deeper understanding of the nurse's role in society

Benefits of service learning to students include developing skills in communication, critical thinking, and collaboration; developing a community perspective and commitment to health promotion and health equity in the community; awareness of diversity and cultural dynamics; and increased student engagement, fostering civic engagement and social justice, developing leadership abilities, and professional development and self-discovery (Groh, Stallwood, & Daniels, 2011; Taylor & Leffers,

2016). Benefits to the community include having control of the service provided and recipients of service becoming better able to serve themselves and be served by their own actions.

As nursing education programs include more community-based learning activities, opportunities to incorporate service learning increase. Meaningful community-based service learning opportunities are based on relationships between the academic unit and the community to be served. For such partnerships to work effectively, there must be a good fit between the academic unit's mission and goals and the needs of the community. A key element of service learning is the community partner's identification of need, according to an integrative review of service learning in nursing education (Taylor & Leffers, 2016).

As is true for any other clinical learning activity, planning for a service-learning activity begins with the teacher's decision that such learning activities would help students to achieve one or more course outcomes. The success of service learning depends on the embedding of this pedagogy in an existing academic course with clearly defined outcomes (Taylor & Leffers, 2016). The teacher should determine how much time to allot to this activity, keeping in mind that the time spent in service learning would replace and not add to the total time available for other clinical activities for that course. An integrative review of service learning in nursing education revealed a wide variation in the duration of student participation, from 3 hours to an entire academic year. Evidence of the minimum amount of time needed for students to achieve course outcomes through service learning is lacking. The time required to establish community partnerships and to orient students to the environment suggests that "multiple opportunities with differentiated outcomes might enhance both the community and the learner outcomes" (Taylor & Leffers, 2016, p. 199).

Before students participate in a service-learning activity, they may prepare a learning contract that includes:

- The name of the community agency or group
- The clients or recipients of that agency's or group's services
- The services to be provided by the student
- A service objective related to a need that has been identified by the community or the community recipient of the proposed service
- A learning objective that is related to a course outcome, goal, or competency that the activity would help the student to achieve

The instructor should identify agencies and groups appropriate for service learning in a specific course from among those with which the educational institution has formed an academic–service partnership. Examples of community settings, programs, and agencies that would be appropriate for service learning include daycare centers, extended care or assisted living centers, senior centers, food delivery programs, the American Red Cross, Head Start, health screening programs, vaccine clinics, health outreach or shelter programs for homeless individuals and families, and camps for children with disabilities or chronic illnesses, among many others.

As another option, a group of students enrolled in the same course could be placed in a community setting to participate in a designated population-based project relevant to the course objectives. For example, Decker, Hensel, and Fasone

(2016) described a service-learning activity in which nursing students implemented a bystander intervention on their college campus. Findings from 118 students over a 2-year period showed that students helped improve campus safety while growing as professionals. The students' service was part of their community clinical nursing course. Benefits of this service-learning activity included:

- Improving campus safety
- Achieving course learning outcomes
- Developing knowledge, skills, and attitudes that reflect the Quality and Safety Education for Nurses competencies, such as minimizing risk of harm
- Developing as leaders and health promoters (Decker et al., 2016)

The role of the clinical teacher as facilitator is crucial to the success of service learning. The teacher needs to structure pre-engagement, on-site, and post-engagement student learning activities to ensure the achievement of desired outcomes (Taylor & Leffers, 2016). Because service learning is more than expecting students to use some of their clinical practice hours for service projects, clinical teachers should plan to spend as much time planning these activities as they do traditional clinical learning activities. Students' reflection on their experiences is an essential component of service learning, differentiating it from a volunteer experience. Therefore, teachers should structure the learning activities to include reflective practices, such as journaling or participation in individual or group debriefing sessions. The teacher must allow time to read and give feedback on students' reflective journal entries about their experiences or to participate in individual or group reflective sessions. Teachers may require students to do presentations about their service-learning projects, which the teachers would observe and evaluate—another time requirement to consider. Faculty members must also continue to interact with members of the community to evaluate the outcomes of service learning from the perspective of the recipients of service and to continually nurture the partnerships that were established.

In an integrative review of service learning in nursing education, students often reported feelings of anxiety or other intense emotion at the start of service learning activities, and they required time to adjust to their engagement with diverse groups in the community or immersion into a new setting. This finding suggests that clinical teachers may need to plan for longer pre-engagement preparation and greater duration and depth of immersion in each service learning activity. Guided reflection on service learning experiences may help students to identify and manage these intense emotions (Taylor & Leffers, 2016).

SUMMARY

This chapter presented a framework for selecting clinical learning assignments. Clinical teachers should select clinical assignments that are related to desired learning outcomes, appropriate to students' levels of knowledge and skill, and challenging enough to motivate learning. Providing comprehensive nursing care to one or more patients is a typical clinical assignment, but it is not always the most appropriate choice.

Clinical teachers typically speak of selecting patients for clinical assignments. However, the primary role of the nursing student in the clinical area is that of learner, not nurse. Caring for patients is not synonymous with learning. Nursing students are *learning to care* for patients; they are not nurses with *responsibility for patient care.* In fact, early responsibility for patient care often creates anxiety that interferes with learning.

Factors affecting the selection of clinical assignments include the learning objectives of the clinical activity; needs of patients; availability and variety of learning opportunities in the clinical environment; and the needs, interests, and abilities of learners. The most important criterion for selection of clinical assignments is usually the desired learning outcome. Each clinical activity should be an integral part of the course or educational program, and it is essential that the clinical teacher, students, and staff members understand the goals of each clinical activity. Learning activities should be selected and structured so that they relate logically and sequentially to the desired outcome.

Individual learner characteristics such as education level; previous experience; aptitude for learning; learning style; and specific needs, interests, and abilities should also influence the selection of clinical assignments. All learners do not have the same needs, so it is unreasonable to expect them to have the same learning assignments on any given day. Students who are able to achieve the objectives of the essential curriculum might quickly receive or choose assignments from the enrichment curriculum that allow them to focus on their individual needs and interests.

Patient needs and care requirements should also be considered when planning clinical assignments. The nursing care activities required by a patient may not present enough of a challenge to one learner and may be too complex for another. Patient wishes regarding student assignment should be respected. Nursing staff members who have provided care to these patients can often help the clinical teacher determine whether student learning needs and specific patient and family needs can both be met through a particular clinical assignment.

Another factor affecting the selection of clinical assignments is the timing and availability of learning opportunities. Ideally, clinical learning activities are scheduled concurrently with relevant classroom content so that learners can apply knowledge to nursing practice immediately. The usual schedule of activities in the clinical facility may determine the optimum timing of learning activities. Some clinical settings are available to both patients and students only at certain times. In other settings, however, scheduling clinical activities during evening or nighttime hours or on weekends provides better learning opportunities.

Alternatives for making clinical assignments include selection by teacher or learner, focus on particular skills or integrative patient care, various student–patient ratio options, management activities, guided observation, and service learning. Advantages and drawbacks of each alternative were discussed.

CNE EXAMINATION TEST BLUEPRINT CORE COMPETENCIES

1. **Facilitate Learning**
   A. Implement a variety of teaching strategies appropriate to
      1. content
      2. setting (i.e., clinical vs. classroom)
      3. learner needs

(continued)

        4. learning style
        5. desired learner outcomes

  E. Practice skilled oral and written (including electronic) communication that reflects an awareness of self and relationships with learners (e.g., evaluation, mentorship, and supervision)

  H. Create opportunities for learners to develop their own critical thinking skills

  K. Demonstrate personal attributes that facilitate learning (e.g., caring, confidence, patience, integrity, respect, and flexibility)

  M. Develop collegial working relationships with clinical agency personnel to promote positive learning environments

  P. Act as a role model in practice settings

2. Facilitate Learner Development and Socialization

  B. Provide resources for diverse learners to meet their individual learning needs

  D. Create learning environments that facilitate learners' self-reflection, personal goal setting, and socialization to the role of the nurse

  E. Foster the development of learners in these areas:
      1. cognitive domain
      2. psychomotor domain
      3. affective domain

  G. Encourage professional development of learners

3. Use Assessment and Evaluation Strategies

  L. Provide timely, constructive, and thoughtful feedback to learners

4. Participate in Curriculum Design and Evaluation of Program Outcomes

  H. Collaborate with community and clinical partners to support educational goals

REFERENCES

Beauvais, A., Foito, K., Pearlin, N., & Yose, E. (2015). Service learning with a geriatric population: Changing attitudes and improving knowledge. *Nurse Educator, 40,* 318–321. doi:10.1097/NNE.0000000000000181

Decker, K., Hensel, D., & Fasone, L. (2016). Outcomes of a bystander intervention community health service-learning project. *Nurse Educator, 41,* 147–150. doi:10.1097/NNE.0000000000000232

Groh, C. J., Stallwood, L. G., & Daniels, J. J. (2011). Service-learning in nursing education: Its impact on leadership and social justice. *Nursing Education Perspectives, 32,* 400–405.

Infante, M. S. (1985). *The clinical laboratory in nursing education* (2nd ed.). New York, NY: Wiley.

Taylor, S. L., & Leffers, J. M. (2016). Integrative review of service-learning assessment in nursing education. *Nursing Education Perspectives, 37,* 194–200.

Woodley, L. K. (2018). Clinical teaching in nursing. In M. H. Oermann, J. C. De Gagne, & B. C. Phillips (Eds.), *Teaching in nursing and role of the educator: The complete guide to best practice in teaching, evaluation, and curriculum development* (2nd ed.). New York, NY: Springer Publishing.

CHAPTER 8

Clinical Simulation

Clinical simulation and manikin-based human patient simulation has evolved and is now a widely accepted and common aspect of clinical nursing education. Since many nursing programs face competition for clinical sites and limited access to clinical facilities, simulation may be the answer for nursing programs struggling to secure clinical placements and provide students with valuable learning experiences (Hayden, Smiley, & Gross, 2014). Simulation activities that mimic reality allow students to develop technical skill proficiency in a safe, nonthreatening environment while contributing to student learning, enhancement of critical thinking, and problem-solving skills.

This use of clinical simulation comes at a time when nurse educators face numerous challenges that impact clinical teaching. A continued interest in nursing as a career has led to more applications to nursing education programs, but the number of nursing faculty members remains inadequate to meet the demand (American Association of Colleges of Nursing, 2014). Educators are faced with capacity limits in classrooms and clinical settings and encounter ongoing struggles as they address this enrollment increase. This situation will continue to remain a concern as large numbers of nurses near retirement. In addition, the health care environment has grown in complexity due to the increasing presence of technology in hospitals and, subsequently, patients with higher acuity levels who are older, frailer, and have greater comorbidity. Patients are also spending less time in the hospital, so students have less exposure to patients in the acute care hospital environment and fewer opportunities to maintain and improve their skills. Finally, a shortage of clinical space, particularly in specialty clinical areas such as obstetrics, pediatrics, and intensive care units, often limits nursing student activities to observation rather than hands-on patient care and may also restrict the number of students placed on those units for clinical learning experiences (Kardong-Edgren, Wilhaus, Bennett, & Hayden, 2012). Nurse educators are thus challenged to prepare students for a complex environment where they must think critically, act quickly, and communicate effectively with multidisciplinary team members. This chapter discusses how simulation can be used to enhance clinical teaching to ensure a better prepared nursing workforce. It also discusses the incorporation of best practice standards into clinical simulation activities.

BACKGROUND

Simulation using a clinical scenario "involves a student or group of students providing care for a patient who is represented by a manikin, an actor, or an SP" (standardized patient; Jeffries, 2012, p. 3) in a realistic clinical environment. Students can demonstrate psychomotor skills, clinical reasoning, clinical judgment, problem solving, and critical thinking through techniques such as role-playing and the use of devices such as interactive videos or manikins. Simulation allows teachers to take specific information—such as a patient's personal characteristics; health information; socioeconomic, family, and community components; and physical, mental, and emotional state—and weave it into a real-life scenario that enhances a student's comprehension of the material because it is meaningful (Jeffries, 2012). In the case of clinical nursing scenarios, simulation provides an opportunity to suspend belief of what is real to produce a low-risk, hands-on opportunity to practice a clinical situation involving patient monitoring, management, communication, and multidisciplinary collaboration.

In the past, simulation activities have been documented in a variety of disciplines, such as medicine, aviation, psychology, and education (Lusk & Fater, 2013). In nursing, simulation has been used for teaching in all clinical areas. Traditionally, medical–surgical and emergency resuscitations were the most commonly used scenarios in nursing programs as identified in the National Council of State Boards of Nursing (NCSBN) National Simulation Survey (Kardong-Edgren et al., 2012). Other specialty areas in nursing education, such as pediatrics, obstetrics, home care, hospice, and palliative care, began using simulation as part of the clinical experience (Guise & Wiig, 2016; Kunkel, Kopp, & Hanson, 2016; Veltri, Kaakinen, Shillam, Arwood, & Bell, 2016). Most recently simulation use with interprofessional education has emerged (Manning, Skiff, Santiago, & Irish, 2016; Pastor, Cunningham, White, & Kolomer, 2016). Simulation may never replace direct student contact with human patients, but it has the potential to make student and teacher time in clinical settings more valuable and cost effective while allowing students to explore diverse learning situations that they may not see in clinical settings.

The use of human patient simulators (HPSs) has become common practice in many nursing education programs. Using simulation-based pedagogy allows students to integrate psychomotor skill performance, critical thinking, clinical judgment, and communication skills while gaining self-confidence prior to entering the clinical setting. In addition, simulation offers an opportunity for evaluation and assessment of student skills with options for remediation and continued learning (Jeffries, Dreifuerst, & Haerling, 2018). The active learning component of simulation also appeals to many of today's millennial generation students, helping them to maintain engagement in the learning process, and retain the material learned.

Various organizations have recognized simulation's value as a teaching technique. The Commission on Collegiate Nursing Education (CCNE) accreditation standards encourages the use of innovative teaching methods and the introduction of technology and informatics to improve student learning (CCNE, 2013). The National League for Nursing (NLN) has also provided long-standing leadership and support for simulation in nursing education, conducting a national multisite multimethod study investigating the innovative use of simulation to teach nursing care of ill adults and children (Forneris & Fey, 2016). NLN's leadership continued with the development of the Simulation Innovation Resource Center (SIRC). SIRC provides education and training about simulation while also allowing participants an opportunity to engage in dialogue with colleagues about simulation and providing resources for the development and integration of simulation into the curriculum (NLN, n.d.). Finally, the NLN Leadership Development Program for Simulation Educators offers an opportunity for experienced simulation nurse educators to examine issues related to research in simulation, curricular integration, and the role of simulation in interprofessional education (NLN, 2017). Another organization, the International Association for Clinical Simulation and Learning (INACSL), has developed simulation standards, publishes a monthly journal focusing on clinical simulation in nursing, offers webinars, and a simulation scholars mentorship program (INACSL, 2015).

The National Council of State Boards of Nursing (NCSBN) simulation study provides sound supporting evidence that high-quality simulation experiences can replicate patient situations and allow students to adequately develop their nursing skills. The findings from this national randomized controlled study suggests that up to 50% high-quality simulation can replace traditional clinical practice experiences and produce comparable educational outcomes in prelicensure programs (Hayden, Smiley, Alexander, Kardong-Edgren, & Jeffries, 2014). Although evidence suggests that simulation prepares students for clinical practice, some states regulate simulation hours and provide guidelines regarding how much clinical time can be replaced by simulation. Other states make these decisions on a case-by-case basis. Or, boards of nursing regulations may be silent and not address simulation use in education at all. Program directors and clinical teachers need to determine regulations that may influence clinical teaching and simulation use decisions (Hayden, Smiley, & Gross, 2014). While nursing experts acknowledge the value of simulation as a teaching–learning approach that mimics reality, experts also emphasize the need for nursing student clinical experiences with real patients, thus encouraging clinical teachers to use all available learning opportunities.

TYPES OF SIMULATORS

There are different levels of sophistication as well as a variety of types of simulators that teachers must consider when planning simulation use in nursing education. The level of simulators, categorized according to the fidelity or how closely it represents a realistic situation, has been described as low, moderate or high. Low-fidelity simulators use static tools, are less precise reproductions, and lack the realism of a clinical situation, but offer opportunities for procedural skill practice. These low-fidelity simulators are sometimes referred to as "task-trainers" (Durham, Cato, & Lasater, 2014). Examples of low-fidelity simulation may involve the use of a disembodied pelvis for catheter insertion simulation or a gel pad for intramuscular injection practice. Moderate-fidelity simulators offer a more realistic reproduction of a clinical situation and provide some feedback to the student. A manikin that produces heart and lung sounds, but does not offer the realism of chest movement, is an example of a moderate-fidelity simulator. Moderate-fidelity simulators allow students to complete an assessment but without interactive features. High-fidelity simulators produce the most lifelike scenarios. These full-size manikins react to student manipulations in real time and in realistic ways, such as speaking, coughing, and demonstrating chest movements and pulses.

SPs represent another type of simulation used in nursing education. This form of simulation uses live actors with scripts that portray patients and require nursing students to engage in nursing care activities with the SP in an environment that simulates patient care areas (Jeffries et al., 2018). Nursing education programs affiliated with academic health centers may have SPs available to them since SPs are commonly used in medical education. Practice with SPs can provide invaluable learning opportunities for students as they refine their communication skills or practice in sensitive or specialized clinical situations such as oncology, mental health, or end-of-life situations. SPs can offer valuable feedback and insight about the patient perspective to the nursing student (MacLean, Kelly, Geddes, & Delta, 2017). Using SPs has also been helpful with health assessment and psychomotor skill development (Ham, 2016; Sarmasoglu, Dinc, & Elcin, 2016; Slater, Bryant, & Ng, 2016) and can be useful as both a teaching–learning strategy or as an evaluation approach. However, for students who do not have this option available, other well-planned simulation experiences can help to meet their needs. Visual and performing arts students, improvisation group members, nursing alumni, or retired professionals (e.g., actors, physicians, nurses, teachers), may be able to role-play as patients, family members, or interdisciplinary health care professionals to enhance simulation realism.

USING SIMULATION AS A TEACHING–LEARNING STRATEGY

Nursing programs are integrating simulation into their curriculum. This integration may be a result of external pressure (visiting prospective students who ask to see the HPSs), administrators who recognize the need, nurse educators who desire to keep up with the technology-driven millennial generation of students, or teachers seeking alternative learning opportunities for students. Still, well-designed research is necessary to demonstrate how the use of simulation creates the desired outcomes in student learning and how simulation can best translate into clinical practice.

The NLN Jeffries Simulation Theory has served as a critical framework to design, implement, and evaluate simulation in nursing (Jeffries, 2016). One component of this theory focuses on simulation design characteristics. Clinical teachers using simulation need to consider the following design characteristics: objectives, fidelity, problem solving, student support, and debriefing. Another component involves outcomes and include learning, skill performance, learner satisfaction, critical thinking, and self-confidence. Finally, clinical teachers using simulation need to consider the facilitator, the participant, and educational practices when using simulation in clinical education (Jeffries, 2016). Teachers need adequate training for the development of appropriate clinical scenarios, implementation of the simulation, and evaluation of the pedagogy. Faculty development related to simulation must be a critical factor to consider when implementing clinical simulation for teaching–learning purposes to ensure that teachers are adequately prepared to implement simulation appropriately.

EDUCATIONAL PRACTICES

Today's millennial generation of nursing students require a teaching pedagogy that is based on active participation, collaboration and group work, incorporates technology, and provides a realistic immersion in the experience (Montenery et al., 2013); simulation meets these needs. By engaging learners directly in the simulation, active learning can occur. Providing constructive feedback during the debriefing session, allowing students to view a recording of their performance, or getting suggestions and critiques from classmates who may be viewing them in a nearby classroom all provide feedback that may enhance student performance (Hallmark, Thompson, & Gantt, 2016).

Acknowledging that students learn through many different styles, simulation allows the incorporation of different teaching strategies to appeal to these diverse needs.

PREPARING FOR SIMULATION

In order to realize the full benefit of clinical simulation, teachers need to ensure that students participating in simulation experiences in clinical nursing laboratories see this as a realistic environment and consider various factors when preparing the clinical scenario for simulation. Specific policies and procedures related to clinical simulation recording and the confidentiality of the recording need to be developed. Students need to be orientated to the manikin and the simulated environment. Additionally, ground rules for professional behavior and attire (e.g., uniform, scrubs, lab coats) and strategies to decrease vulnerability and anxiety are helpful (Durham et al., 2014).

Teachers need to consider many factors and purposively design clinical scenarios that are based on INACSL Standards of Best Practice (2016) used for simulation. Exhibit 8.1 provides a listing of recommendations for inclusion in the clinical scenario design. Program outcomes and course objectives should provide some direction for the type of simulation needed. For example, if a clinical or course objective focuses on client assessment, teachers might decide to create a simulation that has a patient experiencing shortness of breath, decreased oxygen saturation, and abnormal breath sounds. During the simulation, students could use their critical thinking and problem-solving skills to explore the respiratory status of the patient and complete a respiratory assessment.

EXHIBIT 8.1

CLINICAL SCENARIO DESIGN CONSIDERATIONS

- Needs assessment
- Participant preparation and resources
- Prebriefing
- Patient information
- Measurable participant objectives
- Environmental conditions and context
- Fidelity to enhance realism
- Participant roles and expectations
- Progression outline
- Debriefing
- Evaluation

Source: Adapted from INACSL Standards Committee (2016).

CHOOSING FIDELITY

An important planning consideration involves the most appropriate level of fidelity. Teachers should not automatically select a high-fidelity simulator but should consider all aspects of fidelity including physical, conceptual, and psychological. Physical fidelity involves the selection of the simulator and also includes other environmental considerations. When planning the simulation, the teacher should consider the sights, sounds, smells, layout, and props used to create a realistic physical environment. Conceptual fidelity is another important planning consideration. All components of the simulation must fit together appropriately. For example, if the simulation scenario involves a patient having a myocardial infarction, then the subjective and objective data provided to the student should be consistent and reflect the typical activities that would normally occur. The final component of fidelity involves psychological fidelity. Ensuring that the scenario context is realistic and embedding other participants such as family members or health care providers into the simulation will help establish realism (INACSL, 2016; Paige & Morin, 2013).

Basic skills practice can be easily achieved by lower levels of simulation fidelity. Beginning students may be overwhelmed by the high-fidelity manikin. It may be better to introduce novice students to lower level fidelity manikins, allowing them to practice skills before moving on to more complex situations and higher fidelity simulators, while advanced students may require simulations involving complex care or emergent situations that would be best suited for a high-fidelity simulator manikin. The level of technology used in clinical simulation also depends on several other factors: teacher familiarity with the technology, the technology available, and support for use of technology. Clinical teachers should use the resources and expertise available to provide an optimal simulation experience. Nursing education programs that have access to simulation specialists or information technology (IT) support (ideally, designated IT staff members) may have an easier time incorporating simulation into clinical education. In addition, college or university services that support academic excellence with resources and specialists can assist with faculty development, and other departments can help incorporate components that will make the simulation feel more real. Faculty members in a university department of communication may be able to assist nursing clinical teachers with the dialogue component of scenarios. Performing arts faculty members and students can add to the contextual experience by role-playing anxious family members; nursing education colleagues might apply some of their rich clinical experience by portraying a spouse, parent, or child of the HPS.

OTHER PLANNING CONSIDERATIONS

Past simulation and educational experiences, level of student (e.g., first year prelicense students versus advanced practice nurses), and number of clinical students should also be part of the simulation planning considerations. Will all students actively participate in the simulation activities or will a select group of students play an active role serving as the nurse or other health care provider in the simulation scenario while others observe? Have the students participated in simulation activities before or are they new to this experience and need a full orientation to the manikins and simulation environment? Does the simulation build on prior knowledge or is it intended to teach new content? Is the simulation an adjunct for clinical learning, an alternate activity in case of an absence from clinical learning activities, or a replacement for activities at a clinical facility? These factors will impact the amount of time and preparation that may be required for the simulation experience.

Another planning consideration is the focus and purpose of the simulation. Is the simulation planned to provide students with practice opportunities or is the simulation intended to evaluate student performance? Simulated patient experiences are often used for advanced practice nursing students to demonstrate skills needed for practice and are thus used for competency evaluation. Teachers need to consider the high-stakes testing component of simulation as they plan for simulation use. Finally, consider the time for simulation, including lab availability, teacher time, and student time, making sure to include time for introduction, prebriefing, student preparation, simulation implementation, and debriefing. Once these areas have been considered, then further scenario development or selection can occur.

SCENARIO SELECTION

Once some of these preliminary decisions about the simulation have been determined, then teachers can create the scenario. Scenario development incorporates evidence and professional standards, but is at heart a creative process. The use of a simple storyboard template can provide structure without being overwhelming for teachers who are developing their first scenarios. An example of a storyboard for a simple simulation for beginning-level clinical nursing students (see Exhibit 8.2) includes the specific objectives for the simulation activity, the types of cues that the patient and other team members may provide to the students, expected actions, and suggested debriefing and reflection topics. The use of a storyboard template by teachers as they develop scenarios will increase consistency among teachers across a curriculum as well as encourage them to start with basic information (e.g., identifying three to five simulation objectives and learning outcomes). It is important to identify essential learning outcomes, taking into consideration social and demographic trends specific to the geographic area, and incorporating cultural sensitivity, spirituality, and ethical considerations.

EXHIBIT 8.2

EXAMPLE STORYBOARD FOR "HARRY HAS A LOW BLOOD-GLUCOSE LEVEL: A SCENARIO FOR BEGINNING-LEVEL STUDENTS"

Simulation-Specific Objectives
Critical Thinker

1. Interpret subjective and objective symptoms of hypoglycemia.
2. Identify abnormal blood glucose levels.

Evidence-Based Practitioner

3. Demonstrate proper use of a glucometer by obtaining blood sample and recording results.
4. Explain blood glucose results to the patient.

Innovative Professional

5. Demonstrate respect for the patient and family.

(continued)

Simulator Settings/ Other Actions	Verbal Cues	Expected Student Actions	Notes for Reflection
Vital Statistics: T 97.5° F., P 88, R 18, BP 167/88 Report blood glucose below 65.	Harry ■ Oriented to own identity and birth date but is disoriented to time and place. ■ Complains of feeling sweaty and a little strange. ■ Gives permission to have blood sugar checked. Daughter ■ Asks for information about the nurse's actions. ■ Verifies Harry's identity if asked. ■ Expresses concern about father's state if students do not begin to identify patient's condition.	When student enters room: ■ Wash hands, wear gloves appropriately. ■ Introduce self. ■ Identify patient using two identifiers. ■ Inform client of purpose of interaction. ■ Perform brief head-to-toe assessment. ■ Use therapeutic communication during assessment. When student exits the room: ■ Wash hands. ■ Assure that call light is in place. ■ State when a care provider will check on patient next. During care: ■ Check and document blood glucose.	■ How did you know you were caring for the correct patient? ■ What questions did the patient or family have about diabetes? How did it feel when you tried to answer them? ■ Did you check the patient orders? What should you do about the low blood glucose? ■ What do you think you might say to a provider if you call to report a blood glucose level?

Source: Adapted from the Arizona State University College of Nursing and Health Innovation Simulation and Learning Resources Program (2017).

The level of the students, specific course objectives, and teacher clinical expertise all need to be considered when specifying an appropriate learning outcome.

Other suggestions for creating scenarios include reviewing course evaluations, licensure and certification exam results by subject area, communication with clinical facilities, and other program evaluation data to identify essential learning needs of students (Chambers, 2006). Drawing on common situations seen at clinical sites or relying on past clinical cases will help provide ideas for scenario creation. If you are drawing ideas or information from actual patients, make sure case details are generic and that patient privacy is not compromised by revealing too much personal or identifiable information. Sometimes scenarios are a compilation of many patients seen in clinical practice. Incorporate unique aspects of care that can be vividly portrayed in simulations. For example, simulations that use a cluttered, dusty, and insect-infested home during a home health simulation; stressed, arguing parents as part of a pediatric simulation; or a homeless patient with poor literacy skills, comorbidities, and limited support systems can effectively portray challenging situations that nurses face in practice. Regardless of the method used to create scenarios, ensure that they are student-centered, interactive, related to outcomes, and based upon best practices.

Many nursing education programs access or purchase existing scenarios from publishers, simulation manufacturers, other nursing education programs, and national nursing organizations. These already-developed materials aid teachers by providing well-constructed scenarios with the completed template of essential information and support data needed to implement the simulation. When using prepackaged scenarios, it is important to check alignment with course and program outcomes and needs. Sometimes tailoring these scenarios to align with individual program needs may be necessary. Regardless of the origin of the scenario, check to ensure that the scenario uses life-like situations that are appropriate for the level of students and clinical course.

OTHER CONSIDERATIONS

Once the scenario is written, teachers must schedule time with lab staff members (equipment managers and IT experts for programming the equipment) for a rehearsal of the simulation on paper and then in real time. Reviewing scenarios for accuracy, current evidence-based practice guidelines, and unnecessary distracters will ensure the quality of the simulation experience for all and help to identify needed resources (e.g., teacher and staff support, props, space, and time). It is necessary to practice the scenario, and it is ideal if students or teachers are present for a practice session prior to implementing the live scenario with the students. Finally, prepare the manikin or simulated patient with props and include appropriate moulage or a reproduction of special effects so that students can see, feel, smell, and hear in a life-like clinical environment.

Because electronic health record (EHR) use and its relationship to patient safety and prevention of adverse events has been documented (Helwig & Lomotan, 2016), teachers should consider use of this technology as part of simulation. Some nursing programs are using EHRs as a tool to enhance clinical simulation. Students can use the academic EHR to access simulated patient records and document care provided during a simulation, thus giving students an opportunity to develop these essential informatics skills in a safe environment (Mountain, Redd, O'Leary-Kelly, & Giles, 2015). Creating a database of mock patient records as part of the EHR that can be accessed and used during simulation will enhance realism while allowing students to access longitudinal patient data and help ensure that students develop the knowledge and skills needed to function in a technology-rich clinical environment. This hands-on approach of using an EHR during simulation will provide additional practice opportunities and help students make the transition to EHR use in the clinical setting.

IMPLEMENTING SIMULATION

Prebriefing is an important component of simulation. It involves planning, briefing, and facilitating (McDermott, 2016). While planning, the teacher should consider the learner. Factors such as type of program, level in the program, previous clinical experience, previous simulation experience, and prior coursework will all influence learning and impact simulation success (Jeffries, 2016; McDermott, 2016). To adequately prepare for the simulation experience, teachers may plan learning activities that require students to complete an assignment prior to the simulation, such as reading relevant background information on pathophysiology or medications that will be used during the simulation, completing preparation worksheets, reviewing and practicing technical skills, viewing Internet resources, or watching a video or online presentation. Providing students with a brief history of the patient and the diagnosis will then allow students to answer some key questions in preparation for the simulation experience. Exhibit 8.3 provides some sample questions that can be used to prepare for the simulation. Clinical teachers can conduct this presimulation preparation in a variety of ways; students can complete individual written assignments or they can participate in oral discussions with the clinical group. A formal presimulation preparatory group meeting with the students is also an opportunity to review expectations about student performance, remind students about confidentiality of the experience, and obtain signatures for video recording consents.

The simulation should begin with a briefing about the simulation. This is an opportunity for the teacher to assess student preparation for the experience, check on essential student knowledge, review background information about the patient in the simulation, provide instructions, and assign roles for the simulation. It will also be helpful to provide logistical information, set the tone, and clarify expectations before proceeding with the simulation. Teachers should act as facilitators and promote student understanding and answer questions that may arise. Many times the simulation begins with a report or review of background information about the patient in the form of a handoff or change of shift report. It may also include a brief review of

---

EXHIBIT 8.3

SAMPLE PREPARATORY QUESTIONS FOR SIMULATIONS

1. What physical assessments should be completed as a priority for this patient?
2. What questions will you ask the patient so you can fully explore and understand the health problem?
3. What data or information do you still need in order to understand and provide appropriate care for this patient?
4. What lab or diagnostic tests will you review and what might you expect to find?
5. What are the patient's medications (drug classification, dosage, route, administration, nursing implications)?
6. What teaching will be necessary?
7. What might be important to discuss with the family or significant others?
8. What other social, emotional, religious, psychological, or environmental issues need to be considered when planning your care?
9. What will be your priority nursing actions?
10. What other health care providers should be contacted?
11. What nursing interventions will be necessary?

the relevant patient health history. Students begin the scenario and enact the assigned roles, which may include primary nurse, charge nurse, medication nurse, or other supportive staff. Sometimes students or others serve in ancillary or supportive roles that help to enhance the realism of the simulation and add an interprofessional learning opportunity. This is also a chance to collaborate with other disciplines such as students from medicine, speech therapy, respiratory therapy, or dieticians who can serve in their respective roles during the simulation. The teacher, controlling the simulation from a separate room, if feasible, uses the preplanned scenario to respond to student actions during the simulation. Teachers may use either preprogrammed patient vocal responses or spontaneously respond to student questions and actions on behalf of the simulated patient. Teachers should allow students to make mistakes, problem solve throughout the scenario, and find their own way. Many nursing education programs use videorecording capabilities that allow for a recording of all events of the scenarios. These recordings can be used for debriefing after the simulation.

Depending upon clinical group size, learning goals, and time available, teachers may choose to have some students observe the scenario and provide suggestions and insight during debriefing. Students may experience anxiety when they are performing before others during a simulation (Shearer, 2016). The literature suggests strategies that may assist in decreasing anxiety during simulation, including: providing a supportive and respectful learning environment that allows students to make mistakes ensuring adequate preparation, and validating their feelings (Durham et al., 2014; Shearer, 2016). Use of these strategies may help reduce the anxiety during simulation.

DEBRIEFING AND GUIDED REFLECTION

The last, but perhaps most important, area of clinical simulation involves debriefing and providing an opportunity for guided reflection on the simulation. Debriefing has been identified as critical for students' learning and satisfaction with their simulation experience; however, it requires adequate time and some preplanning to be effective. Debriefing encourages reflection, self-awareness, and assists in the transfer of knowledge to practice (INACSL Standards Committee, 2016). Debriefing allows the students to make meaning of the experience, critique performance while reinforcing learning, and figure out how to apply information to practice. Although the importance of debriefing is widely accepted, there are conflicting views on best practice approaches to debriefing (Hall & Tori, 2016). The INACSL Standards of Best Practice can provide some guidance for clinical teachers using debriefing with simulation.

Because debriefing can be critical for student learning, teachers need to carefully plan and consider the methods, format, and approach used while also ensuring that they can effectively facilitate this activity. Exhibit 8.4 provides suggestions for best practices for effective debriefing.

Teachers may choose between a structured or unstructured approach to debriefing. Structured debriefing involves development of prepared questions that can be used to guide the debriefing session. These questions typically arise from simulation objectives and serve as a prompt to focus the debriefing discussion. Caution must be exercised to allow the unfolding of the discussion and to avoid restricting the interactive and reflective activities so crucial in debriefing. Teachers must allow enough flexibility so that they can respond to unexpected developments during simulation and incorporate them into the debriefing activities. On the other hand, unstructured debriefing is a

---

EXHIBIT 8.4

EFFECTIVE DEBRIEFING PRACTICES

1. The debrief is facilitated by a person(s) competent in the process of debriefing.
2. The debrief is conducted in an environment that is conducive to learning and supports confidentiality, trust, open communication, self-analysis, feedback, and reflection.
3. The debrief is facilitated by a person(s) who can devote enough concentrated attention during the simulation to effectively debrief the simulation-based experience.
4. The debrief is based on a theoretical framework for debriefing that is structured in a purposeful way.
5. The debrief is congruent with the objectives and outcomes of the simulation-based experience.

Source: Adapted from INACSL Standards Committee (2016). Reprinted by permission of Elsevier.

---

more spontaneous approach that allows the discussion about the clinical simulation to unfold and go where the participants take it. This free-flowing approach may deviate from the learning objectives, so teachers need to be able to refocus students as needed (Dreifuerst, 2009).

Oral or written format, or a combination of both, may be used to accomplish debriefing. Oral debriefing or discussions about simulation can be public or private. Public debriefing allows observers, typically other clinical students who observed the simulation, to participate in the debriefing process. Student observers and teachers can provide valuable insight and suggestions after watching the simulation. They may notice actions that the students in the nurse's role may not be aware of and can offer insight from their unique perspective of observer. Sometimes the debriefing process can be sensitive and anxiety-provoking, particularly if the student performance is deficient or problems were encountered, or when video playback of the simulation is reviewed. Teachers may choose to complete private debriefing with only those students playing an active role in the simulation. If group debriefing is used then the teacher should facilitate the use of honest, respectful, and supportive feedback. It is also important to demonstrate regard for the student and the emotional aspect of this experience (INACSL, 2016).

Regardless of the approach used for oral debriefing, teachers should anticipate and plan for the amount of time needed to debrief. Time used for debriefing varies and the published literature does not reveal sufficient research to make definitive evidence-based recommendations on this topic. Gore, Van Gele, Ravert, and Mabire (2012) conducted a survey of the INACSL members to identify current simulation practices and found that in the United States, respondents spend equal time on simulation and debriefing; however, international respondents reported debriefings that were twice as long as the simulations. Further research in this area is needed, but as a general guideline for planning purposes, teachers should consider spending at least the same amount of time on debriefing as they do with the simulation.

Oral debriefing typically follows immediately at the conclusion of the scenario. This timing for debriefing is helpful in that students are able to recall recent events and discuss them while they are still current. However, some students may benefit from some additional time to process the simulation events and think about the experience, or they may prefer to privately reflect about the experience in writing rather than orally in a public forum. Journaling activities can be assigned to encourage students to personally reflect on the experience. Electronic activities such as blogging (in a private rather than public format) or threaded electronic discussions can also be used to engage students who are digital natives and promote reflection after simulation. Either structured or unstructured approaches can be used. For example, students can be asked to compose a reflective journal entry that uses a broad prompt, such as, "Write about what you learned from the simulation." Or, they can write more specifically about what went well and what could be improved. Structured prompts could direct students to write about specific examples of actions during the simulation. For example, "What were you thinking when the patient complained of shortness of breath during the simulation? What actions did you take and what else could you have done to address this situation?"

Teachers must also consider the use of technology for the debriefing, such as whether and how to incorporate video playback of the simulation. Conflicting opinions exist regarding debriefing and video use. Gore et al. (2012) reported significant differences between United States and international INACSL respondents regarding the incorporation of videorecording use as part of debriefing. In the United States, participants reported that students were not required to view the simulation video recordings. If teachers and students cannot quickly access pertinent video clips to use for immediate debriefing, training and support are needed. In the meantime, teachers could consider methods to allow students to view the video at another time. Caution should be exercised to prevent inappropriate distribution of the video and potential violation of student confidentiality. Video review can be required as part of the written journaling activities previously discussed. Limited research is available to provide clear guidance about best uses of video replay; however, use of select video snippets of the simulation may help to remind students of what happened during the simulation and could lead to rich debriefing discussions.

Another important debriefing consideration involves the use of a structured framework to guide the debriefing session and promote student reflection. Many teachers report using a semistructured process with an eclectic approach to guide debriefing (Waznonis, 2015). However, frameworks such as Gather, Analyze, Summarize (GAS), Debriefing with Good Judgement, Plus-Delta, Debriefing for Meaning Learning©, or any of the other available frameworks should be used to guide debriefing (INACSL, 2016). Clinical teachers may need training to effectively use these frameworks. Further research is needed to understand the effectiveness of these approaches (Waznonis, 2016).

Once decisions about the method, format, and approach to debriefing are complete, the teacher needs to implement activities that will ensure an appropriate climate for debriefing. The instructor's role during debriefing is that of facilitator, coach, or guide—not lecturer and monopolizer of debriefing conversations. At the beginning of a debriefing session the teacher should orient students to the debriefing process and code of conduct, review the objectives of the simulation, discuss confidentiality, and articulate teacher expectations for students' participation in evaluating themselves and their peers (INACSL, 2016). Teachers must work to establish a trusting environment because students may feel vulnerable and anxious, particularly if video playback is used (Nielsen & Harder, 2013). Sensitive issues need to be openly discussed in a constructive and supportive manner. Once the ground rules of the debriefing session are complete, then discussion about the events and experiences can begin. As students share their impressions and reflections, teachers should listen, redirect discussion as appropriate, and encourage participation. The use of probing open-ended questions will

EXHIBIT 8.5

SAMPLE DEBRIEFING QUESTIONS

- Was there anything you missed on report or was there other information that you needed so you could act more effectively?
- What knowledge do you still need to manage the situation more effectively?
- What areas require further practice?
- What went well?
- What would you do differently the next time? Why?
- Why do you think the patient responded in the manner that he or she did?
- What were you thinking about during the simulation?
- Why did you complete the nursing actions in the order that you did?
- How could you have acted differently to meet the patient's needs more effectively and efficiently?
- What problems did you identify?
- How did you prioritize your care?

help to engage students in reflective conversations. Exhibit 8.5 provides some sample questions that can be incorporated into simulation debriefing. The teacher should use what, how, and why questions to promote student discussion and higher level thinking. Sometimes teachers may need to clarify inaccuracies or correct misinterpretations in a manner that provides positive feedback and specific examples about performance but also gives students suggestions for areas to strengthen or change. Lastly, the teacher should use verbal and nonverbal responses and engage student observers as well as the simulation participants in the analysis and reflection of the events.

The teacher should conclude the debriefing session with some closing statements about what students identified as effective and efficient, areas they need to work on, and take-away learning messages to summarize the experience. Thanking students for their participation and stating the teacher's appreciation for their attention, efforts in enacting the scenario, and shared reflections provides positive reinforcement and shows respect for their efforts. Asking students to identify content that helped them succeed in the scenario and where they received it (classroom, presentations, scenario preparation) will guide the teacher to further course and curricular improvements.

EVALUATING SIMULATIONS

The final aspect of clinical simulation, evaluating simulations, involves multiple components. As the simulation unfolds, teachers can easily identify areas that are working and areas that are problematic. The dynamic process of the simulation allows for some modification during use, but careful note-taking during the scenario, as well as after the debriefing session with students, will document changes necessary to enhance the effectiveness of the simulation for the future. Another method commonly used for simulation evaluation involves asking for student feedback or reactions to the experience. This evaluation can occur in a group debriefing session or individually by each student in a written format. This data, while not directly linked to performance, will provide valuable information about the simulation experience, allowing teachers to consider further revisions and improvements. Reviewing student feedback with teachers and simulation specialists who assisted with the technology component of simulation soon after the scenario is completed provides the best opportunities for change and revision.

There are a variety of ways to assess student performance and determine whether the simulation enabled attainment of the learning objectives. Evaluation methods reflect students' performance and whether they met the objectives and demonstrated the skills and knowledge identified as important outcomes for that scenario. This type of learning can also be assessed with skills checklists, rating scales, or other performance indices. Regardless of the approach used for evaluation, teachers should select valid and reliable tools and determine if formative or summative evaluations will be completed. Student behaviors can be assessed for items such as level of independence, prompting, accuracy, timeliness, and appropriate sequence of activities. Debriefing is enriched with this information because students are provided with concrete, constructive, and immediate feedback in an objective manner.

Sometimes simulation is used during class time to reinforce content and engage the students, in which case it probably involves more than one student with classmates observing (either live or a recording). In this situation, peer observers can be given an assignment that instructs them to observe for specific actions or activities. Because a simulation can often be complex, assigning students specific areas to observe can allow students to focus more effectively. For example, one student can watch the simulation and note safety measures and another student may watch for communication skills; students can then share their impressions and evaluation about these areas during debriefing. Teachers may find it helpful to agree on and detail the behaviors in a particular scenario that best demonstrate achievement of the defined objectives.

Various tools have been used as part of simulation evaluation and research. Adamson, Kardong-Edgren, and Willhaus (2013) reported the use of four tools to evaluate simulation performance and learning: the Sweeny-Clark Simulation Performance Evaluation Tool, the Clinical Simulation Evaluation Tool, the Lasater Clinical Judgment Rubric, and the Creighton Simulation Evaluation Instrument. Widespread use of these tools contributes valuable reliability and validity evidence about their appropriateness for evaluating student performance. Further research is needed to effectively determine how simulation impacts learning, behavior and, ultimately, patient care.

VIRTUAL SIMULATION

An emerging alternative to traditional SP or manikin-based simulation is virtual simulation. Also, known as computer-based, web-based, digital, or e-simulation, this type of simulation combines computer multimedia and animation to simulate nursing scenarios that allow students to interact with patients through a branching patient case. Since the simulation is delivered electronically there are not the usual person, space, cost, or delivery demands found with other types of simulation. Instead a student can engage in the simulated electronic nursing scenarios at a convenient time and place. Multiple students can complete the simulation and actively participate in the nursing case. The student receives immediate performance feedback and can practice in the virtual simulation repeatedly, thus making it ideal for enhanced learning and remediation activities. These virtual simulations also offer a cost-effective alternative to clinical site visits and performance evaluations particularly for online or geographically disbursed students. Although still not widely adopted for clinical teaching this technology is emerging as an attractive option for clinical learning and is expected to grow as more virtual simulations become available (Cant & Cooper, 2014; Foronda & Bauman, 2014; Foronda et al., 2016; Guise, Chambers, & Välimäki, 2011).

CLINICAL SIMULATION INTEGRATION INTO THE CURRICULUM

Simulation activities can be integrated into clinical learning in a variety of ways. First, simulation offers opportunities to prepare students for clinical care by offering practice of psychomotor skills, communication, and problem solving in a simulated environment. By involving a clinical group of students in the simulation activities, students have an opportunity to deliver care, observe performance, reflect on their learning, and critique their practice and that of classmates. Simulation is also used to provide a standardized experience for students. It is particularly useful when the clinical teacher would like all students to have practice with a situation that may not be available to everyone due to variability in patient census or setting constraints. Creating a simulation scenario involving a high-risk, life-threatening, or emergency situation allows all students to experience the same scenario without the potential safety concerns to the patient. Simulation can also be used as a make-up activity to provide additional clinical learning when a student is absent. Or, it can be used for additional review and practice to help remediate at-risk students who are having trouble mastering clinical activities. They can have repeat practice opportunities with simulation. With video-recording capabilities, simulation can be saved and used for other teaching–learning activities such as clinical conferencing. Finally, simulation can be used for evaluation purposes as either a way to ensure all students demonstrate satisfactory performance or for competency assessment.

FUTURE IMPLICATIONS

The use of simulation for clinical teaching continues to evolve. The landmark NCSBN study suggesting that high-quality simulation could be substituted for up to 50% of traditional clinical practice experiences further supports simulation use in nursing education. Along with the INACSL Standards of Best Practice, teachers are provided with further guidance for simulation use. However, further research is indicated, and some suggestions are provided.

- Nurse educators should continue to work with other related professions to conduct interprofessional simulation activities. Evaluate the effectiveness of these interprofessional educational experiences.
- Continued research is needed to demonstrate the efficacy of simulation in nursing education and provide sound evidence-based support for simulation activities.
- Teacher support, resources, and curricular integration require administrative support and affordable simulation software and evaluation systems that streamline faculty efforts. As simulation continues to advance, ongoing faculty training on the latest developments is essential to keep teachers up-to-date on simulation advances.

- More research and support are necessary for the use of EHRs and scenario implementation.
- Simulation research in nursing education needs to move from small-scale, single-site descriptive studies to robust multisite experimental designs using strong methodology, adequate sample sizes, and measurement tools that produce reliable results.

SUMMARY

Clinical simulation has become widely integrated into clinical nursing education. Simulation activities allow students to develop psychomotor skills, clinical reasoning, clinical judgment, problem solving, and critical thinking through techniques such as role-playing and the use of devices such as interactive videos or manikins. In addition, simulation offers an opportunity for evaluation and assessment of student skills with options for remediation and continued practice and refinement. Nursing experts acknowledge the value of simulation as a teaching–learning method that mimics reality but also emphasize the need for nursing student clinical experiences with real patients.

Simulators can be categorized as low, moderate, or high fidelity in relation to how closely they represent a realistic situation. Low-fidelity simulators, sometimes referred to as "task-trainers," lack the realism of a clinical situation but offer opportunities for procedural skill practice. Moderate-fidelity simulators allow students to practice multiple psychomotor skills but without interactive features. High-fidelity simulators produce the most lifelike scenarios. These full-size manikins react to student manipulations in real time and in realistic ways, such as speaking, coughing, and demonstrating chest movements and pulses. Simulations with SPs use live actors with scripts who portray patients, and require nursing students to engage in nursing care activities with the SPs in an environment that simulates patient care areas.

Key elements for nurse educators teaching with simulation include student-centered learning, simulation objectives and focus, simulation fidelity, and guided reflection. Teachers need adequate training for the development of appropriate clinical scenarios, implementation of the simulation, and evaluation of the pedagogy.

Teachers should ensure that students participating in simulation experiences view them as realistic environments by establishing ground rules for professional behavior and attire. Specific policies and procedures related to clinical simulation recording and the confidentiality of the recordings should be developed.

Factors to consider when choosing or preparing clinical scenarios used for simulation include program outcomes and course objectives, the purpose of the activity, the most appropriate level of fidelity, the number and educational level of the students, time available, teacher familiarity with the technology, the technology available, and support for use. Scenario development should incorporate creativity and available scientific evidence for practice, and should be student-centered, interactive, and related to desired outcomes. The use of a simple storyboard template can provide structure for scenario development, such as the example provided in this chapter. Scenarios may also be accessed or purchased from publishers, simulation manufacturers, other nursing education programs, and national nursing organizations. Already-developed scenarios aid inexperienced teachers by providing the completed template of essential information and support data needed to implement the simulation, but it is important to check alignment of the materials with course and program outcomes and needs.

The use of EHRs can be incorporated into scenarios to enhance clinical simulation. Students can use the academic EHR to access simulated patient records and document care provided during a simulation. Creating a database of mock patient records as part of the EHR that can be accessed and used during simulation will enhance realism.

Preparation for using simulation also includes practice sessions prior to implementing the live scenario with the students, and preparing the manikin or SP with props and special effects so that students perceive a life-like clinical environment. Student preparation may include reading relevant background information and a brief patient history and diagnosis, completing preparation worksheets, reviewing Internet resources, viewing a video or online presentation, and answering some key questions in preparation for the simulation activity. This presimulation preparation can be an individual written assignment or oral group discussion.

After a short briefing, students enact their assigned roles and the teacher uses the preplanned scenario to respond to student actions on behalf of the simulated patient. Videorecording allows observation by others during the simulation and provides a recording that can be used for debriefing after the simulation. Debriefing after the simulation activity provides an important opportunity for guided reflection on the positive aspects of the experience to reinforce learning, and encourages critical thinking, making meaning of the experience, and critique of student performance. Suggestions were offered for reducing student anxiety about being observed during simulations. Various options for conducting debriefings were presented, including individual or group, immediate or delayed, structured or unstructured, private or public, and oral or written. The instructor's role during debriefing is that of facilitator, coach, or guide.

The evaluation of clinical simulations involves multiple data sources, including teachers' notes during the simulation and debriefing and group or individual student feedback and reactions to the activity. Teachers can use skills checklists, rating scales, or other performance indices for evaluation purposes. Virtual simulations are emerging as an alternative approach to simulation that can provide students with an electronic repeatable case. As new digital simulations become available, clinical teachers may use this simulation alternative to enhance teaching and learning. There are other ways that clinical simulations can be integrated into the nursing curriculum including for clinical practice and preparation, standardization of clinical learning opportunities, make-up activities, remediation, and evaluation. Further research substantiating educational practices with simulation is needed to guide best practices.

CNE EXAMINATION TEST BLUEPRINT CORE COMPETENCIES

1. **Facilitate Learning**
   A. Implement a variety of teaching strategies appropriate to
      1. content
      3. learner needs

(continued)

      5. desired learner outcomes
      6. method of delivery
   B. Use teaching strategies based on
      1. educational theory
      2. evidence-based practices related to education
   C. Modify teaching strategies and learning experiences based on consideration of learners
      2. past clinical experiences
      3. past educational and life experiences
   D. Use information technologies to support the teaching–learning process
   G. Model reflective thinking practices, including critical thinking
   H. Create opportunities for learners to develop their own critical thinking skills
   I. Create a positive learning environment that fosters a free exchange of ideas
   N. Use knowledge of evidence-based practice to instruct learners
   O. Demonstrate ability to teach clinical skills
   Q. Foster a safe learning environment

2. Facilitate Learner Development and Socialization

   D. Create learning environments that facilitate learners' self-reflection, personal goal setting, and socialization to the role of the nurse
   E. Foster the development of learners in these areas:
      1. cognitive domain
      2. psychomotor domain
      3. affective domain
   F. Assist learners to engage in thoughtful and constructive self- and peer evaluation

3. Use Assessment and Evaluation Strategies

   C. Use a variety of strategies to assess and evaluate learning in these domains:
      1. cognitive
      2. psychomotor
      3. affective
   D. Incorporate current research in assessment and evaluation practices
   E. Analyze available resources for learning assessment and evaluation
   H. Implement evaluation strategies that are appropriate to the learner and learning outcomes
   I. Analyze assessment and evaluation data
   J. Use assessment and evaluation data to enhance the teaching–learning process
   K. Advise learners regarding assessment and evaluation criteria
   L. Provide timely, constructive, and thoughtful feedback to learners

6. Engage in Scholarship, Service, and Leadership

   A. Function as a change agent and leader
      3. Participate in interdisciplinary efforts to address health care and education needs
         a. within the institution
         b. locally
         c. regionally
   B. Engage in scholarship of teaching
      1. Exhibit a spirit of inquiry about teaching and learning, student development, and evaluation methods
      2. Use evidence-based resources to improve and support teaching
      3. Participate in research activities related to nursing education

REFERENCES

Adamson, K. A., Kardong-Edgren, S., & Wilhaus, J. (2013). An updated review of published simulation evaluation instruments. *Clinical Simulation in Nursing, 9,* e393–e405. doi:10.1016/j.ecns.2012.09.004

American Association of Colleges of Nursing. (2014). Nursing shortage. Retrieved from http://www.aacn.nche.edu/media-relations/fact-sheets/nursing-shortage

Arizona State University College of Nursing and Health Innovation Simulation and Learning Resources Program. (2017). *Harry has a low blood-glucose level: A scenario for beginning level students.* Phoenix, AZ: Author.

Cant, R. P., & Cooper, S. J. (2014), Simulation in the internet age: The place of web-based simulation in nursing education: An integrative review. *Nurse Education Today, 34,* 1435–1442. doi:10.1016/j.nedt.2014.08.001

Chambers, K. (2006, June). *Simulation in nursing education: The basics.* Paper presented at the 4th Annual Laerdal® Northeast Simulation User's Group Meeting, Mashantucket, CT.

Commission on Collegiate Nursing Education. (2013). *Standards for accreditation of baccalaureate and graduate degree nursing programs.* Washington, DC: Author.

Dreifuerst, K. T. (2009). The essentials of debriefing in simulation learning: A concept analysis. *Nursing Education Perspectives, 30,* 109–114. doi:10.1043/1536-5026-030.002.0109

Durham, C. F., Cato, M. L., & Lasater, K. (2014). NLN/Jeffries simulation framework state of the science project: Participant construct. *Clinical Simulation in Nursing, 10,* 363–372. doi:10.1016/j.ecns.2014.04.002

Forneris, S. G., & Fey, M. (2016). NLN vision: Teaching with simulation. In P. R. Jeffries (Ed.), *The NLN Jeffries simulation theory.* Philadelphia, PA: Wolters Kluwer.

Foronda, C. L., & Bauman, E. B. (2014). Strategies to incorporate virtual simulation in nursing education. *Clinical Simulation in Nursing, 10,* 412–418. doi:10.1016/j.ecns.2014.03.005

Foronda, C. L., Swoboda, S. M., Hudson, K. W., Jones, E., Sullivan, N., Ockimey, J., & Jeffries, P. (2016). Evaluation of vSIM for Nursing™: A trial of innovation. *Clinical Simulation in Nursing, 12,* 128–131. doi:10.1016.j.ecns.2015.12.006

Gore, T., Van Gele, P., Ravert, P., & Mabire, C. (2012). A 2010 survey of the International Association for Clinical Simulation and Learning membership about simulation use. *Clinical Simulation in Nursing, 8*(4), e125–e133. doi:10.1016/j.ecns.2012.01.002

Guise, V., Chambers, M., & Välimäki, M. (2011). What can virtual patient simulation offer mental health nursing education. *Journal of Psychiatric and Mental Health Nursing, 19,* 410–418. doi:10.1111/j.1365-28500.2011.01797.x

Guise, V., & Wiig, S. (2016). Preparing for organizational change in home health care with simulation based training. *Clinical Simulation in Nursing, 12,* 496–503. doi:10.1016/j.ecns.2016.07.011

Hall, K., & Tori, K. (2016). Best practice recommendation for debriefing in simulation-based education for Australian undergraduate nursing students: An integrative review. *Clinical Simulation in Nursing, 13,* 39–50. doi:10.1016/j.ecns.2016.01.006

Hallmark, B. R., Thomas, C. M., & Gantt, L. (2016). The educational practices construct of the NLN/Jeffries simulation framework: State of the science. *Clinical Simulation in Nursing, 10,* 345–352. doi:10.10166/j.ecns.2013.04.006

Ham, K. (2016). Use of standardized patients to enhance simulation of medication administration. *Nurse Educator, 41,* 166–168. doi:10.1097/NNE.0000000000000248

Hayden, J. K., Smiley, R. A., Alexander, M., Kardong-Edgren, S., & Jeffries, P. (2014). The NCSBN national simulation study: A longitudinal, randomized controlled study replacing clinical hours with simulation in prelicensure nursing education. *Journal of Nursing Regulation, 5*(2), S1–S64.

Hayden, J. K., Smiley, R. A., & Gross, L. (2014). Simulation in nursing education: Current regulations and practices. *Journal of Nursing Regulation, 5*(2), 25–29.

Helwig, A., & Lomotan, E. (2016). Can electronic health records prevent harm to patients? Retrieved from https://www.ahrq.gov/news/blog/ahrqviews/020916.hmtl

International Association for Clinical Simulation and Learning. (2015). About. Retrieved from https://www.inacsl.org/i4a/pages/index.cfm?pageid=3277

International Association for Clinical Simulation and Learning Standards Committee. (2016). International Association for Clinical Simulation and Learning standards of best practice: Simulation SM simulation design. *Clinical Simulation in Nursing, 12,* S5–S12. doi:10.1016/j.ecns.2016.09.005

Jeffries, P. R. (2012). *Simulation in nursing education: From conceptualization to evaluation* (2nd ed.). New York, NY: National League for Nursing.

Jeffries, P. R. (2016). *The NLN Jeffries simulation theory.* Philadelphia, PA: Wolters Kluwer.

Jeffries, P. R., Dreifuerst, K. T., & Haerling, K. A. (2018). Clinical simulations in nursing education: Overview, essentials, and the evidence. In M. H. Oermann, J. C. De Gagne, & B. C. Phillips (Eds.), *Teaching in nursing and role of the educator: The complete guide to best practice in teaching, evaluation, and curriculum development* (2nd ed., pp. 113–134). New York, NY: Springer Publishing.

Kardong-Edgren, S., Wilhaus, J., Bennett, D., & Hayden, J. (2012). Results of the National Council of State Boards of Nursing national simulation survey: Part II. *Clinical Simulation in Nursing, 8*(4), e117–e123. doi:10.1016/j.ecns.2012.01.003

Kunkel, C., Kopp, W., & Hanson, M. (2016). A matter of life and death: End-of-life simulation to develop confidence in nursing students. *Nursing Education Perspectives, 37*, 285–286. doi:10.1097/01.NEP.0000000000000029

Lusk, J., & Fater, K. (2013). Postsimulation debriefing to maximize clinical judgment development. *Nurse Educator, 38*, 16–19. doi:10.1097/NNE.0b013e318276df8b

MacLean, S., Kelly, M., Geddes, F., & Della, P. (2017). Use of simulated patients to develop communication skills in nursing education: An integrative review. *Nurse Education Today, 48*, 90–98. doi:10.1016/j.nedt.2016.09.018

Manning, S. J., Skiff, D. M., Santiago, L. P., & Irish, A. (2016). Nursing and social work trauma simulation: Exploring an interprofessional approach. *Clinical Simulation in Nursing, 12*, 555–564. doi:10.1016/j.ecns.2016.07.004

McDermott, D. (2016). The prebriefing concept: A delphi study of CHSE experts. *Clinical Simulation in Nursing, 12*, 219–227. doi:10/1016/j.ecns.2016.02.001

Montenery, S. M., Walker, M., Sorensen, E., Thompson, R., Kirklin, D., White, R., & Ross, C. (2013). Millenial generation student nurses' perception of the impact of multiple technologies on learning. *Nursing Education Perspectives, 34*, 405–409. doi:10.5480/10-451

Mountain, C., Redd, R., O'Leary-Kelly, C., & Giles, K. (2015). Electronic medical record in the simulation hospital. *Computers, Informatics, Nursing, 33*, 166–171. doi:10.1097/CIN0000000000000144

National League for Nursing. (n.d.). Simulation innovation resource center. Retrieved from http://sirc.nln.org

National League for Nursing. (2017). Faculty programs & resources: Leadership development program for simulation educators. Retrieved from http://www.nln.org/facultyprograms/leadershipinstitute.htm

Nielsen, B., & Harder, N. (2013). Causes of student anxiety during simulation: What the literature says. *Clinical Simulation in Nursing, 9*, e507–e512. doi:10.1016/j.ecns.2013.03.003

Paige, J. B., & Morin, K. H. (2013). Simulation fidelity and cueing: A systematic review of the literature. *Clinical Simulation in Nursing, 9*, e481–e489. doi:10.1016/j.ecns.2013.01.001

Pastor, D. K., Cunningham, R. P., White, P. H., & Kolomer, S. (2016). We have to talk: Results of an interprofessional clinical simulation in delivering bad health news in palliative care. *Clinical Simulation in Nursing, 12*, 320–327. doi:10.1016j.ecns.2016.03.005

Sarmasoglu, S., Dinc, L., & Elcin, M. (2016). Using standardized patients in nursing education: Effects on students' psychomotor skill development. *Nurse Educator, 41*, e1–e5. doi:10.1097/NNE.0000000000000188

Shearer, J. N. (2016). Anxiety, nursing students and simulation: State of the science. *Journal of Nursing Education, 55*, 551–554. doi:10.3928/01484834-20160914-02

Slater, L. Z., Bryant, K., & Ng, V. (2016). Nursing student perceptions of standardized patient use in health assessment. *Clinical Simulation in Nursing, 12*, 368–376. doi:10.1016/j.ecns.2016.04.007

Veltri, L., Kaakinen, J. R., Shillam, C., Arwood, E., & Bell, K. (2016). Controlled post-partum newborn simulation with objective evaluation exchanged for clinical learning. *Clinical Simulation in Nursing, 12*, 177–186. doi:10.1016/j.ecns.2016.01.005

Waznonis, A. (2015). Simulation debriefing practices in traditional baccalaureate nursing programs: National survey results. *Clinical Simulation in Nursing, 11*, 110–119. doi:10.1016/j.ecns.2014.10.002

Waznonis, A. (2016). Faculty descriptions of simulation debriefing in traditional baccalaureate nursing programs. *Nursing Education Perspectives, 37*, 262–268. doi:10.1097/01.NEP.0000000000000065

CHAPTER 9

Technologies for Clinical Teaching

Debra Hagler and Kimberly Day

Artificial boundaries in nursing education have included a boundary between theory and practice, a boundary between knowledge acquisition and knowledge use, and a boundary between classroom and clinical teaching. The call for radical transformation in nursing education outlines the extensive efforts needed to shift the paradigm that is artificially separating knowledge from context (Benner, Sutphen, Leonard, & Day, 2009). Technology is blurring the boundaries between classroom and clinical teaching, which were previously defined by the settings where they occurred rather than what happened in those settings. Preparing students to provide nursing care in a highly technological work environment is a critical responsibility of nurse educators (National League for Nursing, 2015).

Leaders in health professions education have advanced recommendations about the use of technology in education. A panel sponsored by the Josiah Macy Jr. Foundation made six recommendations, beginning with, "In health professions education, technology should be used to support the ongoing development of learners from undergraduate levels through clinical practice; enhance interprofessional learning opportunities; and empower every student, faculty member, and clinician to embrace the role of both teacher and lifelong learner" (Stuart & Triola, 2015, p. 33.) Nursing leaders and educators need to thoughtfully incorporate technology that supports learning the complex skills and developing the competencies demanded of today's health care professionals.

This chapter includes guidelines for selecting educational technology and descriptions of the types of technology useful for clinical teaching. Simulation technology was examined in Chapter 8.

TECHNOLOGY USE IN CLINICAL TEACHING

Clinical courses are incorporating more online and other educational technology, although the range extends from technology as a glitzy add-on resource to incorporation of the technology as the major form of instructional delivery and skill practice. Teachers who adopt online technology learn to think differently about their teaching and reconceptualize what they do, particularly in areas such as managing the learning environment, promoting collegiality and cooperation, and supporting problem solving (Creasman, 2012). Key differences that may come with increased use of online educational technology include:

- Online activities are often asynchronous, meaning that one student's activity occurs independently from the activity of other students and independent of the clinical teacher's presence. Students may be free to interact with course materials when it is convenient for them, often around the clock.
- Online discussions are generally nonlinear, facilitated by discussion boards, blogs, and journals where students can participate in multiple conversations simultaneously.
- Online environments favor the written word, which takes longer for students to compose and may take longer for teachers to review than a face-to-face discussion. However, the written word provides a more relaxed timeline for responding thoughtfully.
- The physical separation of teacher and student may slow communication. A confusing email conversation or discussion board thread can be frustrating without the rapid clarification available during an in-person discussion.
- Students may expect that because clinical activities are available online around the clock, clinical teachers are likewise continuously available to troubleshoot the technology or answer questions about the content. Clinical teachers may have to manage technology support needs and expectations about availability.
- The volume of information available online is seemingly endless. Teachers might be able to keep track of what information is provided in a specific textbook from edition to edition, but keeping track of what new information is available to students online every day is certainly impossible (Creasman, 2012).

Clinical skills for nursing students have traditionally been cultivated through a combination of laboratory activities and direct observation of skilled clinicians in actual clinical practice. Over time, nursing students gradually increase their role and responsibility for the care of patients under the supervision of nurse educators and clinical staff. Today's learners are accustomed to multimedia environments and have come to expect that technology will be integrated into their curricula. Access to infinite online resources for learning supports a change in the clinical teacher's role from the direct provider of information to a facilitator and co-learner.

Simulation and virtual reality-based learning provide learners with experiences in contextually rich environments that encourage reflection. Environments that support learning activities designed to authentically replicate clinical practice settings should be seen and treated as clinical environments. These environments may support and provide a foundation for learning during future clinical experiences. When learners are integrating data and decisions in complex situations, more elaborate technology that includes simulated patient interaction may add a level of realism that engages the student and improves the overall learning experience (Kopp & Hanson, 2012).

Evaluation of textbooks for adoption in a particular clinical course or sharing text selections across courses has taken on a new level of complexity. Considerations for textbook adoption now include whether the book is available in print, as an ebook that students can download on their computers or mobile devices, or both. The availability of additional electronic resources for the cost of the book or for an additional student fee can increase the desirability of a particular text. Supplementary electronic resources may include downloadable test banks, instructor resource manuals, slide sets with elaborate graphics, practice exercises, and simulations. Using publishers' supplementary resources saves teachers time and effort compared with developing new clinical resources. Assigning practice exercises before face-to-face clinical activities can help learners prepare to use their clinical time well.

In some communities, nursing programs and clinical care agencies share online databases for coordinating and negotiating clinical placement scheduling. Requests are entered for clinical specialty rotations and student groups, then reviewed to determine how to best meet the needs of all learners using scheduling that is reasonable and feasible for the agencies. Students may be given access to online orientation modules for individual clinical sites or as a shared resource among many clinical agencies whose leaders have agreed upon collective orientation requirements. Asking students to complete some or all of the educational orientation modules online before arriving at the clinical agency is efficient for the learners, the teachers, and the agency.

Clinical teachers can use social networking sites to facilitate clinical learning. The teacher might establish a Twitter account, separate from his or her own personal account, and use the privacy settings to make tweets visible only to a specific group of students (all of whom must have Twitter accounts, of course). Using this account, the faculty member can teach followers mini-lessons and update them on relevant topics. For example, the teacher may maximize teachable moments that occur outside of the clinical learning environment, such as sharing a new idea from a conference, alerting students to the publication of a relevant article in a current issue of a professional nursing journal, or suggesting that students view a particular television show that relates to content they are studying. The clinical teacher might send a weekly tweet to students with a question or brainteaser related to the competencies they are attempting to master. For students who have clinical learning activities in diverse settings, the clinical teacher may use Twitterchat to conduct post-clinical conferences at a predetermined time. As moderator, the teacher posts questions (designated as Q1, Q2, etc.) to prompt responses from students (labeled R1, R2, etc.) and facilitate discussion among participants. Tools such as Tweetchat, Twchat, Hootsuite, and Tweetdeck can help the teacher as chat host to organize and follow chat content; some of these tools also provide analytics to help the teacher assess the effectiveness of the chat (Miller, 2014; Vikil & Minarcik, 2017).

SELECTING TECHNOLOGY

Clinical teachers who want to incorporate electronic or web-based resources into their courses should consider the course objectives and the characteristics of the learners. Educational technology is a tool; finding the right tool or tools for the purpose is as important in selecting educational technology as it is in performing a health assessment. Some technological tools can serve multiple learning support functions and some learning objectives can be supported by more than one tool. Wenger, White, and Smith (2009) offered general advice for teachers who are considering educational technology:

- Start with simple and inexpensive strategies
- Learn from others who have been there
- Test the tools out before you adopt them
- Watch for what is coming next

Mastering technology that learners will continue to use through their working careers, such as electronic health records (EHRs), may be a worthwhile learning outcome in itself. However, a focus on the specific technology rather than the learning objectives can lead to a misguided instructional effort.

Most educational technology is a resource and a means to an end, a tool rather an intended program outcome. There is no requirement for using the most elaborate possible technology to support clinical learning; expensive and complicated materials and plans may not be a better fit than simple and inexpensive materials and methods for supporting a particular clinical objective. An intensive effort to use a specific non-clinical technology for completion of a single assignment is generally not worthwhile from the perspective of either the students or the teacher. Clinical teachers should take care that even while striving to support students in using new technological learning tools, the teachers do not trade their responsibility of facilitating learning based on the clinical objectives for a full-time role as the technology support specialist and mechanic.

Before choosing a technology to use, the clinical teacher should reflect on the learning objectives and the intended types of interactions to support achieving those objectives. For example, teacher's plan that learners will create a product such as a patient education pamphlet or an electronic clinical portfolio suggests tools such as design or presentation software, while a plan to have learners practice clinical decision making might suggest using human patient simulation, virtual reality simulations, or online case study analysis (Exhibit 9.1).

The role of individual teachers or groups of faculty members who take on the responsibility for implementing technology resources is called *technology steward-ship*. Technology stewards help their community of learners choose, organize, and apply technology to meet the learners' needs. It is not unusual that students show leadership in joining the team of technology stewards, supporting their peers and teachers in beginning use of and in troubleshooting technology. Technology stewards as individuals or teams need a clear understanding of their learning community

EXHIBIT 9.1

SELECTING TECHNOLOGY TO SUPPORT EDUCATIONAL STRATEGIES

Educational Intention	Related Technology
Direct experience	Electronic health records, virtual reality environments, multiplayer online role-playing games, virtual case simulations, high-fidelity simulation
Discussion/Reflection	Online discussion boards, virtual chat, video-conferencing, social media sites
Project production	Software or online sites for design and publishing or producing presentations. Video-recording, posting, and commenting sites
Information access	Websites, mobile applications, massive open online courses, online newspapers and journals, prerecorded or real-time presentations
Drill and practice	Quizzing software, online flashcards and knowledge-based games

members, so that they can respond to both expressed and implied needs in context. It is helpful if stewards are technology experts, but even an awareness of possibilities and available products is sufficient to trigger the process of finding others who can help with the selection and installation of more complex programs or equipment. During adoption of a new technology, stewards serve the leadership functions of managing the direction and pace of the change. Once a new technology is implemented into practice, stewards may support upgrading practices and new applications of the technology in response to emerging needs (Wenger et al., 2009).

Clinical teachers who like to try out new ideas are often natural technology stewards, but a team approach supports successful implementation of more complex systems. Benefits to the clinical teacher of taking on the technology steward role include the satisfaction of moving an initiative forward that does not otherwise have a champion; the impact of improving learning or educational practices; the opportunity for developing leadership, teaching, and technical skills; and enhanced reputation and credibility in both the academic and the practice setting.

How can a busy clinical teacher gain access to educational technology? Teachers can acquire technology through at least seven strategies:

- Use what you have—often teachers do not know what is available unless they ask
- Try free demonstration editions of software or programs
- Build on an enterprise platform—one already owned by the school
- Get a commercial platform that meets current needs
- Build your own custom platform or tool
- Use open-source software
- Patch elements together (Wenger et al., 2009)

ELECTRONIC HEALTH RECORDS

EHRs are used across most health care settings (Choi, Park, & Lee, 2016; Herbert & Connors, 2016). Nursing students need to be prepared for entering electronic documentation and interpreting electronic data, yet many health care agencies have policies preventing students and academic faculty from accessing or entering data in the EHR.

Educators have identified several solutions to support nursing students in learning electronic documentation and data review. Nursing schools can lease or purchase simulated EHRs similar to those found in hospitals and ambulatory health settings; however, simulated EHRs can be costly. An academic institution can develop its own academic electronic health record (AEHR), which requires significant time, technology expertise, and support services (Herbert & Connors, 2016). Nursing programs can also develop a partnership with a specific health care organization to allow the students to complete most of the clinical experiences at the same facility where the students will have access to the EHR. The development of a partnership benefits a nursing program in providing access to an EHR and benefits the hospital by providing new nurses that are already familiar with the electronic documentation process. Orientation to a hospital's EHR can take weeks; completing that orientation as a student before graduation can be a benefit to both the health care organization employing new graduate nurses and the nursing academic program.

The selection of an AEHR requires significant research and thought to meet the needs of the students, faculty, and the curriculum. The AEHR chosen should provide realism for the students learning to read health documents and allow the students to document a simulated or clinical patient's assessment. Faculty should have the opportunity to evaluate the AEHR prior to a purchase decision. The AEHR selected should provide for upgrades and program specific requests, such as integrating barcode technology to increase patient safety and decrease medication errors (Lapkin, Levett-Jones, Chenoweth, & Johnson, 2016).

Educators can plan strategies to help make the implementation of an EHR successful and meaningful for the faculty and the students. An AEHR can be integrated across all levels of the curriculum to complete assignments such as planning care or developing written situation, background, assessment, recommendation (SBAR) reports. Clinical faculty can begin to implement the use of EHRs in nursing programs by having students review the health records developed for simulation patients in the school's AEHR. Students can search the records for the information needed to provide safe patient care, for example, allergies, diagnostic test results, and medications. They also can document the simulation assessment and any interventions performed during the simulation in the AEHR.

Several barriers exist to using AEHRs, including funding the cost of the technology and providing the development time for faculty and students. It is important to have a plan to address the barriers prior to implementing an AEHR. Nursing programs that successfully use EHRs often have a program champion. The program champion is a faculty or staff member familiar with the program who can provide initial training and refresher courses, serving as a resource to both faculty and students as needed. Successful implementation of an EHR also requires strong administrative support (Herbert & Connors, 2016).

MOBILE AND HANDHELD DEVICES

Some clinical settings allow students and clinical teachers to use cell phones and mobile devices while on site, while others do not; it is important to know the clinical site policies regarding mobile devices and remind students to respect the policies. Students in the clinical setting may be able to access some or all of the campus technology applications, such as learning management systems, by using their mobile phones. Mobile technology allows them to access videos for just-in-time review of psychomotor skills (Lee et al., 2016). They may also download their etextbooks on tablets, smartphones, or ereaders to have ready access to resources for current medication or clinical information.

Some faculty members and clinical teachers discourage the use of mobile devices because of the high risk of distraction from patient care. Smartphone use has been shown to increase reaction time, reduce focus, and lower behavioral performance (Cho, Park, & Lee, 2016). When used appropriately, mobile devices can assist in clinical practice, providing resources for more effective and efficient patient care. Mobile technology has become an effective clinical tool supporting evidence based practice and the critical thinking needed for good clinical decisions and care (Sedgwick, Awosoga, Grigg, & Durnin, 2016). Clinical faculty and staff need to help nursing students understand appropriate and inappropriate use of mobile devices.

Faculty may discourage the use of mobile devices in clinical areas because they expect students to be fully prepared for clinical learning activities without consulting information resources during those activities. However, nurses in clinical practice often receive new information that must be evaluated or verified. Learning how to access appropriate resources as needed to plan care is an important goal as students prepare to function without the guidance of instructors. For example, no nurse can be expected to know everything there is to know about every medication that may be ordered for a patient, especially when drugs are newly approved, removed from the market, or have revised indications for use. If a patient's medication order is changed, the nurse providing care to that patient must know how to locate and access the necessary information about the new drug to administer the medication safely or pose a question about the order. Use of mobile devices in the clinical setting can facilitate this process; nursing students need to practice using this technology throughout their educational program so that they will be able to demonstrate this competency on graduation. Clinical teachers can help direct students to credible professional websites for clinical information and help them evaluate information found on other websites.

Concerns related to using mobile technology in nursing clinical education include the expense, lack of technical support and faculty acceptance, absence of structured assignments and/or activities for learning with mobile devices, and constraints on their use in clinical settings. Mobile devices require Internet connectivity, but some clinical agencies do not have or do not allow students or faculty members to use their facility wifi (Strandell-Laine, Stolt, Leino-Kilpi, & Saarikoski, 2015).

The opportunity to use mobile devices during clinical experiences opens the possibility of students inappropriately connecting on social media sites or doing unrelated homework while they are supposed to be engaged in direct care activities. Patients who observe clinical teachers or students using mobile technology for social purposes may be concerned about the unprofessional behavior and the risk to their privacy. The use of mobile devices needs to be closely monitored by the on-site clinical faculty to make sure nursing students are following facility policy and using the technology for appropriate activities. Raman (2015) suggests that nurse educators be supported to learn, then role model, effective use of mobile technology in clinical settings.

BEST PRACTICE RESOURCES

The Internet provides access to numerous libraries and databases of evidence to support effective nursing care and promote health. Government and other public websites provide access to data that can be used to frame the significance of health problems in a given location or target population and provide students with practice in using databases for planning population-based care. Standards of care and policy statements may provide current best practice information. For example, students may visit the Centers for Disease Control and Prevention (CDC) website to prepare for a clinical activity in immunization or disaster preparedness, or to find out more about an emerging disease or condition (CDC, 2017). Searching clinical practice guidelines at the Agency for Healthcare Research and Quality (AHRQ) site helps students locate best practice recommendations for providing care to patients with a specific disease or condition, and to compare clinical guidelines proposed by different expert groups (AHRQ, 2017).

LEARNING OBJECTS

A learning object (LO), also called a reusable learning object (RLO), is a self-contained digital educational resource that may include objectives, content, interactive learning activities, animations, narrated text, visual images, self-assessments, and feedback tools. Frantiska (2016) describes the types of LOs to include tutorial objects (factual information, drill and practice exercises), information objects (reference materials, instructions), and practice objects (case studies, assessments, simulations). LOs may be used independently in support of a smaller, more focused topic or combined with other LOs or activities to teach larger content areas. LOs are often published on the web, embedded in a learning management system, or produced as a podcast or DVD.

A number of open repositories allow educators and their learners to browse for and use LOs that fit particular learning needs and content areas. Some repositories catalog resources that meet specific technical or pedagogical standards while others allow open posting and use.

Repositories such as Multimedia Educational Resource for Learning and Online Training (MERLOT; 2017; www.merlot.org) provide access to simultaneous searches in the databases of multiple other repositories. Some LOs in repositories or independent websites may be covered under Creative Commons licenses (Creative Commons, 2017), which include six standardized levels of copyright permissions to the creative work.

When clinical teachers develop LOs for their own courses, it is important to keep focused on a small area of content, clearly define the scope, and incorporate strategies that facilitate ease of navigation and interactivity. Some teachers use a storyboard approach to help facilitate the development of LOs. Before beginning to create an LO that you may want to make publicly available, review the standards at several online repositories and consider the type of copyright permission you are willing to grant to others for educational or commercial uses.

Common sources of clinical learning activities are the instructor resources and other supplementary materials supplied by publishers based on textbook purchase or an additional fee. There is a wide range of the extent and quality of these resources. Some are only websites with a list of additional recommended readings; some provide application activities and slide sets in concert with each textbook chapter. Test banks that can be uploaded into course learning management system sites are commonly available. Sets of online case simulations can be required for clinical courses, similar to a textbook requirement, and assigned as individual cases throughout the curriculum.

MASSIVE OPEN ONLINE COURSES

Massive open online courses (MOOCs) provide an opportunity for students to attend an online course taught by faculty from a university, non-profit, or for-profit organization, often including nationally known experts. "Massive" describes open enrollment that can exceed 100,000 learners. Some courses begin new sections only at scheduled times, while other MOOCs allow interested learners to begin at any time. The courses have assignments, discussion boards, quizzes, and exams similar to many other online courses taught in colleges and universities. MOOCs ranging from entry level to graduate level courses are commonly used for professional development and continuing education hours (Swigart & Liang, 2016).

MOOCs are free, they have widely varying quality, and only about 10% of students who enroll in MOOCs complete the course (Alraimi, Zo, & Ciganek, 2015; Billings & Kowalski, 2014). However, MOOCs on clinical topics can provide access to organized resources and media that supports just-in-time asynchronous learning. Some universities are now offering credit for MOOC courses, for a fee (Swigart & Liange, 2016).

VIRTUAL REALITY AND GAME-BASED LEARNING

Web, virtual reality, and game-based learning environments can provide important cues and opportunities for students to develop the professional roles and expertise needed for today's complex health care environment (Gould & Bauman, 2012). Teachers can select virtual environments that reflect real-world best practices while allowing for exploration of ethical issues and professional boundaries. Grumme, Barry, Gordon, and Ray (2016) propose that nurses should use virtual environments to prepare for future practice in distance and virtual environments.

Participating in Stories

Nurses have long appreciated the use of stories for teaching and learning. The experience of authoring or being part of a story provides the basic structure for many types of learning games and virtual scenarios. Stories are naturally engaging and highly flexible; they can be told on a moment's notice from a variety of perspectives to emphasize different key messages. Storytelling formats can range from a simple recording to a polished, highly interactive multimedia production.

As Sanford and Emmott (2012) describe, experiencing narrative requires readers to produce rich and complex mental representations. The story offers one of the major means through which the experiences of other people, different cultures, and distant times are conveyed, expanding our virtual experience of the world. Typically, narratives manipulate not only our knowledge of things but also our impressions of how people feel, judge, and react. This ability of a story to help us experience a novel event or a situation from a different perspective provides a way to integrate information across the cognitive, psychomotor, and affective domains. Features common to narratives and stories when used as a teaching method in any format include:

- Specific rather than generic events
- Specific time and place settings
- People involved in the events
- Moment-by-moment thoughts, feelings, and sensory perceptions
- A setting, theme, plot, and resolution
- Audience members feel as if they have entered a different world (Sanford & Emmott, 2012)

Video game and virtual world scholars have come to recognize the power that narratives have in the creation of meaningful learning. Narratives help people recognize patterns and make sense of the world (Walsh, 2011). Pattern recognition marks a critical difference between novices and experts. Through their lived and situated experience, experts come to recognize patterns that lead them to conclusions much more quickly than novices recognize the same patterns.

Narratives provide valuable cues to direct student performance in the virtual world. The teacher can think of the narrative as the background information provided to students during a case-based learning scenario. However, instead of the teacher simply providing the patient's history by reading it aloud to students, the virtual scenario unfolds based on the students' interaction with the environment. Narratives also provide spaces for reflection on the consequences of one's decisions. The virtual world can provide different narrative endings from multiple perspectives based on learners' ongoing interaction with their environment. In this way, students are able to engage in deliberate decision making that will produce varying scenario outcomes. Learners can be encouraged to see the consequences of action or inaction from multiple perspectives. Graduate nursing students assigned avatars in Second Life reported increased ability to relate to people from diverse backgrounds (Tiffany & Hoglund, 2016).

When students care for patients in a clinical setting, they do not have the luxury of revisiting the same clinical encounter to make a better or different decision, but virtual environments allow students to take responsibility for their decisions in a situated and safe context. Teachers can monitor students' progress as the students adjust their behavior and decision making to negotiate outcomes that are more acceptable. For students inhabiting the virtual world, an error simply becomes an opportunity for reflection, learning, and potential behavior change. Shellenbarger and Robb (2015) described using digital storytelling to support nursing students in developing clinical reasoning skills, while nursing graduate students in pediatrics who interacted with virtual patients have reported increased self-efficacy in clinical reasoning (Forsberg, Ziegert, Hult, & Fors, 2016).

Participating in the story assists game players in the negotiation and reconciliation of their virtual and real-world identities. Reflection on the difference in identities represents an opportunity to study aspects of cultural framing of one's self and others (Games & Bauman, 2011). Negotiating responsibilities related to virtual identities within situated narratives can involve sophisticated cognitive effort and critical thinking strategies.

Learning activities in the virtual world can be engineered to emphasize specific curriculum objectives (Gould & Bauman, 2012). For example, a virtual operating room engineered to provide an interactive procedural simulation could introduce and orient students to roles and expectations associated with perioperative nursing. Elements of this environment could include everything from hand antisepsis and gowning to the surgical time-out.

Virtual Learning Environments

Virtual reality and video game–based learning opportunities solve some of the limitations associated with fixed learning spaces such as traditional skills laboratories. Students can access virtual spaces at their convenience without traveling to clinical sites. The virtual environment allows for experiences that simply may not exist in actual clinical environments. As one example, teachers, mentors, and preceptors do not have predictable and reliable access to disasters and crises for teaching purposes. However, students can prepare for disaster management situations through narratives in a virtual-reality scenario without encountering physical danger (Farra, Miller, &

Hodgson, 2015). Where clinical placements are scarce or geographically distant, students can virtually practice public health competencies (Schaffer, 2016).

Many real clinical education settings provide culturally limited environments. Virtual encounters with culture and diversity may provide an opportunity to study aspects of cultural framing of self and other (Games & Bauman, 2011) and prepare learners for actual encounters with patients and colleagues in real clinical settings. Cultural framing in simulations and games helps nursing students learn how to interact in new, different, and often uncomfortable contexts where culture and diversity play important roles (Kastenbaum, Hagler, Brooks, & Ruiz, 2011). Character design and assignment in a game allow individuals to adopt the appearance and persona of cultural groups other than their own and experience others' situations. The ability to try on multiple identities could facilitate behavioral responses from students that represent either cultural competence or cultural clichés and stereotypes (Games & Bauman, 2011; Gould & Bauman, 2012). Facilitated reflection on the experience may help students develop understanding and skills related to culture and diversity that they can bring to future clinical practice.

The virtual environment also may provide an ideal platform for expanding the boundaries of interprofessional multidisciplinary education. Concepts such as values and ethics, roles and responsibilities, communication, and teamwork are generally applicable across health professions (Interprofessional Education Collaborative, 2016). The anonymity of virtual worlds may provide an opportunity to move beyond segregated professional education and collaborate with health care consumers. Moule, Pollard, Armoogum, and Messer (2015) involved nurses, students, and members of a prostate cancer charity to develop virtual patients with prostate cancer.

Implementing student interactions with virtual patients allows each student in the cohort to have a similar experience at a predetermined level of complexity. In a multisite study, undergraduate nursing students conducting a health history with a virtual patient frequently missed opportunities to express empathy to the patient (Strekalova, Krieger, Kleinheksel, & Kotranza, 2017). Data from this type of structured assessment is powerful for curriculum planning.

REFLECTION FOR LEARNING

One of the key strategies that Benner et al. (2009) described as an exemplar of good teaching in any setting is teaching for salience—helping learners reflect on practice to identify what is important in a given situation. Experiences in virtual or other technological environments with the potential to evoke strong emotional responses should include both thoughtful preparation activities and guided debriefing/reflection sessions. Preparation for what to expect and how to behave in a virtual environment reduces student anxiety and focuses attention on the intended outcomes. Debriefing after the experience helps ensure that students and teachers meet targeted learning objectives and encourages further reflection.

Coaching for reflection requires active engagement of the teacher, while reflecting requires active engagement of the learner. Reflection on a technology-based learning activity could be prompted by a list of questions such as, "How do you know?" and "What are the reasons?" considered during a dialogue or in a writing activity such as journaling, blogging, or posting in an online discussion (Ennis, 2010).

Extensive question sets for discussion can be developed as framed around the Universal Intellectual Standards (Elder & Paul, 2010). Ongoing learning can be encouraged by asking what questions remain in the learner's mind after the discussion.

OTHER OUTCOMES

Technology can support learning concepts and development of specific competencies. Regardless of the technology used, careful integration of the activity into the curriculum helps assure a positive program-level learning outcome (Nielsen, Noone, Voss, & Mathews, 2013). Billings and Connors (2012) suggested seven areas of outcomes to evaluate after implementing online technology in the curriculum:

- Access
- Convenience
- Connectedness
- Preparation for real world work
- Socialization to the profession
- Satisfaction with web-based learning
- Proficiency with computer skills, use of learning management system tools

SUMMARY

Technology has blurred the boundaries between classroom and clinical teaching. Students expect technology to be integrated into curricula. Access to online resources supports a change in the clinical teacher's role from the direct provider of information to a facilitator and co-learner.

Clinical teachers can serve as technology stewards in adopting effective tools for teaching and learning. A wealth of resources such as web-based technologies, publishers' supplementary materials, health information technology, mobile or handheld devices, LOs, MOOCs, virtual reality, and game-based learning support exploration and application of clinical concepts. Technology can expand boundaries beyond cultures, professions, and locations.

Learners integrate their personal experiences of technology activities through reflection. Careful curricular integration and ongoing evaluation of technology-supported activities help promote positive learning outcomes.

CNE EXAMINATION TEST BLUEPRINT CORE COMPETENCIES

1. **Facilitate Learning**
    A. Implement a variety of teaching strategies appropriate to
       1. content
       2. setting
       3. learner needs

(continued)

  4. learning style
  5. desired learner outcomes
 B. Use teaching strategies based on
  1. educational theory
  2. evidence-based practices related to education
 C. Modify teaching strategies and learning experiences based on consideration of learners'
  2. past clinical experiences
  3. past educational and life experiences
  4. generational groups (i.e., age)
 D. Use information technologies to support the teaching–learning process
 N. Use knowledge of evidence-based practice to instruct learners

2. Facilitate Learner Development and Socialization

 B. Provide resources for diverse learners to meet their individual learning needs
 D. Create learning environments that facilitate learners' self-reflection, personal goal-setting, and socialization to the role of the nurse
 E. Foster the development of learners in these areas
  1. cognitive domain
  2. psychomotor domain
  3. affective domain

6. Engage in Scholarship, Service, and Leadership

 A. Function as a change agent and leader
  4. Implement strategies for change within the nursing program
  6. Adapt to changes created by external factors

REFERENCES

Agency for Healthcare Research and Quality. (2017). Guidelines and recommendations. Retrieved from http://www.ahrq.gov/professionals/clinicians-providers/guidelines-recommendations/index.html

Alraimi, K. M., Zo, H., & Ciganek, A. P. (2015). Understanding the MOOCs continuance: The role of openness and reputation. *Computers & Education, 80,* 28–38. doi:10.1016/j.compedu.2014.08.006

Benner, P., Sutphen, M., Leonard, V., & Day, L. (2009). *Educating nurses: A call for radical transformation.* San Francisco, CA: Jossey-Bass.

Billings, D., & Connors, H. (2012). *Best practices in online learning.* Retrieved from http://www.electronicvision.com/nln/chapter02/index.htm

Billings, D., & Kowalski, K. (2014). Understanding massively open online courses. *Journal of Continuing Education in Nursing, 45,* 58–59. doi:10.3928/00220124-20140124-14

Centers for Disease Control and Prevention. (2017). *Home page.* Retrieved from http://www.cdc.gov

Choi, M., Park, J. H., & Lee, H. S. (2016). Assessment of the need to integrate academic electronic medical records into the undergraduate clinical practicum: A focus group interview. *Computers, Informatics, Nursing, 34,* 259–265. doi:10.1097/CIN.0000000000000244

Creasman, P. (2012). *IDEA paper # 52: Considerations in online course design.* Manhattan, KS: The IDEA Center. Retrieved from http://www.theideacenter.org/sites/default/files/idea_paper_52.pdf

Creative Commons. (2017). *About the licenses.* Retrieved from http://creativecommons.org/licenses

Elder, L., & Paul, R. (2010). Critical thinking: Competency standards essential for the cultivation of intellectual skills, Part 1. *Journal of Developmental Education, 34*(2), 38–39.

Ennis, R. (2010). A super-streamlined conception of critical thinking. Retrieved from http://www.criticalthinking.net

Farra, S. S., Miller, E. T., & Hodgson, E. (2015). Virtual reality disaster training: Translation to practice. *Nurse Education in Practice, 15,* 53–57. doi:10.1016/j.nepr.2013.08.017

Forsberg, E., Ziegert, K., Hult, H., & Fors, U. (2016). Assessing progression of clinical reasoning through virtual patients: An exploratory study. *Nurse Education in Practice, 16,* 97–103. doi:10.1016/j.nepr.2015.09.006

Frantiska, J. (2016). *Creating reusable learning objects.* Switzerland: Springer.

Games, I., & Bauman, E. (2011). Virtual worlds: An environment for cultural sensitivity education in the health sciences. *International Journal of Web Based Communities, 7,* 189–205. doi:10.1504/IJWBC.2011.039510

Gould, J., & Bauman, E. (2012). Virtual reality in medical education. In S. Tsuda, D. J. Scott, & D. B. Jones (Eds.), *Textbook of simulation, surgical skills and team training* (Chap. 18). Woodbury, CT: Cine-Med.

Grumme, V. S., Barry, C. D., Gordon, S. C., & Ray, M. A. (2016). On virtual presence. *Advances in Nursing Science, 39,* 48–59. doi:10.1097/ANS.0000000000000103

Herbert, V. M., & Connors, H. (2016). Integrating an academic electronic health record: Challenges and success strategies. *Computers, Informatics, Nursing, 34,* 345–354. doi:10.1097/CIN.0000000000000264

Interprofessional Education Collaborative. (2016). *Core competencies for interprofessional collaborative practice: 2016 update.* Washington, DC: Author.

Kastenbaum, B., Hagler, D., Brooks, R., & Ruiz, E. (2011). Simulation: Realistic cultural encounters. *Academic Exchange Quarterly, 15*(2), 27–32.

Kopp, W., & Hanson, M. A. (2012). High-fidelity and gaming simulations enhance nursing education in end-of-life care. *Clinical Simulation in Nursing, 8*(3), e97–e102. doi:10.1016/j.ecns.2010.07.005

Lapkin, S., Levett-Jones, T., Chenoweth, L., & Johnson, M. (2016) The effectiveness of interventions designed to reduce medication administration errors: A synthesis of findings from systematic reviews. *Journal of Nursing Management 24,* 845–858. doi:10.1111/jonm.12390

Lee, N.-J., Chae, S.-M., Kim, H., Lee, J.-H., Min, H. J., & Park, D.-E. (2016). Mobile-based video learning outcomes in clinical nursing skill education: A randomized controlled trial. *Computers, Informatics, Nursing, 34,* 8–16. doi:10.1097/CIN.0000000000000183

Multimedia Educational Resource for Learning and Online Training. (2017). *Search other libraries.* Retrieved from http://fedsearch.merlot.org/fedsearch/fedsearch.jsp

Miller, N. (2014). *Twitter chats 101: A step-by-step guide to hosting or joining a Twitter chat.* Retrieved from https://blog.bufferapp.com/twitter-chat-101

Moule, P., Pollard, K., Armoogum, J., & Messer, S. (2015). Virtual patients: Development in cancer nursing education. *Nurse Education Today, 35,* 875–880. doi:10.1016/j.nedt.2015.02.009

National League for Nursing. (2015). A vision for the changing faculty role: Preparing students for the technological world of health care: A living document. Retrieved from https://www.nln.org/docs/default-source/about/nln-vision-series-(position-statements)/a-vision-for-the-changing-faculty-role-preparing-students-for-the-technological-world-of-health-care.pdf?sfvrsn=0

Nielsen, A. E., Noone, J., Voss, H., & Mathews, L. R. (2013). Preparing nursing students for the future: An innovative approach to clinical education. *Nurse Education in Practice, 13,* 301–309. doi:10.1016/j.nepr.2013.03.015

Raman, J. (2015). Mobile technology in nursing education: Where do we go from here? A review of the literature. *Nurse Education Today, 35*(5), 663–672. doi:10.1016/j.nedt.2015.01.018

Sanford, A. J., & Emmott, C. (2012). *Mind, brain and narrative.* Cambridge, UK: Cambridge University Press.

Schaffer, M. (2016). Second Life® virtual learning in public health nursing. *Journal of Nursing Education, 55,* 536–540. doi:10.3928/01484834-20160816-09

Sedgwick, M. G., Awosoga, O., Grigg, L., & Durnin, J.-M. (2016). A quantitative study exploring undergraduate nursing students' perception of their critical thinking and clinical decision making ability while using apps at the point of care. *Journal of Nursing Education and Practice, 6*(10), 1–7. doi:10.5430/jnep.v6n10p1

Shellenbarger, T., & Robb, M. (2015). Technology-based strategies for promoting clinical reasoning skills in nursing education. *Nurse Educator, 40,* 79–82. doi:10.1097/NNE.0000000000000111

Strandell-Laine, C., Stolt, M., Leino-Kilpi, H., & Saarikoski, M. (2015). Use of mobile devices in nursing student–nurse teacher cooperation during the clinical practicum: An integrative review. *Nurse Education Today, 35,* 493–499. doi:10.1016/j.nedt.2014.10.007

Strekalova, Y. A., Krieger, J. L., Kleinheksel, A., & Kotranza, A. (2017). Empathic communication in virtual education for nursing students: I'm sorry to hear that. *Nurse Educator, 42*, 18–22. doi:10.1097/NNE.0000000000000308

Stuart, G., & Triola, M. (2015). *Enhancing health professions education through technology: building a continuously learning health system.* Proceedings of a conference sponsored by the Josiah Macy Jr. Foundation, April 2015. New York, NY: Josiah Macy Jr. Foundation.

Swigart, V., & Liang, Z. (2016). Digital resources for nursing education: Open courseware and massive open online courses. *International Journal of Nursing Sciences, 3*, 307–313. doi:10.1016/j.ijnss.2016.07.003

Tiffany, J. M., & Hoglund, B. A. (2016). Using virtual simulation to teach inclusivity: A case study. *Clinical Simulation in Nursing, 12*, 115–122. doi:10.1016/j.ecns.2015.11.003

Vikil, R., & Minarcik, J. (2017). Twitter chat saves the day. *American Medical Writers Association Journal, 32*, 28–29.

Walsh, M. (2011). Narrative pedagogy and simulation: Future directions for nursing education. *Nurse Education in Practice, 11*, 216–219. doi:10.1016/j.nepr.2010.10.006

Wenger, E., White, N., & Smith, J. D. (2009). *Digital habitats: Stewarding technology for communities.* Portland, OR: CPsquare.

CHAPTER 10

Cases for Clinical Learning

Clinical practice provides opportunities for students to gain the knowledge and skills needed to care for patients; develop values important in professional practice; and develop higher level thinking skills for analyzing data, deciding on problems and interventions, and evaluating their effectiveness. Ability to apply concepts to clinical situations, solve problems, arrive at carefully thought out decisions, and provide safe, quality care are essential competencies gained through clinical practice. Case method, case study, and unfolding cases are teaching methods that help students meet these learning outcomes. Case method and case study describe a clinical situation developed around an actual or a hypothetical patient for student review and critique. In case method, the case provided for analysis is generally shorter and more specific than in case study. Case studies are more comprehensive in nature, thereby presenting a complete picture of the patient and clinical situation. With unfolding cases, the scenario changes, presenting new data to students for analysis and integration with prior information about the case. Unfolding cases promote students' critical thinking and clinical reasoning skills. Another teaching strategy for developing these cognitive skills, and learning more about best practices for care of a patient, is grand rounds. Grand rounds involve the observation and often interview of a patient or several patients in the clinical setting, or through a webcast of grand rounds conducted elsewhere.

CASES FOR DEVELOPING COGNITIVE SKILLS

With cases, students can apply concepts and theories to clinical situations, identify patient and other types of problems, propose varied approaches for solving them, weigh them against the evidence, and choose the most appropriate approaches. These methods provide experience for students in analyzing clinical situations and thinking through possible decisions.

Problem Solving

The nursing literature contains various perspectives on problem solving, decision making, critical thinking, and clinical judgment. In general, problem solving is the ability to solve clinical problems, some relating to the patient and others that arise from clinical practice. Problem solving begins with recognizing and defining the problem, gathering data to clarify it further, identifying possible approaches, weighing them against evidence, and choosing the best one considering patient needs and responses (Oermann & Gaberson, 2017).

Viewed as a cognitive skill, problem solving can be developed through experiences with patients or through simulated cases. The student does not need to provide hands-on care to develop problem-solving skills. By observing and discussing patients with the clinical educator or preceptor, and by analyzing cases, students gain experience in understanding patient problems and the clinical situation and deciding on approaches to use. Cases expose students to clinical situations that they may not encounter in their own clinical practice.

In clinical practice, nurses make many important decisions when caring for patients. They decide on data to collect and what they mean, problems and their priority, interventions, resources, and effectiveness of interventions. Tanner (2006) referred to this cognitive process as clinical reasoning: the process of generating different alternatives, weighing them against evidence, and deciding on the most appropriate approach to use. With cases, students can practice these skills: they can generate possible alternatives, weigh them against evidence, consider the consequences of each, then arrive at a decision following this analysis.

Critical Thinking

Critical thinking enables the nurse to make reasoned and informed judgments in the practice setting and decide what to do in a given situation. It is purposeful and informed reasoning in clinical practice and in other settings (Alfaro-LeFevre, 2017). Critical thinking is a judgment process. Nurses and other clinicians decide what to believe or do in a particular situation based on available evidence and using the knowledge and skills they acquired through their education and practice; that process also involves weighing the likely consequences of different actions and evaluating their effectiveness (Facione & Facione, 2008).

Critical thinking development can be viewed as a process through which students progress. Elder and Paul (2010) described stages of critical thinking. These include the: (a) unreflective thinker, (b) challenged thinker, (c) beginning thinker, (d) practicing thinker, (e) advanced thinker, and (f) accomplished thinker (Elder & Paul, 2010). These stages were used by nursing faculty members to develop unfolding cases for simulation (West, Holmes, Zidek, & Edwards, 2013).

Critical thinking can also be viewed as reflective thinking about patient problems when the problem is not obvious or the nurse knows what is wrong but is unsure what to do. Through critical thinking, the learner:

- Considers multiple perspectives to care
- Critiques different approaches possible in a clinical situation
- Weighs approaches against evidence and patient responses
- Arrives at sound judgments
- Raises questions about issues to clarify them further
- Resolves issues with a well-thought out approach (Alfaro-LeFevre, 2017; Facione & Facione, 2008; Facione, 2011)

Clinical Judgment

Tanner (2006) developed a model of clinical judgment in nursing that incorporates concepts of problem solving, decision making, and critical thinking. In this model, clinical judgment involves interpreting a patient's needs and problems and deciding on actions and approaches, taking the patient's responses into consideration. The clinical judgment process includes four aspects: (a) noticing, grasping the situation; (b) interpreting, understanding the situation in order to respond; (c) responding, deciding on actions that are appropriate or that no actions are needed; and (d) reflecting, being attentive to how patients respond to the nurse's actions.

This model provides a framework for guiding students' reflections of how they think about clinical situations, interpret them, and arrive at decisions. In simulated cases, students can describe what they would expect to find in the clinical situation in the case (noticing), the meaning of the data in the case, and appropriate interventions or why they would take no action. The model provides a framework for coaching students in how they think about clinical situations.

CASE METHOD AND STUDY

Case method and case study serve similar purposes in clinical teaching: they provide a simulated case for student review and critique. In case method, the case provided for analysis is generally shorter and more specific than in case study.

Case Method

In case method, short cases are developed around actual or hypothetical patients followed by open-ended questions to encourage students' thinking about the case. Short cases are used to avoid directing students' thinking in advance. Depending on how the case is written, case method is effective for applying concepts and other types of knowledge to clinical practice and for promoting development of cognitive skills. With cases, students can analyze patient data, identify needs and problems, and decide on the best approaches in that situation after weighing the evidence. Cases also assist students in relating course content to clinical practice and integrating different concepts and content areas in a particular clinical situation. Examples of case method are presented in Exhibit 10.1.

Case Study

A case study provides an actual or hypothetical patient situation for students to analyze and arrive at varied decisions. Case studies typically are longer and more comprehensive than in case method, providing background data about the patient, family history, and other information for a more complete picture. For this reason, students can analyze case studies in greater depth than with case method and present a more detailed rationale for their analysis. In their critique of the case study, students can describe the concepts that guided their analysis, how they used them in understanding the case, and the literature they reviewed. Examples of case studies are presented in Exhibit 10.2.

EXHIBIT 10.1

EXAMPLES OF CASE METHOD

Mrs. F has moderate dementia. She lets the nurse practitioner do a pelvic examination because she has a "woman's problem." The examination shows an anterior wall prolapse. While helping Mrs. F to get dressed, the nurse practitioner observes that, as soon as the patient stands up, urine begins leaking onto the floor. Mrs. F appears embarrassed.

1. List and prioritize Mrs. F's problems. Provide a rationale for how the problems are prioritized.
2. Develop a plan of care for Mrs. F.

Your patient is admitted from the emergency department with severe headache, right-sided weakness, and aphasia. Her temperature is normal, pulse 120, respirations 16, and blood pressure 180/120.

1. What are possible reasons for these symptoms? Provide an explanation for your answer.
2. What additional data would you collect on admission to your unit? Why is this information important to planning the patient's care?
3. In postclinical conference, as a group develop this case. What information would you include in a report on this patient to the incoming nurse using SBAR (situation, background, assessment, recommendation)?

Mrs. B, 29 years old, is seen for a prenatal checkup. She is in her 24th week of pregnancy. The nurse practitioner notes swelling of the ankles and around Mrs. B's eyes. Mrs. B has not been able to wear her rings for a week because of swelling. Her blood pressure is 144/96.

1. What are possible problems Mrs. B might be facing? List all possible problems given the previously mentioned information.
2. What additional data should be collected at this time? Why?

You are working in a pediatrician's office. Mrs. C brings her son in for a check-up after a severe asthma attack a month ago that required emergency care. When you ask Mrs. C how her son is doing, she begins to cry softly. She tells you she is worried about his having another asthma attack and this time not recovering from it. When the pediatrician enters the examination room, Mrs. C is still crying. The physician says, "What's wrong? Look at him. He's doing great."

1. What would you say to Mrs. C, if anything, in this situation?
2. What would you say to the pediatrician, if anything?
3. Analyze this case in the context of patient-centered case.

You have a new patient, 81 years old, with heart failure. The referral to your home health agency indicates that Mr. A has difficulty breathing, tires easily, and has edema in both legs, making it difficult for him to get around. He lives alone.

1. What are problems you anticipate for Mr. A? Include a rationale for each of these problems.

At your first home visit, you find Mr. A sitting in a chair with his feet on the floor. During your assessment, he gets short of breath talking with you and has to stop periodically to catch his breath.

1. Describe at least three different nursing interventions that could be used in Mr. A's care.
2. Specify outcome criteria for evaluating the effectiveness of the interventions you selected.
3. What would you teach Mr. A? How could you use the teach-back method in this situation?
4. Select one of your interventions and review the evidence on its use. What are your conclusions about the effectiveness of the intervention?
5. Identify one published research study that relates to Mr. A's care. Critique the study and describe whether you could use the findings in caring for Mr. A and similar patients.

(continued)

Mrs. M is a 42-year-old elementary school teacher with a history of inflammatory bowel disease. She calls the clinic for an appointment because of diarrhea that has lasted for 2 weeks. The nurse answering the phone tells Mrs. M to stop taking all of her medications until she is seen in the clinic.

1. Do you agree or disagree with the nurse's advice to Mrs. M? Why?

You have been working in the clinical agency for nearly 6 months. Recently you noticed a colleague having difficulty completing his assignments on time. He also has been late for work on at least three occasions. Today you see him move from one patient to the next without washing his hands.

1. What are your options in this situation?
2. Discuss possible consequences of each option.
3. What would you do? Why is this the best approach?

As you record a patient's vital signs in the electronic medical records, she asks you to show the computer screen to her husband so he can read about the diagnoses they are ruling out.

1. What would you say to this patient?
2. What principles guide your decision? Provide a rationale for your response.

Mrs. J brings her 8-year-old daughter, Laura, into the office for her annual visit. In reviewing the immunization record, the nurse notices that Laura never received the second dose of the measles, mumps, rubella (MMR) vaccine. The nurse tells the mother not to worry; Laura can get the second dose when she is 11 or 12 years old.

1. Do you agree or disagree with the nurse's advice to the mother? Provide a rationale for your decision.

Read the following statements: One in three adults and one in five adolescents are overweight. Being overweight is prevalent among certain ethnic groups.

1. What additional information do you need before identifying the implications of this statement for your community?
2. Why is this information important?

The heart failure clinic at your hospital has been effective in reducing the number of readmissions, but, to save costs, the hospital is closing it. As the nurse practitioner in that clinic, write a report about why the clinic should remain open, with data to support your position. To whom would you send that report and why? Then write a report from the perspective of the hospital administration supporting closure of the clinic.

EXHIBIT 10.2

EXAMPLE OF A CASE STUDY

Mary, 44 years old, is seen in the physician's office with hoarseness and a slight cough. During the assessment, Mary tells the nurse that she also has shortness of breath, particularly when walking fast and going up the stairs. Mary has never smoked. Her vital signs are: blood pressure 120/80; heart rate 88 beats per minute; respirations 32 per minute; and temperature 36.6°C (97.8°F).

Mary is married with two teenage daughters. She works part-time as a substitute teacher. Mary has always been health conscious, watching her weight and eating properly. She tells the nurse how worried she is because she has read about women getting lung cancer even if they never smoked.

1. The physician orders a combined PET/CT scan. What is a PET/CT scan, and why was it ordered for Mary?
2. What would you say to Mary prior to the scan to prepare her for it?

(continued)

3. Identify a potential diagnosis for Mary and add data to the case consistent with that diagnosis. What types of problems would you anticipate for Mary? Describe nursing management for each of those problems.
4. Add data about Mary and her family to the case. Select a family theory and use it to analyze this family. What did you learn about the family, and how will this influence your care?
5. What resources are available in your community for Mary?

Using Cases in Clinical Courses

Short cases, as in case method, and longer case studies can be integrated in clinical courses throughout the curriculum to assist students in applying concepts and knowledge they are learning in their courses to clinical situations of increasing complexity. In beginning clinical courses, teachers can develop cases that present problems that are relatively easy to identify and require standard nursing interventions. At this level, students learn how to apply concepts to clinical situations and think through them. Students can work as a group to analyze cases; explore different perspectives of the case, what students noticed about it, and their interpretations; and discuss possible approaches to use.

In the beginning, the teacher should "think aloud," guiding students through the analysis, pointing out significant aspects of the case and his or her own expectations and interpretations. By thinking aloud, the teacher can model the clinical judgment process step by step through a case. As students progress through the curriculum, the cases can become more complex with varied problems and approaches that could be used in the situation.

Students can analyze cases in a postclinical conference, as an independent activity, or online either individually or in small groups. They can share resources they used to better understand the case. If cases are analyzed individually, further discussion about the case can occur with the clinical group as a whole, or students can post their thoughts and responses online for others to reflect and comment on.

Based on the questions asked about the case, cases can be used to meet many different learning outcomes of a clinical course. For example, if the goal of the case is to guide students in interpreting data, then questions might ask students to identify significant information in the situation and explain what the data mean. Cases are effective as an instructional method, and they can also be graded similar to essay items.

Complexity of Cases for Review

Cases may be of varying levels of complexity. Some cases are designed with the problems readily apparent. With these cases, the problem is described clearly, and sufficient information is included to guide decisions on how to intervene. Brookhart and Nitko (2015) called these cases well structured: They provide an opportunity for students to apply knowledge to a clinical situation and develop an understanding of how it is used in practice. Cases of this type link knowledge presented in class, online, and through readings to practice situations. With well-structured cases, there is usually one correct answer that students can identify based on what they are currently learning in the clinical course or learned in previous courses and experiences.

Well-structured cases are effective for students beginning a clinical course in which they have limited background and experience. These cases give students an opportunity to practice their thinking before caring for an actual patient.

Most patient care situations, however, are not that easily solved. In clinical practice, the problems are sometimes difficult to identify, or the nurse may be confident about the patient's problem but unsure how to intervene. These are problems in Schön's (1990) swampy lowland—ones that do not lend themselves to resolution by a technical and rational approach. These are cases that vary from the way the problems and solutions were presented in class and through readings. For such cases, the principles learned in class may not readily apply, and clinical judgment is required for analysis and resolution.

Brookhart and Nitko (2015) referred to these cases as ill structured, describing problems that reflect real-life clinical situations faced by students. With ill-structured cases, different problems may be possible; there may be an incomplete data set to interpret; or the need and problem may be clear, but multiple approaches may be possible. Exhibit 10.3 presents examples of a well-structured and an ill-structured case.

Developing Cases

Case method and study have two components: a case description and questions to answer about the case or its analysis. In case method, the situations described are typically short and geared to specific outcomes to be met. Case studies include background information about the patient, family history, and complete assessment data to provide a comprehensive description of the patient or clinical situation.

The case should provide enough information for analysis without directing the students' thinking in a particular direction. The case may be developed first, then the questions, or the teacher may draft the questions first, then develop the case to present the clinical situation. Once students have experience in analyzing cases, another strategy is for students to develop a case scenario based on data provided

---

EXHIBIT 10.3

WELL-STRUCTURED AND ILL-STRUCTURED CASES

Well-Structured Case

Mrs. D, 53 years old, reports having bad headaches for the last month. The headaches occur about twice weekly usually in the late morning. Initially, the pain began as a throbbing at her right temple. Her headaches now affect either her right or left eye and temple. The pain is so severe that she usually goes to bed. Mrs. D reports that her neck hurts, and the nurse notes tenderness in the posterior neck on palpation.

1. What type or types of headache might Mrs. D be experiencing?
2. Describe additional data that should be collected from Mrs. D. Why is this information important to deciding what is wrong with Mrs. D?
3. Select two interventions that might be used for Mrs. D. Provide evidence for their use.

Ill-Structured Case

Ms. J, 35 years old, calls for an appointment because she fell yesterday at home. She has a few bruises from her fall and a tingling feeling in her legs. Ms. J had been at the eye doctor's office last week because of double vision.

1. What do you think about this patient?
2. What are possible problems that Ms. J might be experiencing?
3. Plan additional data to collect to better understand those problems and explain why that information is important.

by the teacher. In this method, students need to think about what patient needs and problems might fit the data, which promotes their critical thinking.

The questions developed for the case are the key to its effective use. The questions should be geared to the outcomes to be met. For instance, if the intent of the case method or study is for students to analyze laboratory data, apply physiological principles, and use concepts of pathophysiology for the analysis, then the questions need to relate to each of these. Similarly, if the goal is to improve skill in responding to clinical situations, then the questions should ask about possible actions to take for the situation, including no immediate intervention, and evidence to consider in deciding on actions. With most cases, questions should be included that focus on the underlying thought process used to arrive at an answer rather than the answer alone.

Cases can be written for the development of specific cognitive skills. In designing cases to promote problem solving, the teacher should develop a case that asks students to:

- Identify patient and other problems apparent or expected in the case
- Suggest alternative problems that might be possible if more information were available and identify the information needed
- Identify relevant and irrelevant information in the case
- Interpret the information to enable a response
- Propose different approaches that might be used
- Weigh approaches against the evidence
- Select the best approaches for the case situation
- Provide a rationale for those approaches
- Identify gaps in the literature and evidence as related to the case
- Evaluate the effectiveness of interventions
- Plan alternative interventions based on analysis of the case

An example of a case for problem solving is:

Ms. G, a 56-year-old patient admitted for shortness of breath and chest pain, is scheduled for a cardiac catheterization. She has been crying on and off for the last hour. When the nurse attempts to talk to her, Ms. G says, "Don't worry about me. I'm just tired."

1. What is one problem in this situation that needs to be solved?
2. What assumptions about Ms. G did you make in identifying this problem?
3. What additional information would you collect from the patient and her medical records before intervening? Why is this information important?

Other cases can provide experience with making decisions about clinical situations. A case may present a clinical situation up to the point of a decision, then ask students to analyze the case and arrive at a decision. Or the case may describe a situation and decision, then ask whether students agree or disagree with it. For both of these types, the questions should lead the students through the decision-making process, and students should include a rationale for their responses.

For decision making, the teacher should develop a case that asks students to:

- Identify the decisions needed in the case
- Identify information in the case that is critical for arriving at a decision
- Specify additional data needed for a decision
- Examine alternative decisions possible and the consequences of each
- Arrive at a decision and provide a rationale for it

An example of a case intended for decision making is:

The charge nurse on the midnight shift in a large hospital assigns a nurse new to the unit to work with Ms. P, an experienced RN. Ms. P, however, is irate that she needs to orient a new nurse when she is so busy herself. Ms. P tells the new nurse that she is too busy to work with her tonight. When learning this, the charge nurse reassigns the new nurse to another RN.

1. Do you agree or disagree with the charge nurse's decision? Why?
2. Describe at least two strategies you could use in this situation. What are the advantages and disadvantages of each?
3. How would you handle this situation?

Case method and case study also meet critical thinking outcomes. There are a number of strategies that teachers can use when developing cases that are intended for critical thinking. These are listed in Exhibit 10.4.

EXHIBIT 10.4

STRATEGIES FOR DEVELOPING CASE STUDIES FOR CRITICAL THINKING

Develop	Ask students to
Present an issue for analysis, a question to be answered that has multiple possibilities, or a complex problem to be solved.	Analyze the case and provide a rationale for the thinking process they used for the analysis. Examine the assumptions underlying their thinking. Describe the evidence on which their reasoning was based. Describe the concepts and theories they used for their analysis and *how* they applied to the case.
Have different and conflicting points of view.	Analyze the case from their own points of view and then analyze the case from a different point of view.
Present complex data for analysis.	Analyze the data and draw possible inferences given the data. Specify additional information needed and why it is important.
Present clinical situations that are unique and offer different perspectives.	Analyze the clinical situation, identify multiple perspectives possible, and examine assumptions made about the situation that influenced thinking.
Describe ethical issues and dilemmas.	Propose alternative approaches and consequences. Weigh alternatives and arrive at a decision. Critique an issue from a different point of view.

An example of a case for critical thinking is:

You are a nurse practitioner working in a middle school. Ms. S, a 16-year-old, comes to your office for nausea and vomiting. She says she feels "bloated." She confides in you that she is pregnant and asks you not to tell her parents.

1. What are your options at this time?
2. What option would you choose to implement? Why?
3. Choose another option that you listed for question 1. What are the advantages and disadvantages of that approach over your first choice?

Cases can also be written with the intent to promote clinical judgment skills. Using Tanner's (2006) model of clinical judgment, cases can ask students to:

- Describe what they notice in the clinical situation that demands attention
- Explain the clinical situation based on their prior and current learning
- Interpret the meaning of the data
- Suggest possible courses of action, if any, that would be appropriate
- Provide a rationale for taking no action or to support the proposed actions
- Hypothesize how patients might respond to each of those actions
- Reflect on their own thinking and decisions

An example of a case for this purpose is:

You make a home visit to an 86-year-old patient who lives alone and is having problems concentrating, loss of memory, crying spells, and fatigue. You recommend a follow-up visit with the primary care physician. The patient is diagnosed with depression and treated with a selective serotonin reuptake inhibitor. Two weeks later, you visit the patient and learn she still has fatigue and now also has loss of appetite and difficulty sleeping.

1. What do you notice in this situation?
2. Provide alternative explanations for the patient's current symptoms of fatigue, loss of appetite, and difficulty sleeping.
3. Discuss the case with a peer and compare interpretations. Decide on next steps to be taken by the home health nurse.

Unfolding Cases

A variation of case study is unfolding cases in which the clinical situation changes, thereby creating a simulation for students to analyze. With an unfolding case, instead of having one scenario, the teacher develops the case to expand the information presented to the student. For example, there might be a change in the patient's condition, clinical situation, or setting similar to what might occur with an actual patient. Smallheer (2016) suggested that an unfolding case can be "intentionally unpredictable" to reflect the reality of clinical practice. As an alternative, students can develop the scenario as a reverse case study (Smallheer, 2016).

Day (2011) described the development of unfolding cases for classroom instruction. In this process, the narrative, which is the patient's story, is central and provides the structure for the classroom discussion. With the case, students learn the concepts and content for providing care in that particular clinical situation. The teacher begins by identifying the goals of the class and understanding the learners and their needs; then the teacher specifies the content to be learned, which is taught through the case study as it unfolds. In the next phase the teacher develops the narrative (what should the case do) and decides on the patient situation to achieve the goals and learn the essential content. Unfolding cases are also used frequently in simulation. As the case unfolds in the simulation, students analyze the new information and make decisions about relevant actions to take.

GRAND ROUNDS

Grand rounds involve the observation and often interview of a patient or several patients in the clinical setting, or a webcast of grand rounds conducted elsewhere. Grand rounds provide an opportunity to observe a patient with a specific condition, discuss assessment and interpretation of data, and propose interventions. Rounds are valuable for examining issues facing patients and families, and for exposing students to situations they may not encounter in their clinical experiences. During rounds, students can examine best practices, connect classroom learning and clinical practice, and develop professional skills such as those related to leadership and communication (Lanham, 2011). Grand rounds may involve nursing students and staff members only or be interprofessional.

Nursing grand rounds can also be used for staff education. Grand rounds can be used to keep nurses up to date on new approaches to care, present best practices, explore new evidence and how it might be used in a patient's care, and improve the quality of care. Jennings and Mitchell (2017) used structured, weekly rounds that were conducted at the bedside to improve the care of trauma patients, increase collaboration among staff, and improve nurses' knowledge. Nursing experts and other providers assessed patients and recommended changes to improve care. Grand rounds provide an opportunity for highlighting nurses' clinical expertise and promoting best practices.

Rather than conducting rounds in the clinical setting, faculty members may decide to use webcasts of grand rounds that are available. A number of organizations offer webinars of grand rounds that could be used for staff education and also in nursing education programs.

Grand rounds enable students to:

- Identify patient problems and issues in a clinical situation
- Evaluate the effectiveness of nursing and interdisciplinary interventions
- Share clinical knowledge with peers and identify gaps in their own understanding
- Develop new perspectives about the patient's care
- Gain insight into other ways of meeting patient needs
- Think critically about the nursing care they provide and that given by their peers
- Dialogue about patient care and changes in clinical practice with peers and experts participating in the rounds

Regardless of whether the rounds are conducted in the clinical setting or viewed on a webcast, the teacher should first identify the outcomes that students should meet at the end of the rounds. The outcomes guide the teacher in planning the rounds and their focus. Second, it should be clear why the particular patient or clinical situation was selected for grand rounds. Third, the questions asked after rounds should encourage students to think critically about the patient and care, compare this case to the textbook picture and other patients for whom students have cared, and explore alternative interventions and perspectives of the situation. The final area of discussion should focus on what students have learned from this experience and new insights they have gained about clinical practice. Students might write a short paper reflecting on their learning and new perspectives.

Grand rounds may be conducted by an advanced practice nurse, a staff nurse, the teacher, a student, or another health care provider. Many rounds are interprofessional, with the team assessing the patient and discussing care. For student-led rounds, the teacher is responsible for confirming the plan with the patient. Patients should be assured of their right to refuse participation and should be comfortable to tell those involved in the rounds when they no longer want to continue with it.

For grand rounds in the clinical setting, activities at the patient's bedside should begin with an introduction of the patient to the students, emphasizing the patient's contribution to student learning. If possible, the person conducting the rounds should include the patient and family in the discussion, seeking their perspective of the health problem and input into care. The teacher's role is that of consultant, clarifying information and assisting the student in keeping the discussion on the goals set for the rounds. Students should direct any questions to the teacher prior to and after the grand rounds, and sensitive issues should be discussed when the rounds are completed and out of the patient's presence.

SUMMARY

Cases describe a clinical situation developed around an actual or hypothetical patient for student review and analysis. In case method, the case is generally shorter and more specific than in case study. Case studies are more comprehensive in nature, thereby presenting a complete picture of the patient and clinical situation. In an unfolding case, the clinical situation changes, introducing new information for learners to integrate and analyze.

With these clinical teaching methods, students apply knowledge to practice situations, identify needs and problems, propose varied approaches for solving them considering evidence, decide on courses of action, and evaluate outcomes. As such, cases provide experience for students in thinking through different clinical situations.

Grand rounds involve the observation of a patient or several patients in the clinical setting or in a webcast. Grand rounds may be conducted for nursing students and staff only or by the interprofessional team. Rounds provide an opportunity to observe a patient with a specific condition, review assessment data, discuss interventions and their effectiveness, and make changes in the plan of care. Rounds are also valuable for examining issues facing patients and discussing ways of resolving them. Grand rounds, similar to cases, provide an opportunity for exploring patient problems and varied courses of action, analyzing care and proposing new interventions, and gaining insight into different clinical situations.

CNE EXAMINATION TEST BLUEPRINT CORE COMPETENCIES

1. **Facilitate Learning**

   A. Implement a variety of teaching strategies appropriate to
      1. content
      2. setting (i.e., clinical versus classroom)
      3. learner needs
      4. learning style
      5. desired learner outcomes
   B. Use teaching strategies based on
      1. educational theory
      2. evidence-based practices related to education
   D. Use information technologies to support the teaching–learning process
   G. Model reflective thinking practices, including critical thinking
   H. Create opportunities for learners to develop their own critical thinking skills
   N. Use knowledge of evidence-based practice to instruct learners

2. **Facilitate Learner Development and Socialization**

   E. Foster the development of learners in these areas
      1. cognitive domain
      2. psychomotor domain
      3. affective domain

3. **Use Assessment and Evaluation Strategies**

   C. Use a variety of strategies to assess and evaluate learning in these domains
      1. cognitive
      2. psychomotor
      3. affective

REFERENCES

Alfaro-LeFevre, R. (2017). *Critical thinking, clinical reasoning, and clinical judgment: A practical approach* (6th ed.). St. Louis, MO: Elsevier.

Brookhart, S. M., & Nitko, A. J. (2015). *Educational assessment of students* (7th ed.). Upper Saddle River, NJ: Pearson.

Day, L. (2011). Using unfolding case studies in a subject-centered classroom. *Journal of Nursing Education, 50,* 447–452. doi:10.3928/01484834-20110517-03

Elder, L., & Paul, R. (2010). *Critical thinking development: A state theory.* Retrieved from http://www .criticalthinking.org/pages/critical-thinking-development-a-stage-theory/483

Facione, N. C., & Facione, P. A. (Eds.). (2008). *Critical thinking and clinical reasoning in the health sciences: An international multidisciplinary teaching anthology.* Millbrae: California Academic Press.

Facione, P. A. (2011). *Critical thinking: What it is and why it counts.* Retrieved from http://www .insightassessment.com/CT-Resources/Critical-Thinking-What-It-Is-and-Why-It-Counts

Jennings, F. L., & Mitchell, M. (2017). Intensive care nurses' perceptions of Inter Specialty Trauma Nursing Rounds to improve trauma patient care—A quality improvement project. *Intensive and Critical Care Nursing, 40,* 35–43. doi:10.1016/j.iccn.2017.01.002

Lanham, J. (2011). Nursing grand rounds as a clinical teaching strategy. *Journal of Nursing Education, 50,* 176. doi:10.3928/01484834-20110216-02

Oermann, M. H., & Gaberson, K. B. (2017). *Evaluation and testing in nursing education* (5th ed.). New York, NY: Springer Publishing.

Schön, D. A. (1990). *Educating the reflective practitioner.* San Francisco, CA: Jossey-Bass.

Smallheer, B. A. (2016). Reverse case study: A new perspective on an existing teaching strategy. *Nurse Educator, 41,* 7–8.

Tanner, C. A. (2006). Thinking like a nurse: A research-based model of clinical judgment in nursing. *Journal of Nursing Education, 45,* 204–211.

West, E., Holmes, J., Zidek, C., & Edwards, T. (2013). Intraprofessional collaboration through an unfolding case and the just culture model. *Journal of Nursing Education, 52,* 470–474. doi:10.3928/01484834-20130719-04

CHAPTER 11

Discussion and Clinical Conference

Discussions with learners and clinical conferences provide a means of sharing information, developing critical thinking skills, and learning how to collaborate with others in a group. Discussion is an exchange of ideas for a specific purpose; clinical conference is a form of group discussion that focuses on some aspect of clinical practice. Teachers and students engage in many discussions in planning, carrying out, and evaluating clinical learning activities. Similarly, there are varied types of clinical conferences for use in teaching. Effective conferences and discussions require an understanding of their goals, the types of questions for encouraging exchange of ideas and higher level thinking, and the roles of the teacher and students.

DISCUSSION

Discussions between teacher and student, preceptor and orientee, and nurse manager and staff occur frequently but do not always promote learning. These discussions often involve the teacher telling the learner what to do or not to do for a patient. Discussions, though, should be an exchange of ideas through which the teacher, by asking open-ended questions and supporting learner responses, encourages students to arrive at their own decisions or to engage in self-assessment about clinical practice. Discussions are not intended to be an exchange of the teacher's ideas to the students. In a discussion, both teacher and student actively participate in sharing ideas and considering alternative perspectives.

Discussions give learners an opportunity to interact with one another, critique each other's ideas, and learn from others. For that reason, discussions are an effective method for promoting critical thinking (Berkstresser, 2016). The teacher can ask open-ended and thought-provoking questions, which encourage higher-level thinking if students perceive that they are free to discuss their own ideas and those of others involved in the discussion. The teacher is a resource for students, giving immediate feedback and further instruction as needed. Discussions also provide a forum for students to explore feelings associated with their clinical practice and simulation experiences, clarify values and ethical dilemmas, and learn to interact in a group format. Those outcomes are not as easily met in a large group setting. Over a period of time, students learn to collaborate with peers in working toward solving clinical problems.

Creating a Climate for Discussion

An important role of the teacher is to develop a climate in which students are comfortable discussing concepts and issues without fear that the ideas expressed will affect the teacher's evaluation of their performance and subsequent clinical grade. Similarly, discussions between preceptor and orientee and between manager and staff should be carried out in an atmosphere in which nurses feel comfortable to express their own opinions and ideas and to question others' assumptions. Discussions are for formative, not summative, evaluation; they provide feedback to learners individually or in a small group to guide their learning and thinking. Without this climate for exchanging ideas, though, discussions cannot be carried out effectively, because students fear that their comments may influence their clinical evaluation and grade—or, for nurses, their performance ratings.

The teacher sets an atmosphere in which listening, respect for others' comments and ideas, and openness to new perspectives are valued. Learners need to be free to discuss their ideas with the teacher, who can guide their thinking through careful questioning. Without support from the teacher, students will not participate freely in the discussion nor will they be willing to examine controversial points of view, critique different perspectives of care and decisions, or share misunderstandings with the teacher and peers.

Studies on teacher effectiveness highlight the importance of this interpersonal relationship between teacher and students. Conveying confidence in students and their ability to perform in clinical practice, demonstrating respect for students, being honest and direct with them, and encouraging students to ask questions and participate freely in discussions are important characteristics of effective clinical teaching. Considering the many demands on students as they learn to care for patients, students need to view the teacher as someone who supports them in their learning. This is a critical role of clinical teachers and staff with whom they work.

Guidelines for Discussion

Discussions can be face to face in the clinical setting or conducted online. They can be carried out individually with learners or in a small group. The size of the group for a discussion can range from two to 10 people. A larger group makes it difficult for each person to participate.

The teacher is responsible for planning the discussion to meet the intended outcomes of the clinical course or specific goals to be achieved through the discussion. An effective teacher keeps the discussion focused; avoids talking too much, with students in a passive role; and avoids side-tracking. While the teacher may initiate the discussion, the interaction needs to revolve around the students, not the teacher. Rephrasing students' questions for them to answer suggests that the teacher has confidence in students' ability to arrive at answers and provides opportunities to develop critical thinking skills. Open-ended questions without one specific answer encourage critical thinking among both students and nurses.

The teacher should also be aware of the environment in which the discussion takes place. For discussions that are held face to face with students, chairs should be arranged in a configuration that encourages interaction, such as a circle, semicircle, or U shape. For some discussions, students may be divided into pairs or other small groups. Exhibit 11.1 summarizes the roles of the teacher and students in clinical discussions.

Guidelines for planning a discussion and effectively using it with students in clinical practice are listed as follows:

- Identify the outcomes and goals to be achieved in the discussion considering the time frame.
- Plan questions for structured discussions ahead of time. They may be written for the teacher only or also for students. If not written, the teacher should think about the questions to ask, their order, and important content to discuss prior to beginning the interaction.
- Plan *how* the discussion will be carried out. Will all students in the clinical group participate, or will they be divided into smaller groups or pairs, then share the results of their individual discussions to the clinical group? Will the discussion be held in the clinical setting or conducted online?
- Sequence questions according to the desired outcomes of the discussion.
- Ask open-ended questions that encourage multiple perspectives and different lines of thinking.
- Think about how the questions are phrased before asking them.

EXHIBIT 11.1

ROLES OF TEACHER AND STUDENT IN DISCUSSION

1. Teacher
   - Plans discussion
   - Presents problem, issue, case for analysis, or asks students to do this
   - Develops questions for discussion
   - Facilitates discussion with students as active participants
   - Develops and maintains atmosphere for open discussion of ideas and issues
   - Monitors time
   - Avoids side-tracking
   - Provides feedback

2. Student
   - Prepares for discussion
   - Participates actively in discussion
   - Works collaboratively with group members to arrive at solutions and decisions
   - Examines different points of view
   - Is willing to modify own view and perspective to reach group consensus
   - Reflects on clinical experiences and simulation
   - Identifies implications for own practice and professional development

3. Teacher and Student
   - Summarize outcomes of discussion and learning
   - Identify implications of discussion for other clinical situations

- Ask questions to the group as a whole or ask for volunteers to respond. If questions are directed to a specific learner, be sensitive to his or her comfort in responding and do not create undue stress for the student. If this occurs, the teacher should provide prompts or cues for responding.
- Wait a few seconds between the question and request for students to answer it during face-to-face interactions.
- Give students time to answer the questions. If no one responds, the teacher should try rephrasing the question.
- Reinforce students' answers, indicating why they were or were not appropriate for the question.
- Give nonverbal and verbal feedback to encourage student participation without overusing it.
- Avoid interrupting the learner, even if errors are noted in the line of thinking or information.
- Correct students' errors in thinking when they are finished answering the question. It is critical that the teacher give feedback to students and correct their errors without belittling them. The goal is to focus on the answer and errors in reasoning, not on the student.
- Listen carefully to students' responses and make notes to remember points made in the discussion. The teacher should tell students ahead of time that any notes are for use only during the discussion, not for student evaluation or other purposes. The notes should be destroyed so students are assured of their freedom to respond in discussions.
- Assess own skill in directing discussions and identify areas for improvement.

Discussions may begin with questions raised by the teacher or by students, or discussions may be integrated with other teaching methods, such as case scenarios, simulations, role-play, and media clips. Case scenarios, for instance, may be critiqued and then discussed by students in a clinical conference, either as part of the clinical practicum or online at a later time. Or students may complete a role-play exercise, followed by discussion. Media clips provide an effective format for presenting a clinical situation for analysis and discussion.

These guidelines also apply to online discussions about clinical practice. Instead of a face-to-face postclinical conference as part of the clinical experience, the conference can be held online at a later time (Berkstresser, 2016). With an online discussion or forum, following the clinical experience, students have time for reflection about the care they provided and their interactions with patients, families, and other providers. Students also have time to gather literature and other resources to analyze their approaches and alternate possibilities, with supporting evidence, before participating in the discussion. Online discussions about clinical practice promote learning by allowing students to view and respond to the thinking of their peers, similar to postconference discussions. It is critical that no information is shared about patients and others in the clinical setting, and students need to be told this prior to beginning the course. An online discussion can refer to "a patient" or "a staff member with whom I interacted." Often these discussions are best carried out using generic phrases such as "a patient with heart failure" to avoid any chance of identifying a patient, provider, setting, or specific case.

The teacher can post higher level questions to begin the discussion and specify when students need to post their answers. Similar to a face-to-face discussion, the teacher's role is to facilitate the discussion with prompts and responses to stimulate further thinking but not to dominate with own comments. Consistent with other discussion forums, there needs to be a set time frame for the discussion, for example, 1 week. With online discussions the teacher can prepare questions to help students relate their learning from class and readings to clinical practice, reflect on their care and interactions, identify other perspectives and approaches, and seek further evidence that is relevant to their patient care. Online discussions may also promote affective learning because students may be more comfortable sharing their feelings and values online than in person. For students who are quiet and are hesitant to participate in face-to-face discussions, online ones may build their confidence.

Purposes of Discussion

In a discussion, the teacher has an opportunity to ask carefully selected questions about students' thinking and the rationale used for arriving at decisions and positions about issues. Discussions promote several types of learning depending on the goals and structure:

- Development of problem-solving, critical thinking, and clinical judgment skills
- Debriefing of clinical experiences and following simulations
- Development of cooperative learning and group process skills
- Assessment of own learning
- Development of oral communication skills

Every discussion will not necessarily promote each of these learning outcomes. The teacher should be clear about the intent of the discussion so it may be geared to the particular outcomes to be achieved. For instance, discussions for critical thinking require carefully selected questions that examine alternative possibilities and "what if" types of questions. This same type of questioning, however, may not be necessary if the goal is to develop cooperative learning or group process skills.

Development of Cognitive Skills

An important purpose of discussion is to promote development of problem-solving, critical thinking, and clinical judgment skills. Discussions are effective because they provide an opportunity for the teacher to gear the questioning toward each of these skills. Not all discussions, though, lead to these higher levels of thinking. The key is the type of questions asked by the teacher or discussed among students—questions need to encourage students to examine alternative perspectives and points of view in a given situation and to provide a rationale for their thinking. Exhibit 11.2 presents strategies for directing discussions toward development of higher level cognitive skills.

In these discussions, students can be given a hypothetical or real clinical situation involving a patient, family, or community to critique and identify potential problems. Students can then discuss possible decisions in that situation, consequences of different options they considered as part of their decision making, and other points of view. Discussions are particularly valuable in helping students analyze ethical dilemmas, consider different points of view, and explore their own values and beliefs.

EXHIBIT 11.2

DISCUSSIONS FOR COGNITIVE SKILL DEVELOPMENT

Ask *students to:*

- Identify problems and issues in a real or hypothetical clinical situation.
- Identify possible alternative problems.
- Assess the problem and clinical situation further.
- Differentiate relevant and irrelevant information for the problem or issue being discussed.
- Discuss their own point of view and others' points of view.
- Examine their own assumptions and those of other students.
- Identify different solutions, courses of action, and consequences of each.
- Consider both positive and negative consequences.
- Compare possible alternatives and defend the choice of one particular solution or action over another.
- Take a position about an issue and provide a rationale both for and against that position.
- Identify their own biases, values, and beliefs that influence their thinking.
- Identify obstacles to solving a problem.
- Evaluate the effectiveness of interventions and approaches to solving problems.

Debriefing of Clinical Experiences

Debriefing is the practice of engaging learners in a reflective discussion after a learning experience (Vihos et al., 2017). While debriefing has been examined most frequently in the context of simulation, postclinical conferences are a form of debriefing. These discussions provide an opportunity for students to report on their clinical learning activities, describe and analyze the care they provided and reflect on their practice. In these discussions, students receive feedback from the teacher and also from peers about their decisions and other possible approaches they could use. Debriefing also provides an opportunity to share feelings about clinical practice and interactions with other health care providers.

Debriefing clinical experiences allows students to share feelings and perceptions about their patients and clinical situations in a comfortable environment. In distance education courses, online discussions are critical to provide a way for students to share their experiences with peers and learn from each other and the teacher.

Debriefing also occurs after a simulation and is a critical component of simulation. In the debriefing discussion, the teacher and students examine and reflect on the experience. Through this reflection, guided by the teacher, students develop their clinical reasoning and judgment skills, gain self-awareness, and transfer knowledge to practice (Dreifuerst, 2012; Dufrene & Young, 2014; International Nursing Association for Clinical Simulation and Learning Standards Committee, 2016). However, for reflection to occur, it is important for teachers to consider the types of questions they ask in debriefing (Husebø, Dieckmann, Rystedt, Søreide, & Friberg, 2013). Typically, the educator focuses the debriefing discussions on the intended learning outcomes and goals of the simulation. Other guidelines for debriefing presented in Chapter 8 are relevant for discussions in clinical conferences.

Development of Cooperative Learning Skills

Group discussions are effective for promoting cooperative learning skills. In cooperative learning, students work in small groups to meet particular learning outcomes related to the course. Students are actively involved in their learning and foster the learning of others in the group.

Discussions using cooperative learning strategies begin with the teacher planning the discussion, presenting a task to be completed by the group or a problem to be solved, developing an environment for open discussion, and facilitating the discussion. Students work cooperatively in groups to propose solutions, complete the task, and present the results of their discussions to the rest of the students. Students can work in pairs and share their thinking with the larger group.

Assessment of Own Learning

Discussions provide a means for students to assess their own learning, identify gaps in their understanding, and learn from others in a nonthreatening environment. Students can ask questions of the group and use the teacher and peers as resources for their learning. If the teacher is effective in developing an atmosphere for open discussion, students, in turn, will share their feelings, concerns, and questions as a beginning to their continued development.

Development of Oral Communication Skills

The ability to present ideas orally, as well as in written form, is an important outcome to be achieved by students in clinical courses. Discussions provide opportunities for students to present ideas to a group, explain concepts clearly, handle questions raised by others, and refine presentation style. Participation in a discussion requires formulating ideas and presenting them logically to the group.

Students may make formal presentations to the clinical group as a way of developing their oral communication skills. They may lead a discussion and present on a specific topic related to the outcomes of the clinical course. Discussion provides an opportunity for peers and the teacher to give feedback to students on how well students communicated their ideas to others and to improve their communication techniques.

Exhibit 11.3 presents an assessment form that students may use to rate the quality of presentations and provide feedback on ability to lead a group discussion. This form is not intended for summative or grading purposes, but instead is designed for giving feedback to students following a presentation to the clinical group.

Level of Questions

The level of questions asked in any discussion is the key to directing it toward the intended learning outcomes. In most clinical discussions, the goal is to avoid a predominance of factual questions and focus instead on higher level and open-ended questions. Teachers can use a framework such as Bloom's taxonomy to sequence questions in a discussion or can level those questions in a more general way, beginning with recall (low level) and progressing through clarifying to critical thinking (high level).

EXHIBIT 11.3

EVALUATION FORM FOR RATING PRESENTATIONS IN CONFERENCES

Name
Title of presentation
Rate each of the behaviors listed in the following. Circle the appropriate number and give feedback to the presenter in the space provided.

Behavior	Rating				
	To a limited extent			To a great extent	
Leadership Role in Conference					
Leads the group in discussion of ideas	1	2	3	4	5
Encourages active participation of peers in conference	1	2	3	4	5
Leadership Role in Conference					
Encourages open discussion of ideas	1	2	3	4	5
Helps group synthesize ideas presented	1	2	3	4	5
Comments:					
Quality of Content Presented					
Prepares objectives for presentation that reflect clinical goals	1	2	3	4	5
Presents content that relates to objectives and is relevant for students' clinical practice	1	2	3	4	5
Presents content that is accurate and up to date	1	2	3	4	5
Presents content that reflects theory and research	1	2	3	4	5
Comments:					
Quality of Presentation					
Organizes and presents material logically	1	2	3	4	5
Explains ideas clearly	1	2	3	4	5
Plans presentation considering time demands, needs of clinical group, and type of conference (face to face vs. online)	1	2	3	4	5
Emphasizes key points	1	2	3	4	5
Encourages students to ask questions and reflect on responses	1	2	3	4	5

(continued)

	Rating				
Behavior	To a limited extent			To a great extent	
Answers students' questions accurately	1	2	3	4	5
Quality of Presentation					
Supports alternative viewpoints and encourages their discussion	1	2	3	4	5
Is enthusiastic	1	2	3	4	5
Comments:					

The taxonomy of the cognitive domain, related to knowledge and intellectual skills, was developed by Bloom, Englehart, Furst, Hill, and Krathwohl (1956) many years ago but is still of value today for developing test items and for leveling questions. Learning in the cognitive domain includes the acquisition of facts and specific information, concepts and theories, and higher level cognitive skills (Oermann & Gaberson, 2017). The original cognitive taxonomy includes six levels that increase in complexity: knowledge, comprehension, application, analysis, synthesis, and evaluation. Because these levels are arranged in a hierarchy, recall of specific facts and information is the least complex level of learning, and evaluating clinical situations and making judgments is the most complex. This taxonomy was updated, and the names for the levels of learning were reworded as verbs (Anderson & Krathwohl, 2001). For example, the "knowledge" level was renamed "remembering," and synthesis and evaluation were reordered. In the updated taxonomy, the highest level of learning is "creating," which is the process of synthesizing elements to form a new product.

The cognitive taxonomy is useful in asking questions in a discussion or planning questions for student response, because it levels them along a continuum from ones requiring only recall of facts to higher level questions requiring judgments and synthesis of knowledge. The teacher may begin by asking students factual questions and then progress to questions that are answered based on students understanding, applying knowledge to clinical practice, analyzing data and clinical situations, making judgments based on criteria and standards (evaluation), and synthesizing material from different sources to create a new plan or product.

A description and sample questions for each of the six levels of the updated cognitive taxonomy follow. Sample words for use in developing questions at each level are presented in Exhibit 11.4.

1. *Remembering:* Recall of facts and specific information; memorization of facts.

   "Define the term asystole."
   "What is an example of a cardiac arrhythmia?"

2. *Understanding:* Interpreting; ability to describe and explain.

   "Tell me about your patient's shortness of breath."
   "What does this potassium level suggest?"

EXHIBIT 11.4

QUESTION CLASSIFICATION

Level	Types of Questions	Sample Words for Questions
1. Remembering (knowledge)	Recall, recognition Questions that can be answered by recall of facts and previously learned information	Define, identify, list, name, select
2. Understanding (comprehension)	Interpret, explain Questions that can be answered by explaining and describing	Describe, differentiate, draw conclusions, explain, give examples of, interpret, tell me in your own words
3. Applying	Use, implement Questions that require use of information in new or unfamiliar situations	Apply, relate, use
4. Analyzing	Divide into component parts Questions that ask student to break down material into its component parts, to analyze data and clinical situations	Analyze, compare, contrast, detect, identify reasons and assumptions, provide evidence to support conclusions, relate
5. Evaluating	Make judgments based on criteria Questions that require student to critique or make a judgment based on criteria and standards	Appraise, assess, compare, critique, evaluate, formulate, judge, plan, produce
6. Creating (synthesis)	Develop new ideas and products Questions that ask students to develop new ideas, plans, products	Construct, create, design, develop, propose a plan, suggest a new approach

3. *Applying:* Use of information in a new or unfamiliar situation; ability to transfer knowledge to a new situation.

"What other interventions might be used for your patient? What evidence supports them?"
"Tell me about your patient's problems and related pathophysiological changes. Why are each of these changes important for you to monitor?"

4. *Analyzing:* Ability to break down material into component parts and identify the relationships among them.

"What are possible reasons for the patient's adverse events following transfer from the neonatal intensive care unit?"
"What assumptions did you make about this family that influenced your decisions? What are alternative approaches to consider?"

5. *Evaluating:* Making judgments about value based on criteria and standards; critiquing.

"Take a position for or against not admitting these patients from the emergency department and keeping them in the observation unit instead. Provide a rationale for your position."

"What is the potential impact on patients with this change in the discharge process?"

6. *Creating:* Ability to develop new ideas and materials; combining elements to form a new product or pattern not there before.

"Tell me about your plan to modify the screening questions used for assessing intimate partner violence. Why will these new questions be better than the existing ones? What is your rationale?"

"Develop guidelines for follow-up care of patients with depression following traumatic injuries."

Questions for discussions should be sequenced from low to high level. Low-level questions about patient care and clinical practice can be answered by recalling specific information and explaining it. High-level questions cannot be answered by memory alone and often have more than one answer. Higher level questions ask students to apply information they have learned to patient care or a clinical scenario, analyze a complex clinical situation, evaluate options and alternatives, and create new plans and approaches.

An example of a progression of questions using the taxonomy follows:

Remembering: "Define the gate control theory of chronic pain."

Understanding: "Explain the physiological mechanisms underlying this theory of pain."

Applying: "Tell me about an intervention you are using for your patient and how its use and effectiveness may be explained by the gate control theory."

Analyzing: "Your patient seems more agitated. What additional data have you collected? What are possible reasons for this response?"

Evaluating: "You indicated that your patient's pain continues to increase. What alternative pain interventions do you propose? Why would these interventions be more effective? Describe the evidence you reviewed on these new approaches you are considering for your patient."

Creating: "Develop a pain management plan for your patient now and for his discharge home."

Often clinical teachers do not ask high-level questions of students. The questions asked of students may focus on recall and comprehension rather than higher levels of thinking. If the intent is to improve thinking and clinical reasoning, this goal will not be met with questions that are answered by memorization of facts and specific information.

CLINICAL CONFERENCES

Clinical conferences are discussions in which students share information about their clinical experiences, engage in thinking about and reflecting on clinical practice, lead others in discussions, and give formal presentations to the group. Some clinical conferences involve other disciplines and provide opportunities to work with other health care professionals in planning and evaluating patient care. Conferences serve the same goals as any discussion: develop problem-solving, critical thinking, and clinical judgment skills; reflect on clinical experiences; assess own learning; and develop oral communication skills. The teacher has an important role in clinical conferences in facilitating discussions that help students understand and search for meaning in their clinical experiences (Megel, Nelson, Black, Vogel, & Uphoff, 2013). Guidelines for conducting clinical conferences are the same as for discussion and therefore are not repeated here.

There are many types of clinical conferences. *Preclinical conferences* are small group discussions that precede clinical learning activities. In preclinical conferences, students ask questions about their clinical learning activities, seek clarification about their patients' care and other aspects of clinical practice, and share concerns with the teacher and with peers. Preclinical conferences assist students in identifying patient problems, setting priorities, and planning care; they prepare students for their clinical activities. An important role of the teacher in preclinical conferences is to ensure that students have the essential knowledge and competencies to complete their clinical activities. In many instances, the teacher needs to instruct students further and fill in the gaps in students' learning. Preclinical conferences may be conducted on a one-to-one basis with students or as a clinical group.

Postclinical conferences are held at the conclusion of clinical learning activities. Postclinical conferences provide a forum for analyzing patient care and exploring other options, thereby facilitating critical thinking. Postclinical conferences may be used for peer review and critiquing each other's work. They are not intended as substitutes for classroom instruction with the teacher lecturing and presenting new content to students. A similar problem often occurs with guest speakers who treat the conference as a class, lecturing to students about their area of expertise rather than encouraging group discussion and student reflection.

Clinical conferences can also focus on ethical and professional issues associated with clinical practice. Conferences of this type encourage critical thinking about issues that students have encountered or may in the future. In these conferences, students can analyze events that occurred in the clinical setting, ones in which they were personally involved or learned about through their clinical experience. A student can present the situation to the group for analysis and discussion. The discussion should focus on varied approaches that might be used and how to decide on the best strategy. "What if" questions are effective for this type of conference.

Students and faculty members alike are often fatigued at the end of the clinical practicum. Rather than each student sharing what he or she did in clinical practice, discussions that focus on higher level learning and thinking and that involve each student may be more effective.

Debates provide a forum for analyzing problems and issues in depth, analyzing opposing viewpoints, and developing and defending a position to be taken. In a debate, students should provide a rationale for their decisions. Debates developed around clinical issues give students an opportunity to prepare an argument for or against a particular position and to take a stand on an issue.

Setting for Clinical Conferences

Clinical conferences can be face to face in the clinical or academic setting, or they can be conducted online. With online conferences after the clinical experience, students have time to reflect on their patient care and what they might have done or said differently. One disadvantage is that they might not remember important events to share with the group for discussion.

SUMMARY

Discussions are an exchange of ideas in a small group format. Discussions provide a forum for students to express ideas, explore feelings associated with their clinical practice, clarify values and ethical dilemmas, and learn to interact in a group format. Over a period of time, students learn to collaborate with peers in working toward solving clinical problems.

The teacher is a resource for students. By asking open-ended questions and supporting learner responses, the teacher encourages students to arrive at their own decisions and to engage in self-assessment about clinical practice. The teacher develops a climate in which students are comfortable discussing concepts and issues without fear that the ideas expressed will affect the teacher's evaluation of their performance and subsequent clinical grade.

Discussions promote several types of learning: developing higher level thinking skills; debriefing clinical experiences; assessing own learning; and developing oral communication skills. Debriefing following simulation is a critical aspect of using simulation in nursing education. These discussions typically focus on the intended goals of the simulations and guide students' reflection of the experience.

The level of questions asked in any discussion is the key to directing it toward the intended learning outcomes. In most clinical discussions, the goal is to avoid a predominance of factual questions and focus instead on clarifying and higher level questions. Questions for student response may be leveled along a continuum from ones requiring only recall of facts to higher-level questions requiring evaluating and creating new products and patterns.

Clinical conferences are discussions in which students analyze patient care and clinical situations, lead others in discussions about clinical practice, present ideas in a group format, and give presentations to the group. Conferences serve the same goals as any discussion.

CNE EXAMINATION TEST BLUEPRINT CORE COMPETENCIES

1. **Facilitate Learning**
    A. Implement a variety of teaching strategies appropriate to
       1. content
       2. setting
       3. learner needs
       4. learning style
       5. desired learner outcomes
       6. method of delivery (e.g., face to face, remote, simulation)

(continued)

    B. Use teaching strategies based on
       1. educational theory
       2. evidence-based practices related to education
    C. Modify teaching strategies and learning experiences based on consideration of learners
       1. cultural background
       2. past clinical experiences
       3. past educational and life experiences
       4. generational groups (i.e., age)
    E. Practice skilled oral and written (including electronic) communication that reflects an awareness of self and relationships with learners (e.g., evaluation, mentorship, and supervision)
    F. Communicate effectively orally and in writing with an ability to convey ideas in a variety of contexts
    G. Model reflective thinking practices, including critical thinking
    H. Create opportunities for learners to develop their own critical thinking skills
    I. Create a positive learning environment that fosters a free exchange of ideas
    N. Use knowledge of evidence-based practice to instruct learners

2. Facilitate Learner Development and Socialization

    D. Create learning environments that facilitate learners' self-reflection, personal goal setting, and socialization to the role of the nurse
    E. Foster the development of learners in these areas
       1. cognitive domain
       2. psychomotor domain
       3. affective domain
    F. Assist learners to engage in thoughtful and constructive self- and peer evaluation

REFERENCES

Anderson, L. W., & Krathwohl, D. R. (Eds.). (2001). *A taxonomy for learning, teaching, and assessing: A revision of boom's taxonomy of educational objectives.* New York, NY: Longman.

Berkstresser, K. (2016). The use of online discussions for post-clinical conference. *Nurse Education in Practice, 16*(1), 27–32. doi:10.1016/j.nepr.2015.06.007

Bloom, B. S., Englehart, M. D., Furst, E. J., Hill, W. H., & Krathwohl, D. R. (1956). *Taxonomy of educational objectives. The classification of educational goals. Handbook I: Cognitive domain.* White Plains, NY: Longman.

Dreifuerst, K. T. (2012). Using debriefing for meaningful learning to foster development of clinical reasoning in simulation. *Journal of Nursing Education, 51,* 326–333. doi:10.3928/01484834-20120409-02

Dufrene, C., & Young, A. (2014). Successful debriefing—Best methods to achieve positive learning outcomes: A literature review. *Nurse Education Today, 34*(3), 372–376. doi:10.1016/j.nedt.2013.06.026

Husebø, S. E., Dieckmann, P., Rystedt, H., Søreide, E., & Friberg, F. (2013). The relationship between facilitators' questions and the level of reflection in postsimulation debriefing. *Simulation in Health care, 8*(3), 135–142. doi:10.1097/SIH.0b013e31827cbb5c

International Nursing Association for Clinical Simulation and Learning Standards Committee. (2016). INACSL standards of best practice: Simulation^SM simulation design. *Clinical Simulation in Nursing, 12,* S5–S12. doi:10.1016/j.ecns.2016.09.005

Megel, M. E., Nelson, A. E., Black, J., Vogel, J., & Uphoff, M. (2013). A comparison of student and faculty perceptions of clinical post-conference learning environment. *Nurse Education Today, 33,* 525–529. doi:10.1016/j.nedt.2011.11.021

Oermann, M. H., & Gaberson, K. B. (2017). *Evaluation and testing in nursing education* (5th ed.). New York, NY: Springer Publishing.

Vihos, J., Pollard, L., Bazin, M., Lozza, D., MacDonald, P., Moniz, N., & Spies, D. (2017). Debriefing in laboratory experiences: A quality improvement project. *Nurse Educator.* Advance online publication. doi:10.1097/nne.0000000000000367

Using Preceptors as Clinical Teachers and Coaches

As discussed earlier, the preceptor teaching model is an alternative to the traditional clinical teaching model. It is based on the assumption that a consistent one-to-one relationship between an experienced nurse and a nursing student or novice staff nurse is an effective way to provide individualized guidance in clinical learning as well as opportunities for professional socialization (O'Connor, 2015). Preceptorships have been used extensively with senior nursing students, graduate students preparing for advanced practice roles, and new staff nurse orientees, but they can be used with any level of nursing students (Gubrud, 2016). This chapter discusses the effective use of preceptors as clinical teachers and coaches. The advantages and disadvantages of preceptorships are examined, and suggestions are made for selecting, preparing, evaluating, and rewarding preceptors.

PRECEPTORSHIP MODEL OF CLINICAL TEACHING

A preceptorship is a time-limited, one-to-one relationship between a learner and an experienced nurse who is employed by the health care agency in which the learning activities take place. The clinical teacher may not be physically present during the learning activities; the preceptor provides intensive, individualized learning opportunities that improve the learner's clinical competence and confidence. Regardless of learners' levels of education and experience, preceptorships provide opportunities for socialization into professional nursing roles. They also enhance the personal and professional development of the preceptors (McClure & Black, 2013; Raines, 2012).

The preceptor model is collaborative. The teacher is a faculty member or educator who has overall responsibility for the quality of the clinical teaching and learning. The teacher provides the link between the educational program and the practice setting by selecting and preparing preceptors, assigning students to preceptors, providing guidance for the selection of appropriate learning activities, serving as a resource to the preceptor–student pair, and evaluating student and preceptor performance. The preceptor functions as a role model and provides individualized clinical instruction, coaching, support, and socialization for the learner. The preceptor also participates in evaluation of learner performance, although the teacher has ultimate responsibility for summative evaluation decisions (Ingwerson, 2014; Klein & Ingwerson, 2011; McClure & Black, 2013).

USE OF PRECEPTORSHIPS IN NURSING EDUCATION

In academic programs that prepare nurses for initial entry into practice, preceptorships are usually used for students in their last semester, but providing preceptors for beginning students may have even greater benefits. Beginning students may gain from the individual attention of the preceptor and from assignments that help them to expand their basic skills, develop independence, and improve their self-confidence.

Preceptorships are frequently used in graduate programs that prepare nurses for advanced clinical practice, administration, and education roles. At this level, a preceptorship involves well-defined learning objectives based on the student's past clinical, administrative, and teaching experience. The student observes and participates in learning activities that demonstrate functional role components, allowing rehearsal of role behaviors before actually assuming an advanced practice, administrative, or teaching role. The preceptor must be an expert practitioner who can model the role functions of advanced practice nurses, including decision making, problem solving, leadership, teaching, and scholarship.

In many health care organizations, preceptors participate in the orientation of newly hired staff nurses. Preceptors in these settings act as role models for new staff nurses and support them in their transition into professional practice or socialization into new roles. Preceptors work individually with new staff nurses, but there is wide variation in the scope of the preceptor role. In some settings, the preceptor is a more experienced peer who works side by side with the orientee; in other settings, the preceptor role is more formally that of clinical teacher.

Research findings on the effectiveness of the preceptor teaching model are varied. Generally, studies indicate positive outcomes of students and new staff nurses working with preceptors. Some early studies showed no difference in student performance between students assigned to preceptors and those who were taught according to a traditional clinical teaching model. Some investigators presented anecdotal evidence from preceptors, teachers, and students that preceptorships enhanced student performance. Students who are assigned to preceptors are generally satisfied with the experience because they develop their confidence and independence. However, students may also experience communication and interpersonal problems with their preceptors, and, if these conflicts are not resolved successfully, negative outcomes can result (Killam & Heerschap, 2013). The decision to use preceptors for clinical teaching should be based on the perceived benefits to students, the educational program, and the clinical staff members after a careful evaluation of the potential advantages and disadvantages.

ADVANTAGES AND DISADVANTAGES OF USING PRECEPTORS

The use of preceptors in clinical teaching has both advantages and disadvantages for the involved parties. Effective collaboration is required to minimize the drawbacks and achieve advantages for the educational program, clinical agency, teachers, preceptors, and students.

Preceptorships hold many potential advantages for preceptors and the clinical agencies that employ them. The presence of students in the clinical environment tends to enhance the professional development, leadership, and teaching skills of preceptors. While preceptors enjoy sharing their clinical knowledge and skill, they also appreciate the stimulation of working with students who challenge the status quo and raise questions about clinical practice. The interest and enthusiasm of students is often rewarding to nurses who take on the additional responsibilities of the preceptor role. Students may assist preceptors with research or teaching projects. In agencies that use a clinical ladder, serving as a preceptor may be a means of advancing professionally within the system. The preceptorship model also produces opportunities to recruit potential staff members for the agency from among students who work with preceptors.

The greatest drawback of preceptorships to agencies and preceptors is usually the expected time commitment. Some clinical agencies may not agree to provide preceptors because of increased patient acuity and decreased staff levels, or potential preceptors may decline to participate because of the perception that to do so would add to their workloads. Because of current economic conditions, health care agencies seeking to decrease costs and increase efficiency often make changes in nurses' working conditions, such as increased workloads, decreased number of work hours, decreasing numbers of full-time and increasing numbers of part-time and casual employees, and increased use of technology. These organizational changes do not often facilitate adding the preceptor role to a registered nurse's workload (Gardner & Suplee, 2010). Increased workload, decreased productivity, lack of additional compensation, limited resources, and lack of preparation for teaching are some of the reasons for nurses declining to precept nursing students (Logan, Kovacs, & Barry, 2015).

Students who participate in preceptorships enjoy a number of benefits. They have the advantage of working one-on-one with experts who can coach them to increased clinical competence and performance. Preceptorships also provide opportunities for students to experience the realities of clinical practice, including scheduling learning activities on evening and night shifts and weekends in order to follow their preceptors' schedules. However, following their preceptors' schedules often creates conflicts with students' academic, work, and family commitments. Additionally, a preceptor's patient assignment may not be always appropriate for a student's clinical learning objectives.

Preceptorships offer many advantages for the educational program in which they are used. The use of preceptors provides more clinical teachers for students and thus more intensive, individualized guidance of students' learning activities. Results of one study (Hendricks, Wallace, Narwold, Guy, & Wallace, 2013) comparing preceptored and traditional clinical learning placements for undergraduate prelicensure students showed significantly more clinical practice opportunities for teaching and counseling patients, receiving reports about patients, taking vital signs, documenting care, urinary catheterization, physical assessment, and administration of oral and intravenous medications. However, there were no differences in cognitive performance among students in the two groups. Working collaboratively with preceptors also helps faculty members to stay informed about the current realities of practice; up-to-date clinical information benefits ongoing curriculum development.

Several disadvantages related to the use of preceptors may affect educational programs. Contrary to a common belief, teachers' responsibilities do not decrease when students work with preceptors. Initial selection of preceptors, preparation of preceptors and students, and ongoing collaboration and communication with preceptors and students require as much time or more as the traditional clinical teaching model. The preceptorship model requires considerable indirect teaching time for the development of relationships with agencies and preceptors and the evaluation of preceptors and students. When preceptors are used as clinical teachers, faculty members may be responsible for more students in several clinical agencies and feel uncertain whether students are learning the application of theory and research findings to practice.

SELECTING PRECEPTORS

The success of preceptorships largely depends on the selection of appropriate preceptors; such selection is one of the teacher's most important responsibilities. Most faculty members consider the educational preparation of the preceptor to be important; most academic programs require the preceptor to have at least the degree for which the student is preparing, although insistence on this level of educational preparation does not guarantee that learners will be exposed only to professional role models.

The desire to teach and willingness to serve as a preceptor are important qualities of potential preceptors. Nurses who feel obligated to enact this role may not make enthusiastic, effective preceptors. Additional attributes of effective preceptors, according to Gardner and Suplee (2010), include:

- *Clinical expertise or proficiency, depending on the level of the learner.* Preceptors should be able to demonstrate expert psychomotor, problem-solving, critical thinking, clinical reasoning, and decision-making skills in their clinical practice. Nursing students and new staff nurses need preceptors who are at least proficient clinicians; graduate students need preceptors who are expert clinicians, administrators, or educators, depending on the goals of the preceptorship.
- *Leadership abilities.* Good preceptors are change agents in the health care organizations in which they are employed. They demonstrate effective communication skills and are trusted and respected by their peers.
- *Teaching skill.* Preceptors must understand and use principles of adult learning. They should be able to communicate ideas effectively to learners and give descriptive positive and negative feedback.
- *Professional role behaviors and attitudes.* Because preceptors act as role models for learners, they must demonstrate behaviors that represent important professional values. They are accountable for their actions and accept responsibility for their decisions. Good preceptors demonstrate maturity and self-confidence; their approach to learners is nonthreatening and nonjudgmental. They welcome questions from learners and do not interpret them as criticisms or judgments about the practice setting or care approach. Flexibility, open-mindedness, enthusiasm about working with students, willingness to work with a diverse population of learners, and a sense of humor are additional attributes of effective preceptors.

The selection of preceptor and setting should also take into account the learner's interest in a specific clinical specialty as well as the need for development of particular skills. The teacher may collaborate with nurse managers to select appropriate preceptors. It is wise not to choose preceptors from newly established units or those with recent high staff turnover.

Potential preceptors for nursing students may be found in any clinical setting that meets the requirements of the nursing education program. The staff development or education department is a good first contact with an agency; some agencies ask that all requests for preceptors for nursing students be directed to a specified staff member who can suggest appropriate matches. Students may be able to suggest good potential preceptors from their work experience as nursing assistants or other unlicensed assistive personnel or from their contacts with nursing staff members in their previous clinical learning experiences. Alumni of the nursing education program are a rich source of potential preceptors; many of them would like to give back to their alma mater and are flattered to be asked to preceptor students. They can be recruited at alumni association gatherings, by telephone or email, via professional social media groups, or through an alumni newsletter.

Clinical teachers should carefully screen and select preceptors to ensure that the preceptor complies with program requirements and state board of nursing regulations. Some state boards specify essential preceptor qualifications such as degree requirements, previous work experience, and type of work (Lewallen, DeBrew, & Stump, 2014). Graduate programs need to ensure that preceptors have the appropriate advanced nursing experience and qualifications. Nursing programs offering distance education delivery and are now reaching previously untapped student populations in remote settings face added challenges when planning preceptor experiences. These online programs may need to work with boards of nursing to ensure compliance with appropriate approval processes. When students are working with preceptors at remote or distant sites the board of nursing in those states will need to be are aware of clinical experiences occurring in their jurisdiction and the program must comply with any approval regulations (Lowery & Spector, 2014). The preceptor will need an unencumbered nursing license in the state that patients are located; however, clinical teachers are advised to contact the state board as requirements vary from state to state. Some boards charge an approval processing fee (as much as $750) and some programs may be asked to provide preceptor résumés and proof of preceptor nursing licenses in advance, sometimes as early as a year before the experience (Gormley & Glazer, 2012). It is important to identify possible preceptors early so that appropriate screening can occur and programs can ensure compliance with all regulations are complete before the clinical experience begins. Offering appropriate incentives and rewards to preceptors acknowledges the value of the preceptor's time and effort and can be an effective recruiting tool at a time when employee benefits may be diminishing. A more complete discussion of rewards for preceptors is included later in this chapter. Working with preceptors at clinical sites, particularly those at distant locations or involving advanced practice programs, can be challenging. Developing partnerships with preceptors may be an effective approach to ensure that qualified and adequately prepared preceptors are available for students. Clinical teachers can work closely with the clinical site preceptors to understand the unique aspects of the clinical site, and population served, and ensure that clinical placements align with student needs (Distler, 2015).

PREPARING THE PARTICIPANTS

Thorough preparation of preceptors and students for their roles is key to the success of preceptorships. Teachers are responsible for initial orientation and continuing support of all participants; preparation can be formal or informal.

Preceptor Preparation

Preparation of preceptors may begin with a general orientation, possibly for groups of potential preceptors at the selected agency or for all preceptors working with students from one nursing education program. A preceptorship preparation program acknowledges the need for and commitment to collaboration in nursing education. This preparation supports the learning needs of preceptors enabling them to enact their role effectively and confidently and it may also help to prevent problems (McClure & Black, 2013).

Content of a preceptorship preparation program may include the following information:

- Benefits and challenges of precepting
- Characteristics of a good preceptor
- Facilitating learning
- Principles of adult learning
- Assessment of learner needs
- Communication and conflict resolution
- Clinical teaching methods, including motivating and challenging learners, dealing with difficult learning situations, and when to use coaching techniques
- Evaluation of learning, including how to give effective feedback and use of clinical evaluation tools
- Preceptor's role in developing and implementing an individualized learning contract, if used
- Course and faculty expectations
- Academic program curriculum structure, framework, and goals (McClure & Black, 2013; Raines, 2012)

After preceptors have been selected, they need a specific orientation to their responsibilities. This orientation may take the form of a face-to-face or telephone conference with the teacher. Technology-supported orientation programs using online learning modules or podcasts offer flexibility as well as can be used to provide ongoing support (Blum, 2014; Krampe, L'Ecuyer, & Palmer, 2013). Written guidelines may also be used to supplement the conference. Exhibit 12.1 is an example of written guidelines for preceptors of graduate nursing students. The conference and written guidelines may include information such as:

- *The educational level and previous experience of the student.* Graduate students need learning activities that build on their previous learning and experience in order to produce advanced practice outcomes. Beginning students may not have developed the knowledge and skill to participate in all of the preceptor's activities. Preceptors will find it helpful to understand what courses and content students previously completed so the preceptor can develop realistic performance expectations and select appropriate learning experiences.

- *How to choose specific learning activities based on learning objectives.* The teacher may share samples of learning contracts or lists of learning activities to guide the preceptor's selection of appropriate activities for the student.

- *Scheduling of clinical learning activities.* A common feature of preceptorships is the scheduling of the student's learning activities according to the preceptor's work schedule. Preceptors should be advised of dates on which students and teachers may not be available because of school holidays, examinations, and other course requirements.
- *Contacts.* How and under what circumstances to contact the course faculty member.

New preceptors have learning needs much like those of students and new staff nurses; supportive role models and coaching are essential to success.

Student Preparation

Learners also need to understand the purposes and process of the preceptorship. They need an orientation to the process of planning individual learning activities, an explanation of teacher and preceptor roles, and a review of unit policies specific to student practice. At the beginning of the preceptorship, teachers should clarify evaluation responsibilities and expectations such as dates for learning contract approval, site visits, and conferences with faculty members.

IMPLEMENTATION

Successful implementation of preceptorships depends on mutual understanding of the roles and responsibilities of the participants. The teacher, student, and preceptor collaborate to plan and implement learning activities that will facilitate the student's goal attainment. Key to these processes is frequent, clear, effective communication among the participants.

EXHIBIT 12.1

SAMPLE GUIDELINES FOR A PRECEPTOR OF A GRADUATE NURSING STUDENT

The preceptor is expected to:

- Facilitate the student's entry into the health care organization
- Provide the student with an orientation to the organization and nursing unit
- After receiving the student's goals for the practicum, provide suggestions for how these goals can be accomplished
- Assist the student to identify activities that are consistent with organizational needs and the student's interests, abilities, and learning needs
- Meet with the student at regular intervals to discuss progress and achievement of individual and course objectives
- Provide the student with regular feedback regarding his or her performance
- Communicate regularly with the faculty member regarding the student's progress
- Serve as a role model and facilitate learning opportunities
- At the end of the preceptorship, provide a written evaluation of the student's performance related to goal achievement, clinical knowledge and skill, problem-solving and decision-making skills, communication and presentation skills, and interpersonal skills.

Roles and Responsibilities of Participants

Preceptors

Preceptors are responsible for patient care in addition to clinical teaching of the student. The preceptor is expected to be a positive role model and a resource person for the student. The clinical teaching responsibilities of the preceptor include creating a positive learning climate, including the student in activities that relate to learning goals, and providing feedback to the student and teacher.

Role-model behaviors important for preceptors to demonstrate can be classified into four categories:

- Technical and technology skills—demonstrates nursing care procedures; operation of equipment unique to that clinical setting; use of the electronic health record, and evidence based, current nursing practices
- Interpersonal skills—uses effective communication techniques with patients and family members; interacts with physicians and other health care providers in a collegial, confident manner; displays appropriate use of humor; demonstrates caring attitude toward patients; gives constructive feedback; use questioning techniques
- Clinical reasoning—listens carefully during change-of-shift reports and patient hand-overs and asks pertinent questions about patients' conditions; demonstrates proficient problem solving, critical thinking, clinical reasoning, and incorporates skills of noticing, interpreting, responding, and reflecting as part of clinical decision making (Koharchik, Culleiton, Caputi, & Robb, 2015)
- Professional role behaviors—identifies self to patients at first contact, keeps patient information confidential, encourages discussion of ethical issues, demonstrates enthusiasm about nursing, demonstrates accountability for own actions

Sometimes preceptors experience conflict between the educator and evaluator roles, especially when precepting new staff members. If the learner is unable to perform according to expectations, the faculty member or staff development instructor must be notified so that a plan for correcting the deficiencies may be established.

When preceptors perceive that a student is unable to perform patient care tasks appropriately, they are often tempted to step in and take over by demonstrating the proper technique to the learner. This inclination may be due to the preceptor's concurrent responsibility of a patient care assignment and a genuine desire to share clinical knowledge and skill with the student. However, doing so interferes with both the student's and the patient's perceptions of the student as an "authentic care provider" (Gardner & Suplee, 2010, p. 89).

To support students as they learn to care for patients, preceptors should use a coaching process. In sports, coaches stand on the sidelines; they do not participate in or interfere with the game unless there is a risk of injury (e.g., the soccer coach who sees lightening on the horizon interrupts the game by getting the referee's attention to stop play and clear the field). A good preceptor, using coaching techniques, allows the learner to be in control of the patient situation and stands nearby, monitoring the unfolding situation, offering verbal cues when needed, asking questions to guide the student's problem solving, offering encouragement (e.g., "that's right," "keep going"), and then giving immediate feedback for the student to reflect on (Shellenbarger &

Robb, 2016). The coach's expression of belief in the student's capacity to succeed helps the student develop self-efficacy and self-confidence. Thus, effective coaching can help students feel more confident in their clinical abilities and see themselves as authentic care providers. However, if a student "freezes" because of overwhelming anxiety, an error, inadequate preparation, or an unexpected occurrence, the preceptor may need to intervene if this places the patient at risk. The preceptor may need to temporarily assume responsibility for the task the student was attempting to perform, beginning or taking the next step of the task, and then encouraging the student to continue while continuing to coach from the sidelines.

Students

The student is expected to actively participate in planning his or her own learning activities. Planning may take the form of a learning contract that specifies individualized objectives and clinical learning activities. Because the teacher is not always present during learning activities, the student must communicate frequently with the teacher. Communication may take many forms such as a written reflective journal or an electronic discussion. Written assignments allow students to share experiences with the teacher on a regular basis throughout the semester. The pervasiveness and accessibility of mobile technology allow immediate access to faculty during clinical time. The student must notify the teacher immediately of any problems encountered in the implementation of the preceptorship. Students may experience problems or conflict during their preceptor experiences yet may not report conflict for several reasons: They perceive that they are expected to fit in to the practice setting with minimal disruption. Or, they feel powerless and dependent upon the preceptor's evaluation to complete the clinical practicum successfully. The student's responsibilities also include self-evaluation and evaluation of the preceptor's teaching effectiveness, as will be discussed later in this chapter.

Teachers

As previously discussed, the teacher is responsible for making preceptor selections, pairing students with preceptors, and orienting preceptors and students. Conducting a site visit at the agency prior to student arrival may be helpful for teachers to learn about the patient population served, establish a relationship with the nursing staff, and provide an overview and/or orientation to the program and explain clinical expectations. The teacher is an important resource to preceptors and students to assist in problem solving. The teacher must be alert to any sign of conflict in the student–preceptor relationship and promptly take a proactive role in resolving it. If a conflict cannot be resolved to the satisfaction of student, preceptor, and faculty member, the student's well-being should take precedence, and, if necessary, the student should be reassigned.

Teacher availability is particularly important if a problem arises at the clinical site that the preceptor and student cannot resolve. The teacher must make arrangements for consultation via telephone, email, text messaging, or electronic conferencing. The teacher also arranges individual and group conferences with students and preceptors and visits the clinical sites as needed or requested by any of the participants. During a clinical site visit, the teacher may observe student performance and ask questions of both the preceptor and the student. If problems are identified, the teacher may need to work collaboratively to strategize resolutions. However, teachers may need to initiate remediation plans if potentially unsafe practices are identified (Ingwerson, 2014). Close monitoring by the preceptor and/or faculty may be necessary to ensure patient and student safety is maintained. If students submit reflective journal entries, the teacher responds to them with feedback that helps students to evaluate their progress. Teachers have the responsibility to gather input from the preceptor about the student performance and use that as part of the student's overall evaluation of learner performance. Faculty should also gather input from the student about the effectiveness of the preceptor and the opportunities for learning at the clinical facility.

Planning and Implementing Learning Activities

A common strategy for planning and implementing students' learning activities in the preceptorship model of clinical teaching is the use of an individualized learning contract. A learning contract is an explicit agreement between a teacher and student that clarifies expectations of each participant in the teaching–learning process. It specifies the learning goals that have been established, the learning activities selected to meet the objectives, and the expected outcomes and criteria by which they will be evaluated. In a preceptorship, the learning contract is negotiated among the teacher, student, and preceptor and guides the planning and implementation of the student's learning activities. Even though the learning contract is individualized to meet student and agency needs, it needs to be consistent with course learning outcomes. Exhibit 12.2 is an example of a learning contract format that could be adapted for any level of learner.

As discussed previously, effective communication among the preceptor, student, and teacher is critical to the success of the preceptorship. Communication between teacher and student may be facilitated by the student keeping a reflective journal and sharing it with the teacher on a regular basis. In the journal, the student describes and analyzes learning activities that relate to the objective, reflecting on the meaning and value of the experiences. Journals provide an opportunity for students to review and record their thoughts, impressions, and reactions. They can also assist students to understand and clarify clinical situations, link clinical learning to theory, and examine their thinking and actions while helping to keep the teacher informed of the learning experiences. The journal entries may be recorded in a computer file, on paper, on audiotape, or posted to an online discussion board; the teacher responds via the same medium. Additionally, the student and teacher have telephone, e-mail, or face-to-face contact as necessary for the teacher to give consultation and guidance. Similarly, the teacher and preceptor should have regular contact by telephone, email, text messaging, or face-to-face meetings so that the teacher receives feedback about learner performance and offers guidance and consultation as needed. Results of one study of clinicians who precepted nurse practitioner graduate students from one university (Brooks & Niederhauser, 2010) showed that the majority of preceptors expected two site visits from the students' teachers per semester and that the first site visit should occur in the first 4 weeks of the semester. Preceptors also expected teachers to observe at least two patient encounters per student, suggesting that they wanted the site visits to be more substantive than social.

The realities of clinical and academic cultures present challenges to effective communication among teacher, preceptor, and student. Preceptors often work a variety of shifts, students often have complicated academic and work schedules, and teachers have multiple responsibilities in addition to clinical teaching. Flexibility and commitment to establishing and maintaining communication are essential to overcome these challenges.

EXHIBIT 12.2

LEARNING CONTRACT TEMPLATE

Student Information
    Name and credentials:
    Address:
    Home phone number:
    Mobile phone number:
    email address:

Teacher Information
    Name and credentials:
    Address:
    Office phone number:
    Mobile phone number:
    email address:

Preceptor Information
    Name and credentials:
    Address:
    Office phone number:
    Mobile phone number:
    email address:

Clinical Learning Objectives	Learning Activities and Resources	Evaluation Evidence, Responsibility, and Time Frame

Start date: Completion date:
    Student Signature _____   Date _____
    Preceptor Signature _____   Date _____
    Teacher Signature _____   Date _____

EVALUATING THE OUTCOMES

Students, teachers, and preceptors share responsibility for monitoring the progress of learning and for evaluating outcomes of the preceptorship. Student performance may be evaluated according to the terms specified in the learning contract or through the clinical evaluation methods used by the educational program. Throughout the clinical experiences students should be encouraged to self-assess their performance to identify strengths and areas needing ongoing improvement (Oermann & Gaberson, 2017). If a learning contract is used, student self-evaluation is usually an important strategy for assessing outcomes. As discussed earlier, preceptors are expected to give feedback to the learner and to the teacher, but the teacher has the responsibility for the summative evaluation of learner performance.

An important aspect of evaluation concerns the teaching effectiveness of preceptors. Students are an important source of information about the quality of their preceptors' clinical teaching, but the teacher should also assess the degree to which preceptors were able to effectively guide the students' learning. A modified form of a teaching effectiveness tool used to evaluate clinical teachers may be used to collect data from students regarding their preceptors. Exhibit 12.3 is an example of a form for student evaluation of preceptor teaching effectiveness. Because each preceptor is typically assigned to one student at a time, it is usually impossible to maintain anonymity of student evaluations. Therefore, teachers may wish to share a summary of the student's evaluation, instead of the raw data, with the preceptor.

REWARDING PRECEPTORS

Preceptors make valuable contributions to nursing education programs, and they should receive appropriate rewards and incentives for their participation. At minimum, every preceptor should receive an individualized thank-you letter, specifying some of the benefits that the student received from the preceptorship. A copy of the letter may be sent to the preceptor's supervisor or manager to be used as evidence of clinical excellence at the time of the preceptor's next performance evaluation. Many preceptors prefer nonmaterial rewards such as lighter workloads and support from managers and teachers; however, teachers may not be able to provide all these things as a reward and may use other methods of demonstrating appreciation (Kalischuk, Vendenberg, & Awosoga, 2013).

EXHIBIT 12.3

SAMPLE TOOL FOR STUDENT EVALUATION OF PRECEPTOR TEACHING EFFECTIVENESS

Directions: Rate the extent to which each statement describes your preceptor's teaching behaviors by circling a number following each item, using the following scale:

    4 = to a large extent
    3 = to a moderate extent
    2 = to a small extent
    1 = not at all

1. The preceptor was an excellent professional role model.	4	3	2	1
2. The preceptor guided my clinical problem solving.	4	3	2	1
3. The preceptor helped me to apply theory to clinical practice.	4	3	2	1
4. The preceptor was responsive to my individual learning needs.	4	3	2	1
5. The preceptor provided constructive feedback about my performance.	4	3	2	1
6. The preceptor communicated clearly and effectively.	4	3	2	1
7. The preceptor encouraged my independence.	4	3	2	1
8. The preceptor was flexible and open-minded.	4	3	2	1
9. Overall, the preceptor was an excellent clinical teacher.	4	3	2	1
10. I would recommend this preceptor for other students.	4	3	2	1

Other formal and informal ways of acknowledging the contributions of preceptors for nursing students are:

- A name badge or pin that identifies the nurse as a preceptor
- A certificate of appreciation, signed by the administrator of the nursing education program or the staff development program
- An annual preceptor recognition event, including refreshments and an inspirational speaker
- Free or reduced-price registration for continuing education programs offered by the nursing education program or clinical facility (Andresen & Levin, 2014)
- Documentation of hours for certification renewals
- Free or reduced-rate tuition for one or more academic courses or the opportunity to audit a nursing course
- A free meal
- Campus guest privileges such as library access
- Adjunct or affiliate faculty appointment
- Differential pay or adjustment of work schedule (e.g., exemption from weekend shifts) nomination of preceptors for awards, providing letters of reference, and collaborating on research projects
- A small gift such as a fruit basket, plant, or gift certificate

SUMMARY

The use of preceptors is an alternative to the traditional clinical teaching model based on the assumption that a consistent relationship between an experienced nurse and a nursing student or novice staff nurse is an effective way to provide individualized guidance in clinical learning and professional socialization. Preceptorships have been used extensively with senior nursing students, graduate students preparing for advanced practice roles, and new staff nurse orientees.

A preceptorship is a time-limited, one-to-one relationship between a learner and an experienced nurse. The teacher may not be physically present during the learning activities; the preceptor provides intensive, individualized learning opportunities that improve the learner's clinical competence and confidence. The teacher has overall responsibility for the quality of the clinical teaching and learning and provides the link between the educational program and the practice setting. The preceptor functions as a role model and provides individualized clinical instruction, coaching, support, and socialization for the learner.

Preceptorships are frequently used for students in their last semester of academic preparation for entry into practice and for graduate students preparing for advanced clinical practice, administration, and education roles.

The use of preceptors in clinical teaching has both advantages and disadvantages for the educational program, clinical agency, teachers, preceptors, and students. Benefits for preceptors and their employers include the stimulation of working with learners who raise questions about clinical practice, assistance from students with research or teaching projects, rewards through a clinical ladder system for participation as a preceptor, and opportunities to recruit potential staff members for the agency from among students who work with preceptors. The greatest drawback of preceptorships to agencies and preceptors is usually the expected time commitment.

Students experience the benefits of working one-on-one with clinical experts who can coach them to improved performance as well as opportunities to experience the realities of clinical practice. However, following their preceptors' schedules often creates conflicts with students' academic, work, and family commitments.

Preceptorships offer many advantages to teachers and educational programs. The use of preceptors provides more clinical teachers for students and thus more intensive guidance of students' learning activities. Working collaboratively with preceptors also helps teachers to stay informed about the current realities of practice. Disadvantages include the amount of indirect teaching time required to select, prepare, and communicate with preceptors and students.

Selection of appropriate preceptors is important to the success of preceptorships. Most academic programs require the preceptor to have at least the degree for which the student is preparing. Desire to teach and willingness to serve as a preceptor are very important qualities of potential preceptors. Additional attributes of effective preceptors include clinical expertise or proficiency, leadership abilities, teaching skill, and professional role behaviors and attitudes.

Teachers are responsible for the initial orientation and continuing support of all participants; preparation can be formal or informal. A general orientation for potential preceptors may include information about benefits and challenges of precepting, characteristics of a good preceptor, principles of adult learning, clinical teaching and coaching techniques, evaluation methods, and the structure and goals of the nursing education program. After preceptors have been selected, they need a specific orientation to their responsibilities, including information about the student's educational level and previous experience, choosing specific learning activities based on learning objectives, and scheduling of clinical learning activities. Learners also need an orientation that includes information about the purposes of the preceptorship, the process of planning individual learning activities, and an explanation of teacher and preceptor roles.

Successful implementation of preceptorships depends on mutual understanding of the roles and responsibilities of the participants. The preceptor is expected to be a positive role model and a resource person for the student. The responsibilities of the preceptor include creating a positive learning climate, including the student in activities that relate to learning goals, and providing feedback to the student and teacher. The student usually arranges the schedule of clinical learning activities to coincide with the preceptor's work schedule and is expected to participate actively in planning learning activities. Because the teacher is not always present during learning activities, the student must keep the teacher informed about progress through frequent communication. In addition to making preceptor selections and orienting preceptors and students, the teacher is an important resource to preceptors and students to assist in problem solving. Teachers must make adequate arrangements for communication with participants.

A common strategy for planning and implementing students' learning activities is the use of an individualized learning contract—an explicit agreement between the teacher, student, and preceptor that specifies the learning goals, learning activities selected to meet the objectives, and the expected outcomes and criteria by which they will be evaluated. The learning contract guides the planning and implementation of the student's learning activities.

Students, teachers, and preceptors share responsibility for monitoring the progress of learning and for evaluating outcomes of the preceptorship. Student performance is assessed according to the terms specified in the learning contract or through the clinical evaluation methods used by the educational program, through self-evaluation, and through feedback from preceptors. The teacher is responsible for the summative evaluation of learner performance. Students are an important source of information about their preceptors' clinical teaching effectiveness, but the teacher should also assess the degree to which preceptors were able to effectively guide students' learning.

Preceptors should receive appropriate rewards and incentives for the contributions they make to the educational program. At minimum, every preceptor should receive an individualized thank-you letter, specifying some of the benefits that the student received from the preceptorship. Other formal and informal ways of acknowledging the contributions of preceptors were discussed.

CNE EXAMINATION TEST BLUEPRINT CORE COMPETENCIES

1. **Facilitate Learning**
   A. Implement a variety of teaching strategies appropriate to
      1. content
      2. setting
      3. learner needs
      4. desired learner outcomes
   B. Use teaching strategies based on
      1. educational theory
      2. evidence-based practices related to education
   E. Practice skilled oral and written (including electronic) communication that reflects an awareness of self and relationships with learners (e.g., evaluation, mentorship, and supervision)
   F. Communicate effectively orally and in writing with an ability to convey ideas in a variety of contexts
   H. Create opportunities for learners to develop their own critical thinking skills
   I. Create a positive learning environment that fosters a free exchange of ideas
   N. Use knowledge of evidence-based practice to instruct learners

2. **Facilitate Learner Development and Socialization**
   E. Foster the development of learners in these areas
      1. cognitive domain
      2. psychomotor domain
      3. affective domain
   F. Assist learners to engage in thoughtful and constructive self- and peer evaluation

3. **Use Assessment and Evaluation Strategies**
   C. Use a variety of strategies to assess and evaluate learning in these domains
      1. cognitive
      2. psychomotor
      3. affective
   J. Use assessment and evaluation data to enhance the teaching–learning process
   K. Advise learners regarding assessment and evaluation criteria
   L. Provide timely, constructive, and thoughtful feedback

REFERENCES

Andresen, K., & Levin, P. (2014). Enhancing quantity and quality of clinical experiences in a baccalaureate nursing program. *International Journal of Nursing Scholarship, 11*(1), 137–144. doi:10.1515/ijnes-2013-0053

Blum, C. A. (2014). Evaluating preceptor perception of support using educational podcasts. *International Journal of Nursing Education Scholarship, 11*(1), 1–8.

Brooks, M. V., & Niederhauser, V. P. (2010). Preceptor expectations and issues with nurse practitioner clinical rotations. *Journal of the American Academy of Nurse Practitioners, 22,* 573–579. doi:10.1111/j.1745-7599.2010.00560.x

Distler, J. W. (2015). Online nurse practitioner education: Achieving student competencies. *Nurse Practitioner, 40*(11), 44–49. doi:10.1097/01.NPR.0000472249.05833.49

Gardner, M. R., & Suplee, P. D. (2010). *Handbook of clinical teaching.* Sudbury, MA: Jones & Bartlett.

Gormley, D., & Glazer, G. (2012). Legislative: Nursing distance learning programs and state board of nursing authorizations. *Online Journal of Issues in Nursing, 17*(3). doi:10.3912/OJIN.Vol17No03LegCol01

Gubrud, P. (2016). Teaching in the clinical setting. In D. Billings & J. Halstead (Eds.), *Teaching in nursing: A guide for faculty* (5th ed., pp. 282–302). St. Louis, MO: Elsevier.

Hendricks, S. M., Wallace, L. S., Narwold, L., Guy, G., & Wallace, D. (2013). Comparing the effectiveness, practice opportunities, and satisfaction of the preceptored clinical and the traditional clinical for nursing students. *Nursing Education Perspectives, 34,* 310–314.

Ingwerson, J. (2014). Tailoring the approach to precepting: Student nurse vs. new hire. *Oregon State Board of Nursing Sentinel, 33*(2), 11–13.

Kalischuk, R. G., Vandenberg, H., & Awosoga, O. (2013). Nurse preceptors speak out: An empirical study. *Journal of Professional Nursing, 29*(1), 30–38. doi:10.1016/j.profnurs.2012.04.008

Killam, L. A., & Heerschap, C. (2013). Challenges to student learning in the clinical setting: A qualitative descriptive study. *Nurse Education Today, 33,* 684–691. doi:10.1016/j.nedt.2012.10.008

Klein, T., & Ingwerson, J. (2011). Precepting a student: Your rights and responsibilities. *Oregon State Board of Nursing Sentinel, 30*(3), 6–9.

Koharchik, L., Culleiton, A., Caputi, L., & Robb, M. (2015). Fostering clinical reasoning in nursing students. *American Journal of Nursing, 115*(1), 58–61.

Krampe, I., L'Ecuyer, K., & Palmer, J. L. (2013). Development of an online orientation course for preceptors in a dedicated education unit program. *Journal of Continuing Education in Nursing, 44,* 352–356. doi:10.3928/00220124-20130617-44

Lewallen, L. P., DeBrew, J. K., & Stump, M. R. (2014). Regulations and accreditation requirements for preceptor use in undergraduate education. *Journal of Continuing Education in Nursing, 45,* 386–390. doi:10.3928/00220124-20140826-01

Logan, B., Kovacs, K. A., & Barry, T. L. (2015). Precepting nurse practitioner students: One medical center's efforts to improve the precepting process. *Journal of the American Association of Nurse Practitioners, 27,* 676–682. doi:10.1002/2327-6924.12265

Lowery, B., & Spector, N. (2014). Regulatory implications and recommendations for distance education in prelicensure nursing program. *Journal of Nursing Regulation, 5*(3), 24–33.

McClure, E., & Black, L. (2013). The role of the clinical preceptor: An integrative literature review. *Journal of Nursing Education, 52,* 335–341. doi:10.3928/01484834-20130430-02

O'Connor, A. B. (2015). *Clinical instruction and evaluation: A teaching resource.* Burlington, MA: Jones & Bartlett.

Oermann, M. H., & Gaberson, K. B. (2017). *Evaluation and testing in nursing education.* New York, NY: Springer Publishing.

Raines, D. A. (2012). Nursing preceptors' views of precepting undergraduate nursing students. *Nursing Education Perspectives, 33,* 76–79. doi:10.5480/1536-5026-33.2.76

Shellenbarger, T., & Robb, M. (2016). Effective mentoring in the clinical setting. *American Journal of Nursing, 116*(4), 64–68.

CHAPTER 13

Interprofessional and Collaborative Practice in Clinical Settings

Elizabeth Speakman

To provide comprehensive care, nursing students need to be prepared to work and function in interprofessional health care teams. Clinical practice has always been an important component of nursing education. Within the clinical environment, students link theory to practice and develop their skills and confidence (Cooper, Courtney-Pratt, & Fitzgerald, 2015). Opportunities to develop skill in teamwork must be integrated in nursing programs for students to gain the confidence needed to practice collaboratively and deliver patient-centered care as a nurse. Providing students with deliberate interprofessional clinical opportunities has the greatest potential to move beyond the current practice of silo education and practice in health professions (Speakman, 2014). This chapter examines the need for interprofessional education (IPE), competencies to be developed, and clinical activities for preparing students to work and function in interprofessional health care teams.

DEVELOPMENT AND CHALLENGES OF IPE AND COLLABORATIVE PRACTICE

"Successful collaboration requires that nursing and its members respond to diversity by recognizing, assessing, and adapting the nature of working relationships with individuals, populations, and other health professionals and health workers" (American Nurses Association, 2010, p. 11). This statement captures the spirit of interprofessional health care delivery. Ironically, the notion that better care is delivered by a team versus individual health care providers is not new. In fact, 45 years ago at the Institute of Medicine (IOM) Educating for the Health Team Conference, a panel of experts recommended that students from health care disciplines train together (IOM, 1972). Subsequent reports and white papers concurred and posited that effective team-based care occurs when students are given opportunities to have shared learning experiences and are able to observe these models in action (Committee on Quality Health Care in America, 2001; IOM, 2003; Kohn, Corrigan, & Donaldson, 1999; World Health Organization [WHO], 2010). Yet despite these reports, nurses, physicians, and other health care providers, whose close collaboration is foundational to health care delivery, continued to be educated separately (Wiencek, Lavandero, & Berlinger, 2016).

IPE involves students from two or more professions learning together and about each other's roles to prepare them to collaborate and work together as a team (WHO, 2010). The current resurgence of IPE and its value added, along with academic accreditation standards and hospital guidelines that require students to learn and clinicians to practice team-based care, have had a significant impact on IPE and collaborative practice (CP). The inclusion of IPE in accreditation standards made it a powerful tool in health care education reform (Zorek & Raehl, 2013). This resurgence, however, is not without challenges. Many faculty members feel ill-prepared to deliver IPE and CP curricula because they have had little or no exposure to the concepts of teamwork and communication, and because clinical sites during their training lacked examples of interprofessional team-based care (Hall & Zierler, 2015; Willgerodt & Zierler, 2017). Additionally, health care educators voice their concern about being able to implement IPE and CP curricula because they require collaborating with faculty and students outside of their discipline (Speakman & Hanson-Zalot, 2017).

To promote IPE and CP, the Interprofessional Education Collaborative (IPEC) identified four core competencies, and subset competencies, that all health professionals should possess:

- Values/ethics for interprofessional practice
- Interprofessional communication practices
- Interprofessional teamwork and team-based practice
- Roles and responsibilities for CP

The identification of core competencies was a major asset to the evolution of current IPE and CP curricula. The competencies were general enough to be used in any program (IPEC, 2011), and they created a common language, a deeper understanding of each other's curricula, and a framework to support implementing and evaluating an IPE curriculum. Having a competency-based program that could guide curricular development helped programs meet their IPE accreditation requirements (Hall & Zierler, 2015). These competencies served as curriculum starting points, guideposts, and end points, but most importantly as the intersection point for multiprofessional education programming.

Because interprofessional learning occurs in clinical experiences (Durkin & Feinn, 2017), these competencies were particularly helpful in justifying IPE and CP clinical opportunities. As health care changed, partly with the advent of new insurance mandates and even the use of telehealth care modalities, the IPEC panel recognized the need to update the core competencies and language to ensure that it represented current care delivery (IPEC, 2016). In 2016, IPEC developed a revised set of competencies. Figure 13.1 represents the updated core competencies.

The new IPEC document included broader competencies that offered better approaches to population health. While the competencies were intentionally general and flexible, they ensured that safe, high-quality, accessible care that is patient-centered and patient-focused was still the goal of interprofessional CP (IPEC, 2016).

There were other significant changes. Most importantly, nine additional disciplines joined to support the 2016 competencies, and the competency language was

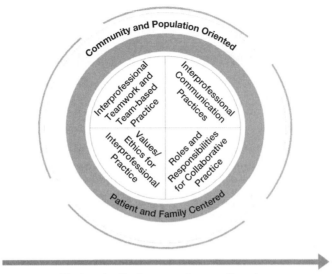

The Learning Continuum pre-licensure through
practice trajectory

FIGURE 13.1 INTERPROFESSIONAL COLLABORATION COMPETENCY DOMAIN.

Source: Reprinted from Interprofessional Education Collaborative (2016). Reprinted with permission from the Interprofessional Education Collaborative.

modified so that professionals from other fields would be able to join the collaboration (IPEC, 2016). The new competencies for IPE and CP included population-health and communities. These additions were especially important to nursing education because nursing curricula examine population health models and use community clinical sites. Furthermore, the new competencies included engaging professionals from health care and other fields. This also was important for nursing as many nursing programs, unlike their counterparts in medicine, are not attached to an academic health center and may not have convenient access to other health professionals. Because a team is a group of individuals who interact, and have a specific skill-set and a shared language, purpose, and goals (Gordon, Mendelhall, & O'Connor, 2013), the new IPEC competencies now offered a variety of settings that supported teamwork. Exhibit 13.1 lists the core competencies for interprofessional CP, updated in 2016.

ROLE OF THE NURSE EDUCATOR IN IPE AND CP

Most registered nurses will acknowledge that their practice includes participating on interprofessional health care teams. Simply put, "extracting nursing from the team is simply impossible" (Speakman & Hanson-Zalot, 2017, p. 2). However, many nurses will also concede that being and feeling like a vital member of the team occurs with experience. Nurses' perceptions about their power cannot be ignored if interprofessional collaboration is going to transform health care. If nurses will be collaborating with other members of the team, their feeling of power and status in the context of their work must be addressed (Hart, 2015). "Nurses, who are the largest group of health care professionals, are positioned to lead and partner in teams that provide services across the continuum" of care (National Academies of Sciences, Engineering, and Medicine, 2015, p. 2).

EXHIBIT 13.1

CORE COMPETENCIES FOR INTERPROFESSIONAL CP: 2016 UPDATE[a]

Competency: Values/Ethics for Interprofessional Practice

Work with individuals of other professions to maintain a climate of mutual respect and shared values.

Values/Ethics Subcompetencies

VE1. Place interests of patients and populations at center of interprofessional health care delivery **and population health programs and policies, with the goal of promoting health and health equity across the life span.**

VE2. Respect the dignity and privacy of patients while maintaining confidentiality in the delivery of team-based care.

VE3. Embrace the cultural diversity and individual differences that characterize patients, populations, and the **health team**.

VE4. Respect the unique cultures, values, roles/responsibilities, and expertise of other health professions and **the impact these factors can have on health outcomes.**

VE5. Work in cooperation with those who receive care, those who provide care, and others who contribute to or support the delivery of prevention and health services **and programs**.

VE6. Develop a trusting relationship with patients, families, and other team members (CIHC, 2010).

VE7. Demonstrate high standards of ethical conduct and quality of care in contributions to team-based care.

VE8. Manage ethical dilemmas specific to interprofessional patient/population-centered care situations.

VE9. Act with honesty and integrity in relationships with patients, families, **communities**, and other team members.

VE10. Maintain competence in one's own profession appropriate to scope of practice.

Competency: Roles and Responsibility for CP

Use the knowledge of one's own role and those of other professions to appropriately assess and address the health care needs of **patients and to promote and advance the health of populations.**

Roles/Responsibilities Subcompetencies

RR1. Communicate one's roles and responsibilities clearly to patients, families, **community members**, and other professionals.

RR2. Recognize one's limitations in skills, knowledge, and abilities.

RR3. Engage **diverse professionals** who complement one's own professional expertise, as well as associated resources, to develop strategies to meet specific **health and healthcare** needs of **patients and populations**.

RR4. Explain the roles and responsibilities of other providers and how the team works together to provide care, **promote health, and prevent disease**.

RR5. Use the full scope of knowledge, skills, and abilities of **professionals from health and other fields** to provide care that is safe, timely, efficient, effective, and equitable.

RR6. Communicate with team members to clarify each member's responsibility in executing components of a treatment plan or public health intervention.

RR7. Forge interdependent relationships with other professions **within and outside of the health system** to improve care and advance learning.

RR8. Engage in continuous professional and interprofessional development to enhance team performance **and collaboration**.

(continued)

RR9. Use unique and complementary abilities of all members of the team to optimize **health and** patient care.

RR10. **Describe how professionals in health and other fields can collaborate and integrate clinical care and public health interventions to optimize population health**

Competency: Interprofessional Communication Practices

Communicate with patients, families, communities, **and professionals in health and other fields** in a responsive and responsible manner that supports a team approach to the promotion and maintenance of health and the **prevention** and treatment of disease.

Interprofessional Communication Subcompetencies:

CC1. Choose effective communication tools and techniques, including information systems and communication technologies, to facilitate discussions and interactions that enhance team function.

CC2. **Communicate** information with patients, families, **community members**, and **health team** members in a form that is understandable, avoiding discipline-specific terminology when possible.

CC3. Express one's knowledge and opinions to team members involved in patient care **and population health improvement** with confidence, clarity, **and** respect, working to ensure common understanding of information, treatment, care decisions, **and population health programs and policies.**

CC4. Listen actively, and encourage ideas and opinions of other team members.

CC5. Give timely, sensitive, instructive feedback to others about their performance on the team, responding respectfully as a team member to feedback from others.

CC6. Use respectful language appropriate for a given difficult situation, crucial conversation, or conflict.

CC7. Recognize how one's uniqueness (experience level, expertise, culture, power, and hierarchy within the **health** team) contributes to effective communication, conflict resolution, and positive interprofessional working relationships (University of Toronto, 2008).

CC8. Communicate the importance of teamwork in patient-centered **care and population health programs and policies.**

Competency: Interprofessional Teamwork and Team Based Practice

Apply relationship-building values and the principles of team dynamics to perform effectively in different team roles to **plan, deliver, and evaluate** patient/population-centered care **and population health programs and policies** that **are** safe, timely, efficient, effective, and equitable.

Team and Teamwork Subcompetencies:

TT1. Describe the process of team development and the roles and practices of effective teams.

TT2. Develop consensus on the ethical principles to guide all aspects of **teamwork**.

TT3. **Engage health and other professionals** in shared patient-centered **and population-focused** problem-solving.

TT4. Integrate the knowledge and experience of **health and** other professions to inform **health and** care decisions, while respecting patient and community values and priorities/preferences for care.

TT5. Apply leadership practices that support CP and team effectiveness.

TT6. Engage self and others to constructively manage disagreements about values, roles, goals, and actions that arise among **health and other** professionals and with patients, **families**, and community members.

TT7. Share accountability with other professions, patients, and communities for outcomes relevant to prevention and health care.

TT8. Reflect on individual and team performance for individual, as well as team, performance improvement.

(continued)

TT9. Use process improvement to increase effectiveness of interprofessional teamwork and team-based **services, programs, and policies**.

TT10. Use available evidence to inform effective teamwork and team-based practices.

TT11. Perform effectively on teams and in different team roles in a variety of settings.

CP, collaborative practice.

aWords in **bold** represent the updated language in 2016 competencies.

Source: Reprinted from Interprofessional Education Collaborative (2016). Reprinted with permission from the Interprofessional Education Collaborative.

The clinical environment is the place where students apply content learned in the classroom to patients. "Clinical placements are a major source of stress for students during their prelicensure nursing education" (Mulcock, Grassley, Davis, & White, 2017, p. 105). Many studies have described students' apprehension in clinical learning activities, and Lundberg (2008) noted that "clinical confidence" occurs when students experience feeling successful after mastering new skills. The nurse educator's responsibility is to prepare students to work in complex health care environments (Moore & Ward, 2017). Part of practice readiness is being comfortable working on and leading health care teams. Because this is difficult to do in the clinical environment, simulation can provide experiences for students from multiple health professions and other fields to learn to work together as a team.

Nursing education has a long and distinguished history of responding to societal needs. Leaders in curriculum reform proposed IPE opportunities long before it was conventional in nursing education. The 2011 IOM *Future of Nursing: Leading Change, Advancing Health* report recommended that "nurses should be full partners, with physicians and other health care professionals, in redesigning health care in the United States" (IOM, 2011, p. 3). This was an endorsement that nurses are integral members and leaders of the health care team. This report highlighted the need for new competencies in nursing education (Stevens, 2013), and although some nursing programs had already experimented in IPE and CP initiatives, this IOM report initiated a growth of IPE and CP in nursing curricula. The subsequent 2015 *Assessing Progress on the IOM Report The Future of Nursing* affirmed these views and also recommended that more attention needs to be given to "interprofessional education, teamwork training, and a better understanding of the roles of all health professionals in creating an optimal health care delivery system" (National Academies of Sciences, Engineering, and Medicine, 2015, p. 4).

Preparing students to meet these demands requires faculty members to rethink and reconceptualize clinical opportunities that support team versus silo approaches to care. Even though the clinical setting is a stressful environment, without IPE and CP clinical experiences as students, how would novice nurses become empowered to be integral members of the team? How would they master the skills needed to work effectively in a team and learn to lead an interprofessional team? When teams are in "name only," the decision making tends to be more competitive, and often members complain that their input is marginalized, ignored, or dismissed. Team members may feel shamed or humiliated when they express their concerns (Gordon et al., 2013). In addition to the traditional outcomes and competencies to be developed in the clinical environment, nurse educators are challenged to add IPE and CP learning activities

STEPS IN DEVELOPING IPE AND CP CLINICAL LEARNING OPPORTUNITIES

Step 1: Understand the Constructs of Team and Teamwork

Before developing IPE and CP initiatives, it is important to understand two constructs: *team* and *teamwork*. The word *team*, whether used as a noun, verb, or adjective, means *to join* or *joining*, as in creating teams or adding to an established team. Those are the two options when developing IPE and CP clinical experiences: students can engage in activities in which they create teams, for example, students from different health professions can work together to solve a unit based problem or as a team to plan an intervention for a patient. In other clinical experiences students can become part of an established team, and learning activities can help them reflect on characteristics of that team, roles of members, and collaboration among team members. Because the 2016 IPEC core competencies generalize team and team composition, clinical teams do not have to solely consist of health care professionals. Any discipline would be appropriate as long as nursing students gain an understanding of how to be a member or leader of a team. For IPE and CP, the construct of *team* is interchangeable and applicable to any setting. When teams effectively communicate, they challenge traditional silo practice (Speakman & Hanson-Zalot, 2017). Engaging students on IPE teams affords them the ability to recognize and address the structures and activities of teamwork (Hart, 2015).

Step 2: Unearth the Details

IPE and CP are not curriculum "add ons"; they are teaching strategies in which content offered in multiple programs is taught simultaneously and in tandem with two or more interprofessional groups. Understanding teamwork is essential as a student. Athletes practice for many more hours then they play. They practice to prepare for untoward events, to get to know others' strengths and weaknesses, and to develop a game plan or vision. They practice effective communication skills; they learn how to strategize and each other's roles. The irony is that we do not have the same expectation of our health care providers who are making critical decisions that might result in life or death. Health care professionals are often unaware of each other's abilities, may have never interacted with another health care practitioner, and have not practiced how to work as a team. Providing students with teamwork learning opportunities is important to develop nurses and other health care professionals who can work effectively in the delivery of care. Students cannot learn teamwork or how to be a member of a team unless they are given opportunities to practice in teams.

Step 3: Recognize Accreditation as an Ally

The profession of nursing has a long history of establishing standards for nursing. The American Society of Superintendents of Training Schools for Nurses (the forerunner of the National League for Nursing [NLN]) was established in 1893 for the sole purpose of maintaining a universal standard of nursing training (Accreditation Commission for Education in Nursing, 2013). Establishing these standards is a way in which the profession of nursing regulates itself and ensures that a high standard of education is offered. Accreditation is a self-assessment reflective process that provides professional and postsecondary institutions the opportunity to identify strengths and areas of improvement that focuses on quality (NLN Commission for Nursing Education Accreditation [CNEA], 2016; Commission on Collegiate Nursing Education, 2013). Today, some health professions programs are required to include IPE as part of their accreditation (Willgerodt et al., 2015). In nursing education, standards for curricula such as the American Association of Colleges of Nursing (AACN) Essentials of Baccalaureate Education for Professional Nursing Practice (2008) and Master's Education in Nursing (2011), and accreditation criteria such as the NLN CNEA standards (2016) support the IPEC competencies. For example, one of the baccalaureate standards, Essential VI, indicates that communication and collaboration among health care professionals are critical to delivering high quality and safe patient care. The AACN master's education standard VII recognizes that the master's-prepared nurse, as a member and leader of interprofessional teams, needs to be able to communicate, collaborate, and consult with other health providers to manage and coordinate care. Accreditation criteria, such as the NLN CNEA, address the need for programs to address quality and safety and prepare students to provide relationship-centered care and engage in teamwork.

Step 4: Develop an IPE/CP Framework

The four core competencies published by the IPEC expert panel justify them as a framework for developing and implementing all IPE and CP learning opportunities in various settings: the classroom, in simulation, and in the clinical environment. While both the classroom and simulation setting can provide ample opportunities for students to master these competencies, they lack the uncertainty of the clinical environment. The clinical environment has a different pace and relies on the use of clinical reasoning and critical thinking for a deeper understanding of the patient condition.

Yet developing IPE and CP clinical experiences is not without challenges. The complexity of interacting with a patient versus a simulation can elevate students' apprehension and challenge how well they work effectively on a team. IPE and CP learning experiences must be effective if they are going to have an impact on students' practice as clinicians (Long, Dann, Wolff, & Brienza, 2014). Moreover, since most health professionals are educated to have different clinical perspectives (Grace & Milliken, 2016), establishing a set framework and standards for effective team-based care is important.

Using the IPEC core competencies as a framework also assists with accreditation compliance. Accreditation requirements are important to promote and advance IPE and can be a powerful tool to promote educational change (Willgerodt et al., 2015; Zorek & Raehl, 2013).

Step 5: Assess IPE and CP Readiness

Understanding if the time is right to implement IPE depends on the readiness of the environment, key personnel, students, and support systems at the clinical facility. The clinical readiness assessment questionnaire in Exhibit 13.2 includes questions that should be considered prior to implementing IPE and CP programs and learning activities in the clinical environment.

EXHIBIT 13.2

QUESTIONS TO ASSESS CLINICAL READINESS FOR INTERPROFESSIONAL AND CP

Have you identified strengths and gaps in the current clinical environment?

Have you prepared an effective data-driven presentation, taking into consideration your audience's interests?

Have you gathered approval from senior leadership for offering IPE and valuing a culture of teamwork and safety across the institution?

Will your institution support the program development and coordination?

Have you assembled a working group of adequate size with faculty representation from all professions that you intend to include in programming?

Have you identified a sufficient number of faculty members who are adept in IPE competencies to serve as instructors for your activities?

Have you organized faculty development activities for interested leaders, faculty members, and staff members to increase their knowledge of IPE and CP?

Have you reviewed all professions' academic calendars and curricula to determine the best positioning of IPE and CP programs?

Have you developed interprofessional clinical programming?

Will your institution revise curricula and allow time in order for learners to attend IPE trainings?

Have you developed an evaluation process for programming?

Have you developed the appropriate structure to revise and improve programming?

Will your institution be able to reinforce and reward positive teamwork behaviors and improvements?

CP, collaborative practice; IPE, Interprofessional education.
Source: Adapted from Speakman, Tagliareni, Sherburne, and Sicks (2016). Copyright 2016 by the National League for Nursing. Reprinted with permission.

Step 6: Develop Clinical Opportunities

The first and most important concept to consider when developing an IPE and CP activity is that it is a teaching strategy, not a new content area. Because collaborative clinical learning opportunities foster collective intelligence through better communication and problem solving (Speakman, 2014), implementing these opportunities is analogous to using a problem-based learning or case study method. No content has to be sacrificed to teach the principles of team-based care. The second notion is to recognize that not every student will have the exact same IPE or CP experience, just like not every student has the exact same clinical experience. However, by debriefing in postclinical conference, the clinical teacher can help students share their IPE or CP experiences, learning from one another how team-based care can and is implemented in different settings with different team members.

CLINICAL LEARNING ACTIVITIES

There are varied clinical learning activities to develop competencies in teamwork and collaboration. Three examples of clinical activities are observation of teams, interprofessional clinical rounding, and teach-back.

Clinical Observation

Most if not all inpatient and outpatient clinical environments have interprofessional health care teams already in place. Rehabilitation, surgery, obstetrics, psychiatry services, to name a few, generally have well-formed interprofessional teams. The purpose of this clinical learning activity is to embed students in already assembled teams so they can observe how a team-in-action provides patient-centered care. Exhibit 13.3 describes this learning activity for students. Students should be asked to reflect on the experience and be prepared to share in postclinical conference or a written assignment.

Interprofessional Clinical Rounding

Interprofessional clinical rounding fuses traditional uni-professional bedside rounding with a clinical model of multiple professionals collectively developing an integrated plan of care (Lyons et al., 2013). Clinical rounding occurs daily on most inpatient clinical units and as team conferences in many outpatient facilities. An example of an interprofessional clinical rounding experience for students is in Exhibit 13.4. Students

---

EXHIBIT 13.3

CLINICAL OBSERVATION EXEMPLAR

Purpose of Activity

The purpose of the clinical observation is to increase a student's exposure to team-based care as applied to real patients

Learning Objectives

- Describe the roles and expertise of different health professionals on the health care team
- Identify the benefits of and challenges related to working on an interprofessional CP team
- Analyze the role each profession plays in developing team-based solutions

Description of the Activity

- Students witness and evaluate firsthand how the team of health care providers attends to the potential dilemmas and solutions related to the patient.

Coordination Needs

Prior to Event:

- Determine a date and practice team
- Orient practice team to the activity
- Conduct pretest or preactivity surveys (optional)

After the Event:

- Debrief with students in postclinical conference; ask them to share their experience
    1. How did the team collaborate?
    2. Did the team respect each other's contributions?
    3. Did the discussion reflect shared decision-making?
    4. Was the patient or significant other part of the team discussion?
- Conduct and analyze posttest or postactivity surveys (optional)

CP, collaborative practice.
Source: Adapted from Speakman et al. (2016). Copyright 2016 by the National League for Nursing. Reprinted with permission.

EXHIBIT 13.4

INTERPROFESSIONAL CLINICAL ROUNDING EXEMPLAR

Purpose of Activity

- The purpose of this learning activity is to provide a real-time, CP learning opportunity for nursing and other health professions students and to expose them to patient-centered CP.

Learning Objectives

- Recognize how a patient's plan of care is determined through collaboration among team members during interprofessional clinical rounds
- Formulate a patient presentation and a recommended plan of care as members of an interprofessional team
- Present patient assessments (e.g., collecting vital signs and social and health factors) and report on patients' statuses as members of an interprofessional team

Description of the Activity

- Students conduct preliminary rounds on the patients, under the guidance of their preceptors or clinical instructors. During preliminary rounds, the nursing students should interact with the patients, assess vital signs, and check in with the nursing staff for any overnight updates.
- The interprofessional students then meet together in person prior to the team rounds to review patients' current plans of care, study results, anticipated discharge dates, and interprofessional plans for discharge.
- The students collaborate to create patient presentations and then join the practice team for rounding, under the guidance of their preceptors or clinical instructors.
- Multiple student professions can be included in the rounding and should correlate with the professions that are involved in the patient care within the specific team or unit.
- With proper security in place, there may be opportunities for some student professions to participate virtually if they are unable to leave their regular duties during the rounding event.

Coordination Needs

Prior to Event:

- Obtain permission from a clinical team or unit to have students participate in interprofessional clinical rounding
- Secure a point of contact from each profession with whom you can coordinate
- Determine a date and specific location for the rounding to take place with the practice team
- Coordinate with nursing clinical instructors and preceptors and physician residents for students to complete preactivity rounds, conduct a meeting, and join the team on their rounds

During the Event:

- Direction given by the team leaders, e.g., the nurse practitioner or attending physician

After the Event:

- Debrief with students in postclinical conference; ask them to share their experiences
    1. How did the team collaborate?
    2. Did the team respect each other's contributions?
    3. Did the discussion reflect shared decision-making?
    4. Was the patient or significant other part of the team discussion?
- Conduct and analyze posttest or postactivity surveys (optional)

CP, collaborative practice.
Source: Adapted from Speakman et al. (2016). Copyright 2016 by the National League for Nursing. Reprinted with permission.

should have an opportunity to discuss their observations and share their experiences with rounding, focusing on interactions among team members, and how effectively the team functioned. This can be done in a postclinical conference, as an online discussion, in a written reflection, or through other strategies.

Teach-Back

The teach-back method evaluates patients' understanding by asking them to restate information they were given (Centrella-Nigro & Alexander, 2017; Agency for Healthcare Research and Quality, 2015). Using the principles of health literacy, interprofessional teams of students can collaborate to confirm patients' comprehension by asking the patient to reiterate the information they were taught. A description of a teach-back learning activity for students for interprofessional collaboration is in Exhibit 13.5.

EXHIBIT 13.5

TEACH-BACK EXEMPLAR

Purpose of Activity

The purpose of this learning activity is for students of nursing and other disciplines to work together on patient education using the teach-back method.

Learning Objectives

- Describe the roles of interprofessional team members in a clinical setting
- Participate as a member of an interprofessional team to develop a patient-centered plan of care
- Demonstrate interprofessional communication skills and discuss how to apply patient-centered interprofessional principles during a team-based clinical experience
- Discuss the scope and challenges presented by low health literacy

Description of the Activity

- The students are given the patient assessment data prior to the activity for their review.
- To begin the activity, the students meet with the clinical instructor or preceptor on the unit to learn the teach-back method.
- Students review the data in a team huddle.
- After the huddle, the nursing students conduct an oral health history with the selected patient, assessing the patient's health history, health literacy, and learning needs.
- Then the nursing students collaborate with a student from another discipline to identify the appropriate teaching plan to meet the patient's needs.
- The students debrief with their clinical instructor or preceptor for confirmation on the plan and for any additional teach-back coaching before gathering the appropriate teaching materials.
- The students then meet with the patient.
- Using the teach-back method, students employ appropriate strategies for effective communication and education to ensure the patient understanding.
- Students debrief with the clinical instructor or preceptor.

Potential Student Collaborations

Inpatient Setting:

Nursing and pharmacy students—medication reconciliation
Nursing and occupational therapy students—safety assessment
Nursing and physical therapy students—home exercise instructions

(continued)

Nursing and medical students—discharge Instructions
Nursing and dental students—oral hygiene assessment
Nursing and dietitian students—dietary reconciliation

Outpatient Setting:

Nursing and law students—HIPAA and Patient Bill of Rights
Nursing and social work students—accessing health resources and social programs
Nursing and community health worker students—accessing community resources

Coordination Needs

Prior to Event:

■ Determine a date and clinical location that teach-back is most feasible
■ Send students the patient assessment data via email.

During the Event:

■ Students meet with their team member and develop a teach-back
■ Students then receive feedback and reflection from the preceptors or clinical instructors

After the Event:

■ Debrief with students in postclinical conference; ask them to share their experiences
  1. How did the team collaborate?
  2. Did the team respect each other's contributions?
  3. Did the discussion reflect shared decision-making?
  4. Was the patient or significant other part of the team discussion?
■ Conduct and analyze posttest or postactivity surveys (optional)

Source: Adapted from Speakman et al. (2016). Copyright 2016 by the National League for Nursing. Reprinted with permission.

SUMMARY

Unlike the classroom setting, the clinical setting is where faculty members model "thinking-in-action." These opportunities are the perfect setting for students from multiple professions to learn from, about, and with each other (WHO, 2010). More importantly, if students are not given the opportunity to practice in interprofessional teams as students, they are not likely to practice in interprofessional teams. The reality is that even well-meaning academic institutions are still choosing to educate students using the old health care system model (Speakman & Arenson, 2015). Clinical teachers are ill prepared to create IPE and CP opportunities because many have not had these experiences as students. Simply put, regardless of how many IPE and CP learning experiences a student has outside of the clinical environment, if the culture in the clinical environment is not team-based, then students will only learn and mimic what they experience. If health care professionals acknowledge the value of interprofessional patient care, then they need to provide these clinical learning opportunities in the clinical setting. More importantly, team-based care impacts patient care; in fact, recent publications have correlated interprofessional team-based care to enhanced patient outcomes (Cox & Naylor, 2013; National Academies of Sciences, Engineering, and Medicine, 2015).

Clinical nurse educators provide an environment where students can test their thinking and prepare students for practice. Nursing students must learn a significant amount of information if they are going to be prepared to practice in the complex clinical environment (Mulcock et al., 2017). Therefore, developing IPE and CP clinical learning opportunities supports students' transition into practice and prepares them to care for patients who have complex clinical needs.

CNE EXAMINATION TEST BLUEPRINT CORE COMPETENCIES

1. **Facilitate Learning**

   A. Implement a variety of teaching strategies appropriate to
      1. content
      2. setting
      3. learner needs
      4. learning style
      5. desired learner outcomes
   B. Modify teaching strategies and learning experiences based on consideration of learners':
      1. cultural background
      2. past clinical experiences
      3. past educational and life experiences
   C. Practice skilled oral and written (including electronic) communication that reflects an awareness of self and relationships with learners (e.g., evaluation, mentorship, and supervision)
   D. Communicate effectively orally and in writing with an ability to convey ideas in a variety of contexts
   E. Create opportunities for learners to develop their own critical thinking skills
   F. Create a positive learning environment that fosters a free exchange of ideas
   G. Act as a role model in practice settings

2. **Facilitate Learner Development and Socialization**

   A. Foster the development of learners in these areas:
      1. cognitive domain
      2. psychomotor domain
      3. affective domain
   F. Assist learners to engage in thoughtful and constructive self- and peer evaluation
   G. Encourage professional development of learners

3. **Use Assessment and Evaluation Strategies**

   L. Provide timely, constructive, and thoughtful feedback to learners

REFERENCES

Accreditation Commission for Education in Nursing. (2013). History of nursing accreditation. Retrieved from http://www.acenursing.org/acen-history-of-accreditation

Agency for Healthcare Research and Quality. (2015). Use the teach-back method: Tool #5. Retrieved from http://www.ahrq.gov/professionals/quality-patient-safety/qualityresources/tools/literacy-toolkit/healthlittoolkit2-tool5.html

American Association of Colleges of Nursing. (2008). *The essentials of baccalaureate education for professional nursing practice.* Washington, DC: Author.

American Association of Colleges of Nursing. (2011). *The essentials of master's education in nursing.* Washington, DC: Author.

American Nurses Association. (2010). *Nursing's social policy statement: The essence of the profession.* Washington, DC: Author.

Canadian Interprofessional Health Collaborative. (2010). *A national interprofessional competency framework.* Retrieved from www.cihc.ca/resources/publications

Centrella-Nigro, A. M., & Alexander, C. (2017). Using the teach-back method in patient education to improve patient satisfaction. *Journal of Continuing Education in Nursing, 48,* 47–52. doi:10.3928/00220124-20170110-10

Commission on Collegiate Nursing Education. (2013). *Standards for accreditation of baccalaureate and graduate nursing programs.* Washington, DC: Author. Retrieved from http://www.aacn.nche.edu/ccne-accreditation/Standards-Amended-2013.pdf

Committee on Quality Health Care in America, Institute of Medicine. (2001). *Crossing the quality chasm: A new health system for the 21st century.* Washington, DC: National Academies Press.

Cooper, J., Courtney-Pratt, H., & Fitzgerald, M. (2015). Key influences identified by first year undergraduate nursing students as impacting on the quality of clinical placement: A qualitative study. *Nurse Education Today, 35,* 1004–1008. doi:10.1016/j.nedt.2015.03.009

Cox, M., & Naylor, M. (2013). *Transforming patient care: Aligning interprofessional education with clinical practice redesign.* New York, NY: Josiah Macy Jr. Foundation.

Durkin, A. E., & Feinn, R. S. (2017). Traditional and accelerated baccalaureate nursing students' self efficacy for interprofessional learning. *Nursing Education Perspectives, 38,* 23–28. doi:10.1097/01.NEP.0000000000000101

Gordon, S., Mendenhall, P., & O'Connor, B. B. (2013). *Beyond the checklist: What else health care can learn from aviation teamwork and safety.* New York, NY: Cornell University Press.

Grace, P., & Milliken, A. (2016). Educating nurses for ethical practice in contemporary health care environments. *Hastings Center Report, 46*(S1), S13–S17. doi: 10.1002/hast.625

Hall, L. W., & Zierler, B. K. (2015). Interprofessional education and practice guide No. 1: Developing faculty to effectively facilitate interprofessional education. *Journal of Interprofessional Care, 29,* 3–7. doi:10.3109/13561820.2014.937483

Hart, C. (2015). The elephant in the room: Nursing and nursing power on an interprofessional team. *Journal of Continuing Education in Nursing, 46,* 349–355. doi:10.3928/00220124-20150721-01

Institute of Medicine. (1972). *Education for the health team.* Washington, DC: National Academy of Science.

Institute of Medicine. (2003). *Health professions education: A bridge to quality.* Washington, DC: National Academies Press.

Institute of Medicine. (2011). *The future of nursing: Leading change, advancing health.* Washington, DC: National Academies Press.

Interprofessional Education Collaborative. (2016). *Core competencies for interprofessional collaborative practice: 2016 update.* Washington, DC: Author.

Interprofessional Education Collaborative Expert Panel. (2011). *Core competencies for interprofessional collaborative practice: Report of an expert panel.* Washington, DC: Author.

Kohn, L. T., Corrigan, J. M., & Donaldson, M. S. (Eds.). (1999). *To err is human: Building a safer health system.* Washington, DC: National Academies Press.

Long, T., Dann, S., Wolff, M. L., & Brienza, R. S. (2014). Moving from silos to teamwork: Integration of interprofessional trainees into a medical home model. *Journal of Interprofessional Care, 28,* 473–474. doi:10.3109/13561820.2014.891575

Lundberg, K. M. (2008). Promoting self-confidence in clinical nursing students. *Nurse Educator, 33,* 86–89. doi:10.1097/01.NNE.0000299512.78270.d0

Lyons, K. J., Giordano, C., Speakman, E., Isenberg, C., Antony, R., Hanson-Zalot, M., . . . Papastrat, K. (2013). Jefferson interprofessional clinical rounding project. *Journal of Allied Health, 42,* 197–201.

Moore, S. C., & Ward, K. S. (2017). Nursing student perceptions of structural empowerment. *Nursing Education Perspectives, 38,* 32–33.

Mulcock, P. M., Grassley, J., Davis, M., & White, K. (2017). Beyond the dedicated education unit: Using cognitive load theory to guide clinical placement. *Journal of Nursing Education, 56,* 105–109. doi:10.3928/01484834-20170123-07

National Academies of Sciences, Engineering, and Medicine. (2015). *Assessing progress on the IOM report the future of nursing.* Washington, DC: National Academies Press.

National League for Nursing Commission for Nursing Education Accreditation. (2016). *Accreditation standards for nursing education programs.* Washington, DC: Author. Retrieved from http://www.nln.org/docs/default-source/accreditation-services/cnea-standards-final-february-201613f2bf5c78366c709642ff00005f0421.pdf?sfvrsn=8

Speakman, E. (2014). Creating an infrastructure and culture of empowerment. *Clinical Scholars Review, 7*(2), 90–91.

Speakman, E., & Arenson, C. (2015). Going back to the future: What is all the buzz about interprofessional education and collaborative practice. *Nurse Educator, 40,* 3–4. doi:10.1097/NNE.0000000000000104

Speakman, E., & Hanson-Zalot, M. (2017). Introduction to interprofessional education and collaborative practice: Setting the foundation. In E. Speakman (Ed.), *Interprofessional education and collaborative practice: Creating a blueprint for nurse educators* (pp. 1–10). Philadelphia, PA: Wolters Kluwer.

Speakman, E., Tagliareni, M. E., Sherburne, A., & Sicks, S. (2016). *Guide to effective interprofessional education experiences in nursing education. National League for Nursing Toolkit.* Retrieved from http://www.nln.org/docs/default-source/default-document-library/ipe-toolkit-krk-012716.pdf?sfvrsn=6

Stevens, K. (2013). The impact of evidence-based practice in nursing and the next big ideas. *Online Journal of Issues in Nursing, 18*(2). doi:10.3912/OJIN.Vol18No02Man04

Wiencek, C., Lavandero, R., & Berlinger, N. (2016). From the team to the table: Nursing societies and health care organizational ethics. *Hastings Center Report, 46*(S1), S32–S34. doi:10.1002/hast.629

Willgerodt, M. A., Blakeney, E. A-R., Brock, D. M., Liner, D., Murphy, N., & Zierler, B. (2015). Interprofessional education and practice guide No. 4: Developing and sustaining interprofessional education at an academic health center. *Journal of Interprofessional Care, 29,* 421–425. doi:10.3109/13561820.2015.1039117

Willgerodt, M. A., & Zierler, B. K. (2017). Faculty development in interprofessional education and interprofessional collaborative practice. In E. Speakman (Ed.), *Interprofessional education and collaborative practice: Creating a blueprint for nurse educators* (pp. 21–32). Philadelphia, PA: Wolters Kluwer.

World Health Organization. (2010). *Framework for action on interprofessional education and collaborative practice.* Geneva, Switzerland: Author.

Zorek, J., & Raehl, C. (2013). Interprofessional education accreditation standards in the USA: A comparative analysis. *Journal of Interprofessional Care, 27,* 123–130. doi:10.3109/13561820.2012.718295

Evaluation Strategies in Clinical Teaching

CHAPTER 14

Written Assignments

Written assignments enable students to learn about concepts relevant to clinical practice, develop higher level thinking skills, and examine values and beliefs that may affect patient care. Written assignments about clinical practice combined with feedback from the teacher provide an effective means of developing students' writing abilities. Although writing assignments may vary with each clinical course, depending on the outcomes of the course, assignments may be carefully sequenced across courses for students to develop their writing skills as they progress through the nursing program. The teacher is responsible for choosing written assignments that support the learning outcomes of the course and meet other curriculum goals.

PURPOSES OF WRITTEN ASSIGNMENTS

Written assignments for clinical learning have four main purposes: (a) assist students in understanding concepts, theories, and other content that relate to care of patients; (b) develop higher level thinking skills; (c) examine their own feelings, beliefs, and values generated from their clinical learning experiences; and (d) develop writing skills.

In choosing written assignments for clinical courses, the teacher should first consider the outcomes to be met through the assignments and the competencies that students need to develop in the course and nursing program. Writing assignments should build on one another to progressively develop students' skills. Another consideration is the number of assignments to be completed. How many assignments are needed to demonstrate mastery? It may be that one assignment well done is sufficient for meeting the outcomes of the clinical course, and students may then progress to other learning activities. Teachers should avoid using the same written assignments repeatedly throughout a clinical course and should instead choose assignments for specific learning outcomes.

Promote Understanding

In written assignments, students can describe concepts, theories, and other information relevant to the care of their patients and can explain how that knowledge guides their clinical decisions and judgments. Assignments for this purpose need a clear focus to prevent students from merely summarizing and reporting what they read. Shorter assignments that direct students to apply particular concepts to clinical practice may be of greater value in developing higher level thinking skills than longer assignments for which students summarize readings without any analysis of them.

Examples of written assignments to promote understanding of concepts and other information related to clinical practice are:

- Compare, in no more than three pages, two interventions appropriate for your patient in terms of their rationale and evidence. How will you evaluate their effectiveness?
- Read a research article related to care of one of your patients, critique the article, report on the analysis, and explain why the research findings are or are not applicable to the patient's care.
- Compare data collected from your patient with the description of that condition in your textbook or other readings. What are similarities and differences? Why?
- Develop a concept map (a graphic arrangement of key concepts related to your patient's care) and provide a written description of the relationships among the concepts in your map.
- Investigate the process used in your clinical setting for handoff. Write a summary report. How does the handoff process relate to concepts you learned in your course about communicating patient information between providers?

Develop Higher Level Thinking Skills

Written assignments provide an opportunity for students to analyze patient and other problems they have encountered in clinical practice, evaluate their interventions, and propose new approaches. In writing assignments, students can analyze data and clinical situations, identify additional assessment data needed for decision making, identify patient needs and problems, propose approaches, compare interventions based on evidence, and evaluate the effectiveness of care. Writing assignments are particularly valuable for learning about evidence-based practice (EBP). Students can search for and examine the evidence underlying different interventions and make decisions about the best approaches to use with their patients. Students can identify assumptions they made about patients' responses that influenced their clinical decisions, critique arguments, take a stand about an issue and develop a rationale to support it, and draw generalizations about patient care from different clinical experiences.

Assignments geared to critical thinking should give students freedom to develop their ideas and consider alternative perspectives. If the assignment is too restrictive, students are inhibited in their thinking and ways of approaching the problem.

Written assignments for developing higher level thinking skills can be short, ranging from one to two paragraphs to a few pages. In developing these assignments, the teacher should avoid activities in which students merely report on the ideas and thinking of others. Instead, the assignment should ask students to consider an alternative point of view or a different way of approaching an issue. Short assignments also provide an opportunity for teachers to give prompt feedback to students.

The writing assignment should focus on meeting a particular learning outcome and should have specific directions to guide students' writing. For example, students may be asked to prepare a one-page paper comparing the physiological processes of asthma and bronchitis. Rather than writing on everything they read about asthma and bronchitis, students can focus their papers on the physiology of these two conditions.

Examples of written assignments for developing higher level cognitive skills follow:

- Describe in one paragraph significant information you collected from your patient and why it is important to your decisions about approaches to use with that patient.
- Select one need or problem you identified for your patient and provide a rationale for it. What is one alternative need or problem you might also consider and why? Complete this assignment in two typed pages.
- Identify a near miss (close call) or an unsafe practice that you experienced or observed in your clinical setting. Analyze what went wrong and practices that should have been used. Prepare a response integrating the concept of just culture.
- Identify an issue affecting your patient, family, or community. Analyze that issue from two different points of view. Provide a rationale for actions to be taken from both perspectives. How would you approach this issue and why?
- Identify a procedure you performed in your clinical setting. Find the policy. Was your performance consistent with that policy? Why or why not? Are there deviations or workarounds you observed on the unit with that procedure? Write a report about what you learned.
- Identify a patient you cared for in this or a prior course. Briefly describe the patient. What were the most important contributors to that person's health? How do they relate to the social determinants of health?

Examine Feelings, Beliefs, and Values

Written assignments help learners examine feelings generated from caring for patients and reflect on their beliefs and values that might influence that care. Journals, for instance, provide a way for students to record their feelings about a patient or clinical activity and later reflect on these feelings. Assignments may be developed for students to identify their own beliefs and values and analyze how they affect their interactions with patients, families, and staff. Value-based statements may be given to students for written critique, or students may be asked to analyze an ethical issue, propose alternative courses of actions, and take a stand on the issue.

Examples of writing assignments that help students explore their feelings, beliefs, and values are:

- Identify an issue that affects patient care. Read about the issue, and write an editorial that describes how you would address the issue either as a nurse manager or in the role of a bedside nurse.
- In your journal, write about your feelings about caring for your patient and other patients in this setting. In what way do those feelings influence your care?

- A peer tells you she forgot to give her patient the scheduled pain medications but is not telling her preceptor because the patient never complained of pain. What would you say to this individual? Why did you choose this approach?
- Think about the community in which your patients live. How does that community influence their health?

Develop Writing Skills

An important outcome of writing assignments is the development of skill in communicating ideas in written form. Assignments help students learn how to organize thoughts and present them clearly. This clarity in writing develops through planned writing activities integrated in the nursing program. As a skill, writing ability requires practice, and students need to complete writing assignments across clinical courses. All too often, writing assignments are not sequenced progressively across courses or levels in the program; students, then, do not have the benefit of building writing skills sequentially.

Learning to write effectively is the responsibility of the entire faculty and requires more than taking an English course or writing one term paper in a clinical nursing course. Students need an opportunity to write about nursing in varied contexts. Through writing assignments in nursing courses, students learn to disseminate their ideas and explain and persuade (Oermann, 2013). This is referred to as writing in the discipline (Writing Across the Curriculum [WAC] Clearinghouse, 2017a). By writing multiple types of papers with feedback from the teacher, students learn the writing style and conventions of the field. For example, in a prelicensure clinical course students might write a brief evidence summary to support a nursing intervention, whereas at the graduate level the writing assignment may be a systematic review of the evidence. Through writing in the discipline students begin to think like a nurse and communicate clearly within the field. Generally these papers are formal papers that adhere to the format and style of the field (WAC Clearinghouse, 2017b). These assignments should be sequenced across the nursing curriculum to improve students' writing skills. Students can begin with short assignments related to the clinical course, such as summarizing data they collected on a patient or preparing a report on how their assessment or nursing care related to their readings or what they learned in class. In later assignments, students can complete literature reviews, EBP papers, critiques of research studies related to clinical practice, analyses of quality and safety problems on the unit, and term papers. In this way, the writing assignments become more complex and build students' writing skills; they also provide variety for students.

A benefit of this planned approach to teaching writing is faculty feedback, provided through drafts and rewrites of papers. Drafts are essential to foster development of writing skill. Drafts should be critiqued by faculty members for accuracy of content, development of ideas, organization, clarity of expression, and writing skills such as sentence structure, punctuation, and spelling (Oermann & Hays, 2016).

Small group critique of each others' writing is appropriate particularly for formative purposes. Small group critique provides a basis for subsequent revisions and gives feedback to students about both content and writing style. Although students may not identify every error in sentence structure and punctuation, they can provide valuable feedback on content, organization, how the ideas are developed, and clarity of writing. In a study with graduate students, peer review of the draft of the final assignment was an effective strategy to improve the quality of the paper and student understanding of the content (Schlisselberg & Moscou, 2013). Peer review should be used for giving feedback only, not for determining a grade for the assignment.

TYPES OF WRITING ASSIGNMENTS FOR CLINICAL LEARNING

Many types of writing assignments are appropriate for enhancing clinical learning. Some assignments help students learn the content they are writing about but do not necessarily improve writing skill, and other assignments also promote competency in writing. For example, structured assignments such as care plans provide minimal opportunity for freedom of expression, originality, and creativity. Other assignments, though, such as term papers on clinical topics, promote understanding of new content and its use in clinical practice as well as writing ability.

Types of written assignments for clinical learning include concept map, short written assignments, nursing care plan, analysis of cases, EBP papers, teaching plan, reflective journal, group writing, and electronic portfolio.

Concept Map

A concept map is a graphic or pictorial arrangement of key concepts related to a patient's care, which shows the interrelationships of those concepts. By developing a concept map, students can visualize how assessment data, problems, interventions, medications, and other aspects of a patient's care relate to one another. Concept maps are also useful for teaching in the classroom and online courses. Students can develop a concept map for organizing ideas, brainstorming, linking concepts together, planning and evaluating care, and learning collaboratively (Daley, Morgan, & Black, 2016; Spencer, Anderson, & Ellis, 2013). They can also be used to teach concepts rather than focusing on content.

Concept maps have many uses in clinical learning. First, students may complete a concept map from their readings to assist them in applying new information to their patients. The readings that students complete for clinical practice, and in nursing courses overall, contain vast amounts of facts and specific information; concept maps help students process this information in a meaningful way, linking new and existing ideas.

Second, concept maps are useful in helping students prepare for clinical practice. They can be developed prior to or at the beginning of a clinical experience as a way of organizing assessment information, relating it to the patient's needs and problems, and planning nursing care. In preclinical conferences, students can present the maps for feedback from the teacher and from peers. Students can modify the maps as they provide care for patients.

Third, concept maps may be developed collaboratively by students in clinical conferences. For this purpose, students may present a patient for whom they have provided care, and the clinical group then develops a concept map about that patient's care. Or the clinical group may develop a concept map about conditions they are learning about in the course. As another strategy, students can present the concept maps they developed for their patients, and the group can analyze and discuss them. Critiquing each others' concept maps enhances students' thinking, learning from one another, and group process; it also allows for feedback from the teacher and peers.

Concept maps are organized with specific concepts written under more general ones (Daley, Morgan, & Black, 2016). Students first identify relevant concepts for their patients' care and then analyze the interrelationships among these concepts. Different types of lines can be used to illustrate the connections among the concepts.

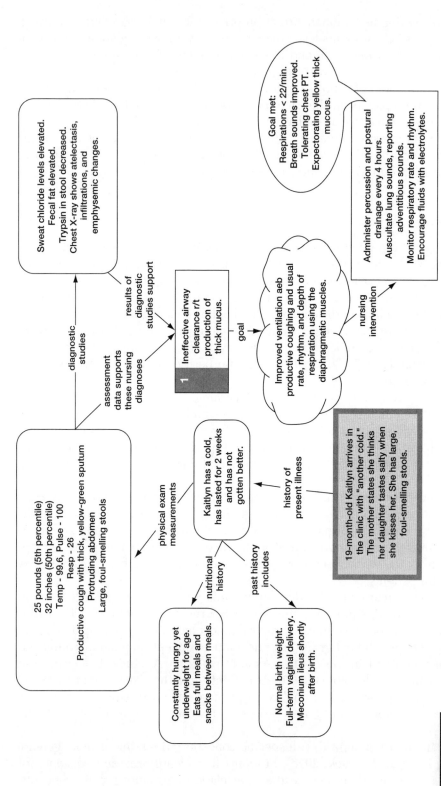

FIGURE 14.1   THIS CONCEPT MAP DEPICTS THE PLAN OF CARE FOR A 19-MONTH OLD WHO HAS BEEN DIAGNOSED WITH CYSTIC FIBROSIS. AEB, AS EVIDENCED BY; PT, PHYSICAL THERAPY; R/T, RELATED TO.

Source: Developed by Deanne Blach (2017). Reprinted with permission.

Figure 14.1 provides an example of a concept map. Concept maps are most appropriately used for formative evaluation, although students could write papers or present on the concepts in the maps, their interrelationships, and rationale, which could then be graded.

Short Written Assignments

Short written assignments in clinical courses are valuable for promoting higher level thinking and helping students apply what they are learning in class to clinical practice. Short assignments avoid students' reporting on and summarizing what others have written without thinking critically about the content themselves. With a short assignment, students can analyze patient problems, compare interventions with their evidence, explore decisions that might be made in a clinical situation, analyze an issue and approaches, and analyze a case scenario. Sample assignments are found in Exhibit 14.1.

Nursing Care Plan

Nursing care plans enable students to analyze patients' health problems and design plans of care. With care plans, students can record assessment data, identify patient needs and problems, select evidence-based interventions, and identify outcomes to

---

EXHIBIT 14.1

EXAMPLES OF SHORT WRITTEN ASSIGNMENTS FOR CLINICAL COURSES

- The unit clerk is slow about notifying nursing staff when patients use their call bells. It appears that only the assigned staff will answer the call bells; other nurses and staff who happen to be close by the patient's room will not respond. Develop a quality improvement project to address this issue.
- Select an intervention or treatment you used in patient care. Search for evidence related to that intervention or treatment. What were your sources of evidence? Summarize the strength of the evidence and discuss what it means for patient care.
- Read the article on loneliness. In no more than one page, explain how you would use that concept in an assessment.
- Describe patient-centered care and key attributes.
- In what ways did your patient's needs and problems compare to the description in your textbook?
- Your patient had a knee replacement and reports too much pain to go to physical therapy. Two hours ago, the prior nurse recorded in the electronic medical record that the patient "had no pain and walked twice around the room." What are two different ways of approaching this situation? What would you do and why?
- Your patient is readmitted with heart failure. He is agitated, and his respiratory rate is increasing rapidly. He is receiving oxygen by nasal cannula at 2 L/min. What additional data would you collect? What would you do next? Provide a rationale for your answer.
- Identify a decision you made in clinical practice involving either patients or staff. Describe the situation and why you responded that way. Propose another approach that could have been used.
- Describe the process on your unit for handoff at the end of the shift. What changes would you propose in that process and why?

be measured. Care plans should be usable—they should guide students' planning of their patients' care, be realistic, and be able to be implemented in the health care setting.

Completing a written care plan may help the student identify nursing and other interventions for specific problems, but whether that same care plan promotes problem-solving learning and higher level thinking is questionable. Often students develop care plans from their textbook or the literature without thinking about the content. Even if the care plan is an appropriate written assignment for the course outcomes, the question remains as to how many care plans students need to complete in a clinical course to meet the learning goals. Once the goals have been achieved, then other written assignments may be more effective for clinical learning.

Cases

Case scenarios describe a clinical situation developed around an actual or a hypothetical patient for student review and critique. In case method, the case provided for analysis is generally shorter and more specific than in case study. Case studies are more comprehensive, thereby presenting a complete picture of the patient and clinical situation. After analyzing the case, students complete written questions about it; questions may be answered individually or by small groups of students. Cases were discussed in detail in Chapter 10.

EBP Papers

Assignments in clinical courses can guide students' learning about EBP and its use in patient care. Clinical assignments that are integrated in courses throughout the nursing program prepare students with the skills they need to search for and use evidence in their future practice. Through these assignments, students can learn the steps of the EBP process, beginning with recognizing the need for evidence to guide decisions and writing a clinical question, through evaluating the outcomes of practice decisions and disseminating evidence (Melnyk & Fineout-Overholt, 2015; Melnyk, Fineout-Overholt, Stillwell, & Williamson, 2010). These steps can be used as a framework for planning learning activities for students and assignments in clinical courses. By using a framework such as this one or another EBP model, teachers can plan assignments for each clinical course in the curriculum, systematically developing students' understanding and skills and avoiding repetition of assignments. Exhibit 14.2 provides sample clinical assignments for learning about EBP and steps in the process.

Teaching Plan

Teaching plans enable students to apply concepts of learning and teaching to patients, families, communities, and populations. This is another type of written assignment that may be completed individually or in small groups. After developing the teaching plan, students may use it as a basis for their teaching or might role play teaching in the laboratory, simulation, or post conference. There are many formats for teaching plans, but typically the assignment should provide experience for students in writing objectives, planning content to teach, identifying instructional strategies to use such as teach-back, and selecting realistic, evaluation strategies.

EXHIBIT 14.2

SAMPLE CLINICAL ASSIGNMENTS FOR LEARNING ABOUT EBP

Develop Questions About Clinical Practice

Write a clinical question using PICOT (patient, intervention, comparison, outcome, and time) format.

Think about a patient for whom you cared this week. Identify a question you had about that patient's care and write the question in PICOT format. List two sources of information you could consult to answer that question with a rationale for why these are appropriate. Discuss your question with a peer during postclinical conference. Is your question specific enough to guide a search? If not, revise it.

Identify a change in practice needed on your unit. Why is it needed? What led you to this decision? Write a short paper (no more than one page).

Search for Evidence

Conduct a search using your PICOT question. Identify key words or terms to search for an answer. Go to the Cumulative Index to Nursing and Allied Health Literature (CINAHL) and modify your key words as needed. Complete the search in CINAHL, mapping out your search strategy. Summarize your findings. What would you do differently with this search the next time? Write a two- to three-page paper on this search and what you found.

Conduct the same search in PubMed (MEDLINE). What are the differences, if any, in the results of your search? What did you learn about these two databases? Present in clinical conference.

Conduct a search using your PICOT question. For this search, start with PubMed Clinical Queries and describe your search strategy and results. Then continue your search in CINAHL. What evidence did you find related to your PICOT question?

Identify a bibliographic database other than CINAHL or PubMed that you might use in your clinical practice—for example, PsycINFO. Identify a clinical question that could be answered by searching in that database. Conduct the search and summarize your results. How could you use these results in clinical practice? What did you learn about this database? Present in the discussion board.

Critically Appraise the Evidence

Identify a PICOT question or a change in practice that might be indicated. Search for evidence and record your search strategy and results. What studies are relevant for inclusion in your review and why? Critique the evidence (consider validity, relevance, and applicability). Summarize your findings and develop a written proposal for use of this evidence to guide practice or why a practice change is not indicated.

Review clinical research studies in an area of nursing practice related to the course. Critically appraise those studies and synthesize findings. What are issues in implementing those findings in your clinical setting? What would you propose to facilitate implementation? Prepare a paper on your review and analysis.

Discuss how you can use the Cochrane Database of Systematic Reviews in your patient care. Select a nursing intervention and locate information about this intervention in Cochrane. Write a three- to four-page report on your findings.

Select one of your PICOT questions and searches. Critique the evidence you found in that search. Use an established evidence hierarchy and rate the strength of the evidence. Discuss the implications of the evidence for nursing practice.

Use the Evidence in Clinical Practice

How do the nurse's clinical expertise and the patient's preferences and values interface with evidence-based practice (EBP)? Should the evidence be weighed more heavily in decisions than patient preferences? Lead a discussion on this topic in the discussion board.

(continued)

List interventions for one of your patients. What is the evidence base for each of these? Provide a rationale for their use based on the strength of the evidence. Include the sources of information you used to determine the evidence base. What evidence is missing, and what do you propose?

Review your patient's care. Select one problem not adequately met with current practices. Search for evidence to suggest a change in practice, evaluate the evidence, and write a paper about how you would change practice based on your review. What would you do differently the next time you care for that patient or patients with similar problems?

Select an intervention and find evidence using resources from the Joanna Briggs Institute. Describe the evidence you located. Did it help you make a decision about the effectiveness of the intervention? Why or why not? How would you use this information in your clinical practice? Prepare a short paper.

Evaluate Outcomes of Practice Decisions

For a practice change or evidence-based intervention you proposed in an earlier assignment, plan how you would evaluate its effect on patient outcomes. Present in online discussion forum.

Identify a question you had about your patient's care. Go to the National Guideline Clearinghouse. What EBP guidelines are relevant for this patient? If you implemented one of these guidelines in your clinical setting, what outcomes would you measure?

Implement one evidence-based intervention in patient care and evaluate its outcomes. Write a short (no more than two pages) report on your findings.

Reflective Journals

Journal writing assists students in relating theory to clinical practice, linking their classroom and online instruction to care of patients, and reflecting on their clinical learning activities. When students reexamine their clinical decisions and propose alternative actions, journaling also encourages the development of higher level thinking skills and clinical judgment. Assignments in which students write in journals about their reflections and experiences in clinical practice can achieve many outcomes; some of these are listed in Exhibit 14.3. Reflective journals also can be

EXHIBIT 14.3

USES OF REFLECTIVE JOURNALS

- Reflect on clinical practice experiences and their meaning.
- Document feelings related to clinical practice and reflect on their meaning personally and professionally.
- Describe perceptions of patients, families, communities, and experiences with other health care providers.
- Develop values and affective skills.
- Analyze ethical issues.
- Assess one's own knowledge and clinical performance.
- Identify gaps in learning and how to improve clinical performance.
- Analyze one's own actions and decisions following a clinical experience.
- Communicate with the clinical teacher, preceptor, and others involved in learning experience.

used with simulation. Bussard (2015a, 2015b) found that reflective journaling following simulations promoted the development of clinical judgment among prelicensure nursing students.

Through a reflective journal, students can:

- Find meaning in their clinical experiences
- Integrate theory and practice
- Examine their own values and develop values for professional practice
- Develop effective communication skills
- Learn about the perspectives of others, including patients, families, nurses, and interprofessional team members
- Reflect on one's own role and the roles and responsibilities of others, including interprofessional teams
- Develop thinking and clinical judgment skills

There are different ways of structuring journals, and the decision should be based on the intended outcomes of using the journal in the clinical course. The first step for the teacher is to identify the learning outcomes to be met through journal writing, such as reflecting on clinical decisions or describing feelings in caring for a patient, and then how journal entries should be made. Students should have written guidelines for the journal activity (Ruiz-Lopez et al., 2015). Often the guidelines include open-ended questions to guide students' thinking and reflection. Journals can be done electronically with course management systems, e-mail, blogs, and by using software for this purpose. Electronic journaling makes it easier for teachers to provide prompt feedback, dialogue with students, and store the journals.

Journals are not typically graded but provide an opportunity for giving feedback to learners and developing a dialogue with them. Students have greater freedom in recording feelings, ideas, and responses when the journal is used only for feedback. Faculty members are responsible for providing thoughtful and prompt feedback similar to any written assignment. Ruiz-Lopez et al. (2015) suggested providing constructive feedback to students over short time periods.

Group Writing

Not all writing assignments need to be done by students individually. There is much to be gained with group writing exercises as long as the groups are small and the exercises are carefully focused. Short written assignments, such as analyzing an issue and reporting in writing the outcomes of the analysis or developing a care plan as a group, may be completed in clinical conferences or done online in small groups. These group assignments provide opportunities for students to express their ideas to others in the group and work collaboratively to communicate the results of their thinking as a group in written form.

Electronic Portfolio

A portfolio provides an opportunity for students to present projects they completed in their clinical courses over a period of time. Portfolios can be prepared using hard copies of documents, but in most cases, it is more efficient to develop an electronic portfolio or e-portfolio. These can be prepared using commercially available software, or students can upload their e-portfolios in the course management system or at a website for this purpose. Portfolios may include evidence of student learning for a series of clinical learning activities over the duration of a clinical course or for documenting competencies in terms of overall course or program outcomes (Oermann & Gaberson, 2017).

There are two types of portfolios: best-work and growth and learning progress (Brookhart & Nitko, 2015). Best-work portfolios include materials and products developed by students in clinical practice that demonstrate their learning and achievement. These portfolios reflect the best work of the students in the clinical course. In contrast, growth and learning progress portfolios include materials and products in the process of being developed. These portfolios serve as a way of monitoring students' progress in clinical practice (Oermann & Gaberson, 2017). With both types of e-portfolios, the teacher reviews them periodically and provides feedback on the materials and products in the portfolio.

The content of the e-portfolio depends on the goals to be achieved. Students may include in their portfolios any materials they developed individually or in a group that provide evidence of their achieving the outcomes of the clinical course or demonstrating the clinical competencies. Examples of these materials are:

- Documents that students developed for patient care
- Teaching plans and materials
- Papers written about clinical practice
- Selected journal entries
- Reports of group work and products
- Reports and observations made in the clinical setting
- A self-assessment
- Reflections of their patient care experiences and meaning to them
- Other products that demonstrate their clinical competencies and what they learned in the course

Exhibit 14.4 presents a process for developing an e-portfolio for a clinical course.

EXHIBIT 14.4

DEVELOPING A PORTFOLIO FOR CLINICAL LEARNING

Step 1: Identify the purpose of the e-portfolio.

- Why is an e-portfolio useful in the course? What goals will it serve?
- Will the portfolio serve as a means of assessing students' development of clinical competencies, focusing predominantly on the growth of the students? Will the portfolio provide evidence of the students' best work in clinical practice, including products that reflect their learning over a period of time? Or, will the portfolio meet both demands, enabling the faculty member or clinical teacher to give feedback to students on the process of learning and projects on which they are working, as well as providing evidence of their accomplishments and achievements in clinical practice?

(continued)

- Will the e-portfolio be used for formative or summative evaluation? Or both?
- Will the e-portfolio provide assessment data for use in a clinical course? Or, will it be used for curriculum and program evaluation?
- What is the role of the students, if any, in defining the focus and content of the e-portfolio?

Step 2: Identify the type of entries and content to be included in the e-portfolio.

- What types of entries are required in the e-portfolio, for example, products developed by students, descriptions of projects with which the students are involved, descriptions of clinical learning activities and reflections about them, observations made in clinical practice and analysis of them, and papers completed by the students, among others?
- In addition to required entries, what other types of content and entries might be included in the e-portfolio?
- Who determines the content of the e-portfolio and the types of entries? Teacher only? Student only? Or both?
- Will the entries be the same for all students or individualized by the student?
- What is the minimum number of entries to be considered satisfactory?
- How should the entries in the e-portfolio be organized, or will the students choose how to organize them?
- Are there required times for entries to be made in the e-portfolio, and when should it be submitted to the teacher for review and feedback?
- Will teacher and student meet to discuss the e-portfolio, or will feedback be provided only in written form?

Step 3: Decide on the evaluation of the e-portfolio entries, including criteria for evaluation of individual entries and the portfolio overall.

- How will the e-portfolio be integrated within the clinical evaluation grade and course grade, if at all?
- What criteria will be used to evaluate, and perhaps score, each type of entry and the e-portfolio as a whole?
- Will only the teacher evaluate the e-portfolio and its entries? Will only the students evaluate their own progress and work? Or, will the evaluation be a collaborative effort?
- Should a rubric be developed for scoring the e-portfolio and individual entries?

Source: Adapted from Oermann and Gaberson (2017). Copyright ©2017 by Springer. Reprinted with permission.

EVALUATING WRITTEN ASSIGNMENTS

Written assignments may be evaluated formatively or summatively. Formative evaluation provides feedback to students for their continued learning but not for grading purposes. Periodic assessment of drafts of papers and work in progress is formative in nature and is not intended for arriving at a grade. Summative evaluation of completed writing assignments is designed for grading the assignment, not for giving feedback to the student.

For written assignments that are not graded, the teacher's role is to give prompt and sufficient feedback for students to learn from the assignment. If the assignment will be graded at a later time, however, then criteria for grading should be established and communicated to the learner. Any assignment that will eventually be graded should have clear, specific, and measurable criteria for evaluation. Some writing assignments, such as journals, do not lend themselves to grading and instead are best used for formative evaluation only.

Drafts

If drafts of written assignments are to be submitted, the teacher should inform students of each required due date. Feedback should be given on the quality of the content, as reflected in the criteria for evaluation, and on writing style if appropriate for the assignment. Students need specific suggestions about revisions, not general statements such as "unclear introduction." Instead, tell students exactly what needs to be changed; for instance, "The introduction is about noise reduction strategies rather than the problem on the unit with noise. Revise the introduction to explain the problem with noise on the unit, supporting data on noise levels, and why we need strategies to reduce noise for both patients and staff." Drafts of written assignments are important because they serve as a means of improving writing and thinking about the content. Prompt, clear, and specific feedback about revisions is essential to meet this purpose. Feedback is typically provided in written form but can also be given using various technology tools. Drafts in most instances are used for feedback and are therefore not graded.

Criteria for Evaluation

The criteria for evaluation should relate to the learning outcomes to be met with the assignment. For example, if students write a short paper to meet the objective, "Compare interventions for nausea associated with chemotherapy," criteria should relate to the appropriateness and evidence for the interventions selected for critique, how effectively the student compared them, the rationale developed for the analysis, and the like.

General criteria for evaluating written assignments in clinical courses are presented in Exhibit 14.5. These criteria need to be adapted based on the type of assignment and its intent. For assignments that are graded, students should have the criteria for evaluation and scoring protocol or rubric before they begin writing so they are clear about how the assignment will be assessed.

Grading Assignments

In grading written assignments, a scoring protocol should be developed based on the criteria established for evaluation. The protocol should include the elements to be evaluated and points allotted for each one. The scoring protocol must be used in the same way for all students. This is an important principle in grading written assignments to assure consistency across papers and to focus the evaluation on the specific criteria. Some teachers tend to be more lenient, and others tend to be more critical in their review of papers. A scoring protocol helps the teacher base the grade on the established criteria rather than some other standard. Teachers will be more consistent in grading papers if they first establish specific criteria for evaluation, then develop a scoring protocol based on these criteria, and then use that scoring protocol in the same way for each student.

For some papers, a scoring rubric can be developed to guide the evaluation. A rubric lists the criteria to be met in the paper or characteristics of the paper and the points given for their evaluation. Exhibit 14.6 shows an example of how a rubric for scoring papers is developed using the general criteria in Exhibit 14.5. There are different types of rubrics. With a holistic rubric, the teacher scores the paper as a whole without assessing individual parts of the paper. An analytic rubric guides the assessment of separate parts of the paper and then sums them for a total score. For short written assignments in clinical courses, a protocol for scoring them is sufficient. However, for longer assignments, the teacher should develop a more detailed rubric for use in evaluating them.

Written assignments that are graded should be read anonymously if at all possible. This is sometimes difficult with small groups of students. Nevertheless, students can record on their papers their student numbers rather than their names.

EXHIBIT 14.5

GENERAL CRITERIA FOR EVALUATING PAPERS IN CLINICAL COURSES

Content

Content is relevant to patient or clinical situation.
Content is accurate.
Significant information is presented.
Concepts and theories are used appropriately for analysis.
Content is comprehensive.
Content reflects current research and evidence.
Hypotheses, conclusions, and decisions are supported.

Organization

Content is organized logically.
Ideas are presented in logical sequence.
Paragraph structure is appropriate.
Headings are used appropriately to indicate new content areas.

Process

Process used to arrive at approaches, decisions, judgments, and so forth is adequate.
Consequences of decisions are considered.
Sound rationale is provided.
For papers analyzing issues, rationale supports position taken.
Multiple perspectives and new approaches are considered.

Writing Style

Ideas are described clearly.
Sentence structure is clear.
There are no grammatical errors.
There are no spelling errors.
Appropriate punctuation is used.
Writing does not reveal bias.
Length of paper is consistent with requirements.
Literature used in paper is up to date (within the past 3–5 years)
References are cited appropriately throughout paper.
References are accurate and prepared according to required format.

EXHIBIT 14.6

SAMPLE SCORING RUBRIC FOR PAPERS IN CLINICAL COURSES

Content		
Content relevant to patient or clinical situation, comprehensive, and in-depth 5	Content relevant to patient or clinical situation with critical information included 4–3	Some content not relevant to patient or clinical situation, critical information missing, lacks depth 2–1
Content accurate 5	Most of content accurate 4–3	Major errors in content 2–1
Sound background developed from peer-reviewed articles and wide range of information sources 5	Textbook and websites predominant sources of information for developing background 4–3	Background not developed, limited support for ideas 2–1
Current research and evidence synthesized and integrated effectively 10–7	Current research and evidence summarized 6–4	Limited research and evidence in paper, not used to support ideas 3–1
Organization		
Purpose of paper well developed and clearly stated 3	Purpose apparent but not developed sufficiently 2	Purpose poorly developed, not clear 1
Content well organized and logically presented, organization supports arguments and development of ideas 10–7	Clear organization of main points and ideas 6–4	Poorly organized, content not developed adequately 3–1
Effective conclusions based on analysis 3	Conclusions based on summary of content, limited analysis 2	Poor conclusions, not based on content in paper 1
Writing Style and Format		
Sentence structure clear, smooth transitions, correct grammar and punctuation, no spelling errors 10–7	Adequate sentence structure and transitions; few grammar, punctuation, and spelling errors 6–4	Poor sentence structure and transitions; errors in grammar, punctuation, and spelling 3–1

(continued)

Writing Style and Format		
Professional appearance of paper, all parts included, length consistent with requirements	Paper legible, some parts missing or too short or too long considering requirements	Unprofessional appearance, missing sections, paper too short or too long considering requirements
3	2	1
References used appropriately, references current, no errors in references, correct use of APA style	References used appropriately but limited, most references current, some citations or references with errors or some errors in APA style	Few references and limited breadth, old references (not classic), errors in references, errors in APA style
6–5	4–3	2–1
Total score _____ (sum points for total score; maximum score 60)		

There is a tendency in evaluating papers and other written assignments, similar to essay items, for the teacher to be influenced by a general impression of the student. This is called the halo effect. The teacher may have positive or negative feelings about the student or other biases that may influence evaluating and grading the assignment.

Another reason to read papers anonymously is to avoid a carryover effect, in which the teacher carries an impression of the quality of one written assignment to the next one that the student completes. If the student develops an outstanding paper, the teacher may be influenced to score subsequent written assignments at a similarly high level; the same situation may occur with a poor paper. The teacher therefore carries the impression of the student from one written assignment to the next. If there are multiple questions that students answered as part of a written assignment, the previous scores should be covered to avoid being biased about the quality of the next answer. In addition, the teacher should evaluate all students' answers to one question before proceeding to the next question (Oermann, 2013; Oermann & Gaberson, 2017).

All written assignments should be read twice before scoring. In the first reading, it is important to note errors in content, omission of major content areas, problems with organization, problems with the process used for approaching the issue, and problems with writing style. Comments can be recorded on the student's paper with suggestions for revision. After reading through all of the papers, then the teacher should begin a second reading for scoring purposes. Reading the papers twice gives the teacher a sense of how students approached the assignment. This is important because, in some cases, the scoring protocol may need to be revised.

Papers and other types of written assignments should be read in random order. After the first reading, the teacher can shuffle the papers so they are read in a random order the second time. Papers read early may be scored higher than those read near the end (Oermann & Gaberson, 2017). Teacher fatigue may also set in and influence the grading of papers. Although this section discusses grading written assignments, the teacher should remember that many writing assignments will not be graded.

SUMMARY

Written assignments for clinical learning have four main purposes: to learn about concepts, theories, and other content related to clinical practice; develop thinking skills; examine values and beliefs that may affect patient care; and develop writing skills. Not all writing assignments achieve each of these outcomes. The teacher decides first on the outcomes to be met, then plans the writing assignment with these outcomes in mind.

Short written assignments can be used in clinical courses to encourage students' independent thinking and avoid their summarizing what others have written. In developing these assignments, the teacher should not ask students to merely report on the ideas of others; instead, the assignment should ask students to consider an alternative point of view or a different way of approaching an issue. Short assignments also provide an opportunity for faculty members to give prompt feedback to students.

Written assignments help learners examine feelings generated from caring for patients and reflect on their beliefs and values that might influence that care. They also help students learn how to organize thoughts and present them clearly. Some faculty members have developed writing-to-learn programs in which written assignments are sequenced across the nursing curriculum.

Many types of written assignments can be used for clinical learning. Concept map, short written assignment, nursing care plan, cases, EBP papers, teaching plan, reflective journal, group writing, and e-portfolio were presented in this chapter.

Written assignments may be evaluated formatively or summatively. Formative evaluation provides feedback to students for their continued learning but not for grading purposes. Periodic assessment of drafts of papers and work in progress is formative in nature and is not intended for arriving at a grade. Summative evaluation of completed writing assignments is designed for grading the assignment, not for giving feedback to the student.

In grading written assignments, a scoring protocol or rubric should be developed based on the criteria established for evaluation. The scoring protocol and rubric are used in the same way for all students. Many written assignments, though, are best if assessed formatively and not graded.

CNE EXAMINATION TEST BLUEPRINT CORE COMPETENCIES

1. **Facilitate Learning**

    A. Implement a variety of teaching strategies appropriate to
        1. content
        2. setting
        3. learner needs

(continued)

      4. learning style
      5. desired learner outcomes
      6. method of delivery
  B. Use teaching strategies based on
      1. educational theory
      2. evidence-based practices related to education
  E. Practice skilled oral and written (including electronic) communication that reflects an awareness of self and relationships with learners (e.g., evaluation, mentorship, and supervision)
  F. Communicate effectively orally and in writing with an ability to convey ideas in a variety of contexts
  G. Model reflective thinking practices, including critical thinking
  H. Create opportunities for learners to develop their own critical thinking skills
  I. Create a positive learning environment that fosters a free exchange of ideas
  N. Use knowledge of evidence-based practice to instruct learners

2. **Facilitate Learner Development and Socialization**

  A. Foster the development of learners in these areas
      1. cognitive domain
      3. affective domain
  F. Assist learners to engage in thoughtful and constructive self and peer evaluation

3. **Use Assessment and Evaluation Strategies**

  C. Use a variety of strategies to assess and evaluate learning in these domains
      1. cognitive
      3. affective
  D. Incorporate current research in assessment and evaluation practices
  G. Use assessment instruments to evaluate outcomes
  J. Use assessment and evaluation data to enhance the teaching-learning process
  K. Advise learners regarding assessment and evaluation criteria
  L. Provide timely, constructive, and thoughtful feedback

REFERENCES

Brookhart, S. M., & Nitko, A. J. (2015). *Educational assessment of students* (7th ed.). Upper Saddle River, NJ: Pearson.

Bussard, M. E. (2015a). Clinical judgment in reflective journals of prelicensure nursing students. *Journal of Nursing Education, 54*, 36–40. doi:10.3928/01484834-20141224-05

Bussard, M. E. (2015b). The nature of clinical judgment development in reflective journals. *Journal of Nursing Education, 54*, 451–454. doi:10.3928/01484834-20150717-05

Daley, B. J., Morgan, S., & Black, S. B. (2016). Concept maps in nursing education: A historical literature review and research directions. *Journal of Nursing Education, 55*, 631–639. doi:10.3928/01484834-20161011-05

Melnyk, B., & Fineout-Overholt, E. (Eds.). (2015). *Evidence-based practice in nursing and healthcare: A guide to best practice* (3rd ed.). Philadelphia, PA: Wolters Kluwer Health.

Melnyk, B. M., Fineout-Overholt, E., Stillwell, S. B., & Williamson, K. M. (2010). Evidence-based practice: Step by step: The seven steps of evidence-based practice. *American Journal of Nursing, 110*(1), 51–63. doi:10.1097/01.NAJ.0000366056.06605.d2

Oermann, M. H. (2013). Enhancing writing in online education. In K. H. Frith & D. J. Clark (Eds.), *Distance education in nursing* (3rd ed., pp. 145–162). New York, NY: Springer Publishing.

Oermann, M. H., & Gaberson, K. B. (2017). *Evaluation and testing in nursing education* (5th ed.). New York, NY: Springer Publishing.

Oermann, M. H., & Hays, J. (2016). *Writing for publication in nursing* (3rd ed.). New York, NY: Springer Publishing.

Ruiz-Lopez, M., Rodriguez-Garcia, M., Villanueva, P. G., Marquez-Cava, M., Garcia-Mateos, M., Ruiz-Ruiz, B., & Herrera-Sanchez, E. (2015). The use of reflective journaling as a learning strategy during the clinical rotations of students from the faculty of health sciences: An action-research study. *Nurse Education Today, 35*(10), e26–e31. doi:10.1016/j.nedt.2015.07.029

Schlisselberg, G., & Moscou, S. (2013). Peer review as an educational strategy to improve academic work: An interdisciplinary collaboration between communication disorders and nursing. *Work, 44,* 355–360. doi:10.3233/WOR-121512

Spencer, J. R., Anderson, K. M., & Ellis, K. K. (2013). Radiant thinking and the use of the mind map in nurse practitioner education. *Journal of Nursing Education, 52,* 291–293. doi:10.3928/01484834 -20130328-03s

Writing Across the Curriculum Clearinghouse. (2017a). Basic principles of WAC. Retrieved from http://wac.colostate.edu/intro/pop3a.cfm

Writing Across the Curriculum Clearinghouse. (2017b). What is writing in the disciplines? Retrieved from http://wac.colostate.edu/intro/pop2e.cfm

CHAPTER 15

Clinical Evaluation and Grading

Nursing practice requires the development of higher level cognitive skills, values, psychomotor and technological skills, and other competencies for care of patients across settings. Through clinical evaluation, the teacher arrives at judgments about students' competencies—their performance in practice. After establishing a framework for evaluating students in clinical practice and exploring one's own values, attitudes, and biases that may influence evaluation, the teacher identifies a variety of methods for collecting data on student performance. Clinical evaluation methods are strategies for assessing learning outcomes in clinical practice. Some evaluation methods are most appropriate for use by faculty members or preceptors who are onsite with students and can observe their performance; other evaluation methods assess students' knowledge, cognitive skills, and other competencies but do not involve direct observation of their performance. This chapter describes the process of clinical evaluation in nursing, methods for evaluating clinical performance, and how to grade students in clinical courses.

CONCEPT OF CLINICAL EVALUATION

Clinical evaluation is a process by which judgments are made about learners' competencies in practice. This practice may involve care of patients, families, and communities; other types of learning activities in the clinical setting; simulation activities; performance of varied skills in learning laboratories; or activities using multimedia. Most frequently, clinical evaluation involves observing performance and arriving at judgments about the student's competence. Judgments influence the data collected— that is, the specific types of observations made to evaluate the student's performance— and the inferences and conclusions drawn from the data about the quality of that performance. Teachers may collect different data to evaluate the same outcomes, and when presented with a series of observations about a student's performance in clinical practice, there may be minimal consistency in their judgments about how well that student performed.

Clinical evaluation is not an objective process; it involves subjective judgments of the teacher and others involved in the process. The teacher's values influence evaluation. This is most apparent in clinical evaluation, where teachers' values influence the observations they make of students and the judgments they make about the quality of their performance. Thus, it is important for teachers to be aware of their own values that might bias their judgments of students. For example, if the teacher prefers students who initiate discussions and participate actively in conferences, this value should not influence the assessment of students' competencies in other areas. The teacher needs to be aware of this preference to avoid an unfair evaluation of other dimensions of the students' clinical performance. Or, if the teacher is used to the fast pace of most acute care settings, when working with beginning students or someone who moves slowly, the teacher should be cautious not to let this prior experience influence expectations of performance. Clinical nurse educators and preceptors should examine their values, attitudes, and beliefs so that they are aware of them as they teach and assess students' performance in practice settings.

Clinical Evaluation Versus Grading

Clinical evaluation is not the same as grading. In evaluation, the teacher makes observations of performance and collects other types of data, then compares this information to a set of standards to arrive at a judgment. From this assessment, a quantitative symbol or grade may be applied to reflect the evaluation data and judgments made about performance. The clinical grade, such as pass–fail or A through F, is the symbol to represent the evaluation. Clinical performance may be evaluated and not graded, such as with formative evaluation or feedback to the learner, or it may be graded. Grades, however, should not be assigned without sufficient data about clinical performance.

Norm- and Criterion-Referenced Clinical Evaluation

Clinical evaluation may be norm- or criterion-referenced. In norm-referenced evaluation, the student's clinical performance is compared with that of other students, indicating that the performance is better than, worse than, or equivalent to that of others in the comparison group or that the student has more or less knowledge, skill, or ability than the other students. Rating students' clinical competencies in relation to others in the clinical group—for example, indicating that the student was "average"—is a norm-referenced interpretation.

In contrast, criterion-referenced clinical evaluation involves comparing the student's clinical performance to predetermined criteria, not to the performance of other students in the group. In this type of clinical evaluation, the criteria are known in advance and used as the basis for evaluation. Indicating that the student has met the clinical outcomes or achieved the clinical competencies, regardless of how other students performed, represents a criterion-referenced interpretation.

Formative and Summative Clinical Evaluation

Clinical evaluation may be formative or summative. Formative evaluation in clinical practice provides feedback to learners about their progress in meeting the outcomes of the clinical course or in developing the clinical competencies. The purposes of formative evaluation are to enable students to develop further their clinical knowledge, skills, and values; indicate areas in which learning and practice are needed; and provide a basis for suggesting additional instruction to improve performance. With this type of evaluation, after identifying the learning needs, instruction is provided to move students forward in their learning. Feedback is critical to learning in the clinical setting: The teacher provides specific information that fills in gaps in learning and helps students improve their performance. Formative evaluation, therefore, is diagnostic; it should not be graded (Brookhart & Nitko, 2015). For example, the clinical teacher or preceptor might observe a student perform wound care and give feedback on changes to make with the technique. The goal of this assessment is to improve subsequent performance, not to grade how well the student carried out the procedure.

Summative clinical evaluation, however, is designed for determining clinical grades because it summarizes competencies the student has developed in clinical practice. Summative evaluation is done at the end of a period of time—for example, at midterm or at the end of the clinical practicum—to assess the extent to which learners have achieved the clinical outcomes or competencies. Summative evaluation is not diagnostic; it summarizes the performance of students at a particular point in time. For much of clinical practice in a nursing education program, summative evaluation comes too late for students to have an opportunity to improve performance. At the end of a course involving care of children, for instance, there may be behaviors the student would not have an opportunity to practice in subsequent courses.

Any protocol for clinical evaluation should include extensive formative evaluation and periodic summative evaluation. Formative evaluation is essential to provide feedback to improve performance while practice experiences are still available.

FAIRNESS IN CLINICAL EVALUATION

Considering that clinical evaluation is not objective, the goal is to establish a fair evaluation system. Fairness requires that:

1. The teacher identify his or her own values, attitudes, beliefs, and biases that may influence the evaluation process.
2. Clinical evaluation be based on predetermined outcomes or competencies.
3. The teacher develop a supportive clinical learning environment.

Identify One's Own Values

Teachers need to be aware of their personal values, attitudes, beliefs, and biases that may influence the evaluation process. These can affect both the data collected about students and the inferences made. In addition, students have their own sets of values and attitudes that influence their self-evaluations of performance and their responses to the teacher's evaluations and feedback. Students' acceptance of the teacher's guidance in clinical practice and information provided to them for improving performance is affected by their past experiences in clinical courses with other faculty members. Students may have had problems in prior clinical courses, receiving only negative feedback and limited support from the teacher, staff members, and others. In situations in which student responses inhibit learning, the teacher may need to intervene to guide students in more self-awareness of their own values and the effect they are having on their learning.

Base Clinical Evaluation on Outcomes or Competencies

Clinical evaluation should be based on preset outcomes, clinical objectives, or competencies that are then used to guide the evaluation process. Without these, neither the teacher nor the student has any basis for evaluating clinical performance. What are the outcomes of the clinical course (or, in some nursing education programs, the clinical objectives) to be met? What clinical competencies should the student develop? These outcomes or competencies provide a framework for faculty members to use in observing performance and for arriving at judgments about achievement in clinical practice. For example, if the competencies relate to developing communication skills, then the learning activities—whether in the patient care setting, as part of a simulation, or in the skills laboratory—should assist students in learning how to communicate. The teacher's observations and subsequent assessment should focus on communication behaviors, not on other competencies unrelated to the learning activities.

Develop a Supportive Learning Environment

It is up to the teacher to develop a supportive learning environment in which students view the teacher as someone who will facilitate their learning and development of clinical competencies. Students need to be comfortable asking the clinical educator and staff members questions and seeking their guidance rather than avoiding them in the clinical setting. A supportive environment is critical for effective assessment because students need to recognize that the teacher's feedback is intended to help them improve performance.

Many factors influence the development of a supportive learning environment. The clinical teacher needs to plan learning activities that foster student learning and development. Staff members need to be supportive of students and work collaboratively with them and with the teacher and other faculty from the nursing program. Most of all, there has to be trust and respect between the teacher and students.

FEEDBACK IN CLINICAL EVALUATION

For clinical evaluation to be effective, the teacher should provide continuous feedback to students about their performance and how they can improve it. Feedback is the communication of information to students, based on the teacher's assessment, that enables students to reflect on their performance, identify continued learning needs, and decide how to meet them (Bonnel, 2008). Feedback may be verbal, by describing observations of performance and explaining what to do differently, or visual, by demonstrating correct performance.

Feedback should be accompanied by further instruction from the teacher or by working with students to identify appropriate learning activities. The ultimate goal is for students to progress to a point at which they can judge their own performance, identify resources for their learning, and use those resources to further develop competencies.

Students must have an underlying knowledge base and beginning skills to judge their own performance. Sometimes students are not able to perform at the expected level because they lack the prerequisite knowledge and skills for developing the new competencies. As such, it is important to begin the clinical instruction by assessing whether students have learned the necessary concepts and skills and, if not, to start there.

Principles of Providing Feedback as Part of Clinical Evaluation

There are five principles for providing feedback to students as part of the clinical evaluation process. First, the feedback should be precise and specific. General information about performance, such as, "You need to work on your assessment" or "You need more practice in the simulation laboratory," does not indicate what behaviors need improvement or how to develop them. Instead of using general statements, the teacher should indicate what specific areas of knowledge are lacking, where there are problems in critical thinking and clinical judgments, and what particular competencies need more development. Rather than saying to a student, "You need to work on your assessment," the student would be better served if the teacher identified the specific areas of data collection omitted and the physical examination techniques that need improvement. Specific feedback is more valuable to learners than a general description of their behavior.

Second, for procedures, use of technologies, and any psychomotor skills, the teacher should provide both verbal and visual feedback to students. This means that the teacher should explain first, either orally or in writing, where the errors were made in performance and then demonstrate the correct procedure or skill. This should be followed by student practice of the skill with the teacher guiding performance. By allowing immediate practice, with the teacher available to correct problems, students can more easily use the feedback to further develop their skills.

Third, feedback about performance should be given to students at the time of learning or immediately following it. Providing prompt and rich feedback is equally important when teaching graduate students, nurses, and other learners regardless of their educational level. The longer the period of time between performance and feedback from the teacher, the less effective is the feedback. As time passes, neither student nor teacher may remember specific areas of clinical practice to be improved. This principle holds true whether the performance relates to cognitive learning, a procedure or clinical skill, or an attitude or value expressed by the student, among other areas.

Whether working with a group of students in a clinical setting, communicating with preceptors about students, or teaching an online course, the teacher needs to develop a strategy for giving focused and immediate feedback to students and following up with further discussion as needed. Recording short notes about observations of students' performance for later discussion with individual students helps the teacher remember important points about performance.

Fourth, students need different amounts of feedback and positive reinforcement. In beginning practice and with clinical situations that are new to learners, most students will need frequent and extensive feedback. As students progress through the program and become more competent, they should be able to assess their own performance and identify personal learning needs. Some students will require more feedback and direction from the teacher than others.

One final principle is that feedback should be diagnostic. After identifying areas in which further learning is needed, the teacher's responsibility is to guide students so that they can improve their performance. The process is cyclical—the teacher observes and assesses performance, gives students feedback about that performance, and then guides their learning and practice so they can become more competent.

RELATIONSHIP OF EVALUATION TO CLINICAL OUTCOMES AND COMPETENCIES

There are different ways of specifying the outcomes to be achieved in clinical practice, which in turn provide the basis for clinical evaluation. These may be stated in the form of outcomes to be met or as competencies to be demonstrated in clinical practice. Regardless of how these are stated, they represent what is evaluated in clinical practice.

In some nursing programs there are general outcomes that each clinical course addresses. For example, with this model, each course would have an outcome on communication. In a beginning clinical course, the outcome might be, "Identifies verbal and nonverbal techniques for communicating with patients." In a later course in the curriculum, the communication outcome might focus on the family and working with caregivers—for example, "Develops interpersonal relationships with families and caregivers." Then, in a community health course, the outcome might be, "Collaborates with other health care providers in care of patients in the community and the community as client."

As another approach, some teachers state the outcomes broadly and then indicate specific behaviors students should demonstrate to meet those outcomes in a particular course. For example, the outcome on communication might be stated as, "Communicates effectively with patients and others in the health system." Examples of behaviors that indicate achievement of this outcome in a course on care of children include, "Uses appropriate verbal and nonverbal communication based on the child's age, developmental status, and health condition" and "Interacts effectively with parents, caregivers, and others." Generally, the outcomes or competencies are then used for developing the clinical evaluation tool or form, which is discussed later in the chapter.

Regardless of how the outcomes are stated for a clinical course, they need to be specific enough to guide the evaluation of students in clinical practice. An outcome such as, "Use the nursing process in care of children" is too broad to guide evaluation. More specific outcomes such as, "Carries out a systematic assessment of children reflecting their developmental stage," "Evaluates the impact of health problems on the child and family," and "Identifies resources for managing the child's care at home" make clear to students what is expected of them in clinical practice.

Competencies are the knowledge, skills, and attitudes that students need to develop in clinical practice; they are the basis for the evaluation (Sullivan, 2016). For nurses in practice, these competencies reflect the expected level of performance to care for patients in the health care setting. Competencies for nurses are assessed as part of the initial employment and orientation to the health care setting and on an ongoing basis.

Caution should be exercised in developing clinical outcomes and competencies to avoid having too many for evaluation, considering the number of learners for whom the teacher is responsible, types of clinical learning opportunities available, and time allotted for clinical learning activities. In preparing outcomes or competencies for a clinical course, teachers should keep in mind that they need to collect sufficient data about students' performance of each outcome or competency specified for that course. The clinical outcomes or competencies need to be realistic and useful for guiding the assessment.

CLINICAL EVALUATION METHODS

There are many evaluation methods for use in nursing education. Some methods, such as journals, are most appropriate for formative evaluation, while others are useful for either formative or summative evaluation.

Selecting Clinical Evaluation Methods

There are several factors to consider when selecting clinical evaluation methods to use in a course. First, the evaluation methods should provide information on student performance of the clinical competencies associated with the course. With the evaluation methods, the teacher collects data on performance to judge whether students are developing the clinical competencies or have achieved them by the end of the course. For many outcomes of a course, different strategies can be used, thereby providing flexibility in choosing methods for evaluation. In planning the evaluation for a clinical course, the teacher reviews the outcomes or competencies to be developed and decides which evaluation methods will be used for assessing them, recognizing that most methods provide information on more than one outcome or competency.

Second, there are many different clinical evaluation strategies that might be used to assess performance. Varying the methods maintains student interest and takes into account learners' individual needs, abilities, and characteristics. Some students may be more proficient in methods that depend on writing, while others prefer strategies such as conferences and other discussions. Using multiple evaluation methods in clinical courses takes into consideration these differences among students. It also avoids relying on one method, such as a rating scale, for determining the entire clinical grade.

Third, the teacher should select evaluation methods that are realistic considering the number of students to be evaluated, available practice or simulation activities, and constraints such as the teacher's or preceptor's time. Planning for an evaluation method that depends on patients with specific health problems or particular clinical situations is not realistic considering the types of experiences with actual or simulated patients available to students. Some methods are not appropriate because of the number of students who would need to use them within the time frame of the course. Others may be too costly or require resources not available in the nursing education program or health care setting.

Fourth, evaluation methods can be used for formative or summative evaluation. In the process of deciding how to evaluate students' clinical performance, the teacher should identify whether the methods will be used to provide feedback to learners (formative) or for grading (summative). In clinical practice, students should know ahead of time whether the assessment by the teacher is for formative or summative purposes. Some of the methods designed for clinical evaluation provide feedback to students on areas for improvement and should not be graded. Other methods, such as rating scales and written assignments, can be used for summative purposes and can therefore be included as part of the course or clinical grade.

Fifth, before finalizing the plan for how students will be evaluated in a course, the teacher should review the purpose and number required of each assignment completed by students. What are the purposes of these assignments, and how many are needed to demonstrate competency? In some clinical courses, students complete an excessive number of written assignments. Students benefit from continuous feedback from the teacher, not from repetitive assignments that contribute little to their development of clinical knowledge and skills. Instead of daily or weekly care plans or other assignments, which may not even be consistent with current practice, once students develop the competencies, they can progress to other, more relevant learning activities.

Sixth, in deciding how to evaluate clinical performance, the teacher should consider the time needed to complete the evaluation, provide feedback, and grade the assignment. Instead of requiring a series of written assignments in a clinical course, the same outcomes might be met through discussions with students, cases analyzed by students in postclinical conferences, group writing activities, and other methods requiring less teacher time and accomplishing the same purposes. Considering the demands on nursing faculty members, it is important to consider one's own time when planning how to evaluate students' performance in clinical practice.

Observation

The main strategy for evaluating clinical performance is observing students in clinical practice, simulation and learning laboratories, and other settings. In a survey of 1,573 faculty members representing all types of prelicensure nursing programs (diploma, 128; associate degree, 866; baccalaureate, 563; and entry-level master's, 8), observation of student performance was the predominant strategy used across programs ($n = 1,289$, 93%; Oermann, Yarbrough, Ard, Saewert, & Charasika, 2009).

Although observation is widely used, there are threats to its validity and reliability. First, observations of students may be influenced by the teacher's values, attitudes, and biases, as discussed earlier. There may also be overreliance on first impressions, which might change as the teacher or preceptor observes the student over a period of time and in different situations. Altmiller (2016) emphasized that feedback about performance should be an unbiased reflection of observations and events. In any performance assessment, there needs to be a series of observations made before drawing conclusions about performance.

Second, in observing performance, there are many aspects of performance on which the teacher may focus attention. For example, while observing a student administer an intravenous medication, the teacher may focus mainly on the technique used for its administration, ask limited questions about the purpose of the medication, and make no observations of how the student interacts with the patient. Another teacher observing this same student may focus on other aspects.

Third, the teacher may arrive at incorrect judgments about the observation, such as inferring that a student is inattentive during conference when, in fact, the student is thinking about the comments made by others in the group. It is important to discuss observations with students, obtain their perceptions of their behavior, and be willing to modify one's own inferences when new data are presented. In discussing observations and impressions with students, the teacher can learn about their perceptions of performance.

Fourth, every observation in the clinical setting reflects only a sampling of the learner's performance during a clinical activity. An observation of the same student at another time may reveal a different level of performance.

Finally, similar to other clinical evaluation methods, the outcomes or competencies guide the teacher on what to observe. They help the teacher focus the observations of performance. However, all observed behaviors should be shared with the students.

Notes About Performance

It is difficult, if not impossible, to remember the observations made of each student for each clinical activity. For this reason, teachers need a device to help them remember their observations and the context in which the performance occurred. There are several ways of recording observations of students in clinical settings, simulation and learning laboratories, and other settings: narrative notes about performance, checklists, and rating scales.

The teacher can make notes that describe the observations made of students in the clinical setting; these are sometimes called anecdotal notes. In a study by Hall (2013), 92.4% of faculty members reported using anecdotal notes for record keeping about students' performance. Some teachers include only a description of the observations and then, after a series of observations, review the pattern of the performance and draw conclusions about it. Other teachers record their observations and their judgment about how well the student performed. Notes about the student's performance should be recorded as close to the time of the observation as possible; otherwise, it is difficult to remember what was observed and the context (e.g., patient and clinical situation) of that observation. In the clinical setting, notes can be handwritten or recorded using some technology.

Notes about the observations made in clinical practice and the quality of the student's performance should be shared with students frequently; otherwise, they are not effective for feedback. Considering the issues associated with observations of clinical performance, the teacher should discuss observations with the students and be willing to incorporate their own judgments about the performance. These notes are also useful in conferences with students—for example, at midterm and at the end of term—for reviewing a pattern of performance over time.

Checklists

A checklist contains specific behaviors or activities to be observed with a place for marking whether they were present during the performance (Brookhart & Nitko, 2015). A checklist often lists the steps to be followed in performing a procedure or demonstrating a skill. Some checklists also include errors in performance that are commonly made. Checklists not only facilitate the teacher's observation of procedures and behaviors performed by students and nurses learning new technologies and procedures, but they also provide a way for learners to assess their own performance. With checklists, learners can review and evaluate their performance prior to assessment by the teacher.

For common procedures and skills, teachers can often find checklists already prepared that can be used for evaluation, and some nursing textbooks have accompanying skills checklists. When these resources are not available, teachers can develop their own checklists but should avoid including every possible step, which makes the checklist too cumbersome. Instead, the focus should be on critical behaviors and where they fit into the sequence.

Rating Scales

Rating scales, also referred to as clinical evaluation tools or instruments, provide a means of recording judgments about the observed performance of students in clinical practice. A rating scale has two parts: (a) a list of outcomes or competencies the student is to demonstrate in clinical practice and (b) a scale for rating their performance of them.

Rating scales are most useful for summative evaluation of performance; after observing students over a period of time, the teacher draws conclusions about performance, rating it according to the scale provided with the instrument. Rating scales may also be used to evaluate specific activities that students complete—for example, rating a student's presentation of a case in clinical conference. Other uses of rating scales are to: (a) help students focus their attention on critical behaviors to be performed in clinical practice; (b) give specific feedback to students about their performance; and (c) demonstrate growth in clinical competencies over a designated time period if the same rating scale is used.

The same rating scale can be used for multiple purposes. Exhibit 15.1 shows sample competencies from a rating scale that is used midway through a course; in Exhibit 15.2, the same competencies are used for the final evaluation, but the performance is rated as satisfactory or unsatisfactory as a summative rating.

EXHIBIT 15.1

SAMPLE COMPETENCIES FROM RATING SCALE FOR FORMATIVE EVALUATION

Maternal–Newborn Nursing
Midterm Progress Report

Name _____   Date _____

Objective	Yes	No	Not Obs.
1. Provides patient-centered care to mothers and newborns			
A. Assesses the individual needs of mothers and newborns			
B. Plans care to meet the patient's needs			
C. Implements nursing interventions based on evidence			
D. Evaluates the outcomes of care			
E. Includes the family in planning and implementing care for the mother and newborn			
2. Participates in health teaching for maternal-newborn patients and families			

(continued)

Objective	Yes	No	Not Obs.
A. Identifies learning needs of mothers and families			
B. Identifies processes for improving the quality of health teaching in the setting			

Not Obs., not observed.

EXHIBIT 15.2

SAMPLE COMPETENCIES FROM SAME RATING SCALE FOR FINAL EVALUATION

Maternal–Newborn Nursing
Clinical Performance Evaluation

Name _____   Date _____

Objective	S	U
1. Provides patient-centered care to mothers and newborns		
A. Assesses the individual needs of mothers and newborns		
B. Plans care to meet the patient's needs		
C. Implements nursing interventions based on evidence		
D. Evaluates the outcomes of care		
E. Includes the family in planning and implementing care for the mother and newborn		
2. Participates in health teaching for maternal-newborn patients and families		
A. Identifies learning needs of mothers and families		
B. Identifies processes for improving the quality of health teaching in the setting		

S, satisfactory; U, unsatisfactory.

Types of Rating Scales

Many types of rating scales are used for evaluating clinical performance. The scales may have multiple levels for rating performance, such as 1 to 5 or exceptional to below average, or have two levels, such as pass–fail. Types of scales with multiple levels for rating performance include:

■ Letters: A, B, C, D, E or A, B, C, D, F
■ Numbers: 1, 2, 3, 4, 5

- Qualitative labels: excellent, very good, good, fair, poor; exceptional, above average, average, below average
- Frequency labels: always, usually, frequently, sometimes, never

A short description included with the letters, numbers, and labels for each of the outcomes or competencies rated improves objectivity and consistency (Brookhart & Nitko, 2015). For example, if teachers use a scale of exceptional, above average, average, and below average or a scale based on the numbers 4, 3, 2, and 1, short descriptions of each level in the scale could be written to clarify the performance expected at each level. For the clinical outcome "Collects relevant data from patient," the descriptors might be:

Exceptional (or 4): Differentiates relevant from irrelevant data, analyzes multiple sources of data, establishes comprehensive database, identifies data needed for evaluating all possible patient problems.

Above average (or 3): Collects significant data from patients, uses multiple sources of data as part of assessment, identifies possible patient problems based on the data.

Average (or 2): Collects significant data from patients, uses data to develop main patient problems.

Below average (or 1): Does not collect significant data and misses important cues in data; unable to explain relevance of data for patient problems.

Most rating scales for clinical evaluation have two levels, such as pass–fail and satisfactory–unsatisfactory. A survey of nursing faculty members from all types of programs indicated that most faculty members ($n = 1,116$, 83%) used pass–fail in their clinical courses (Oermann et al., 2009). Exhibit 15.3 is an example of a clinical evaluation tool that has two levels for rating performance: satisfactory–unsatisfactory. This tool is based on the Quality and Safety Education for Nurses (QSEN) competencies (QSEN, 2014). Competencies on this form could also be rated as pass–fail.

Issues With Rating Scales

One problem in using rating scales is apparent by a review of the sample scale descriptors. What are the differences between above average and average or between a 2 and a 1? Is there consensus among faculty members using the rating scale about what constitutes different levels of performance for each outcome, competency, or behavior evaluated? This problem exists even when descriptions are provided for each level of the rating scale. Teachers may differ in their judgments of whether the student collected relevant data, whether multiple sources of data were used, whether the database was comprehensive, if all possible nursing diagnoses were considered, and so forth.

Scales based on frequency labels are often difficult to implement because of limited experiences for students to practice and demonstrate a level of skill rated as "always, usually, frequently, sometimes, and never." How should teachers rate students' performance in situations in which they practiced the skill perhaps once or twice? Even two-dimensional scales such as pass–fail present room for variability among clinical nurse educators.

EXHIBIT 15.3

CLINICAL EVALUATION TOOL WITH TWO LEVELS FOR RATING PERFORMANCE (BASED ON QSEN COMPETENCIES)

NICHOLLS STATE UNIVERSITY
DEPARTMENT OF NURSING
BSN PROGRAM

Clinical Performance Evaluation Tool
NURS 225 Level I

Self Evaluation _____
Faculty Evaluation _____

Student Name _____

Faculty _____   Course: NURS 225   Semester _____

Student must obtain a Satisfactory "S" grade in all competencies at the Final Evaluation to pass the Course.

Core Competencies	Midterm			Final	
	S	NI	U	S	U
Focusing on wellness, health promotion, illness and disease management across the lifespan in a variety of settings while recognizing the diverse uniqueness of individuals, providing directed care to individuals with well-defined health alterations, the student at the end of N225, should be able to:					
I. Patient-Centered Care					
a. Develop an individualized plan of care with a focus on assessment and planning utilizing the nursing process					
b. Demonstrate caring behaviors					
c. Conduct a comprehensive assessment while eliciting patient values, preferences, and needs					
d. Respect diversity of individuals					
e. Assess the presence and extent of pain and suffering					
f. Demonstrate beginning competency in skills					

(continued)

Core Competencies	Midterm			Final	
	S	NI	U	S	U
II. Teamwork and Collaboration					
a. Develop effective communication skills (orally and through charting) with patients, team members, and family					
b. Identify relevant data for communication in pre- and postconferences					
c. Identify intra- and interprofessional team member roles and scopes of practice					
d. Establish appropriate relationships with team members					
e. Identify need for help when appropriate to situation					
III. Evidence-Based Practice					
a. Locate evidence-based literature related to clinical practice and guideline activities					
b. Reference clinical related activities with evidence-based literature					
c. Value the concept of evidence-based practice in determining best clinical practice					
IV. Quality Improvement					
a. Deliver care in timely and cost effective manner					
b. Seek information about processes/ projects to improve care					
c. Value the significance of variance reporting					
V. Safety					
a. Demonstrate effective use of technology and standardized practices that support safety and quality					
b. Implement strategies to reduce risk of harm to self or others					
c. Demonstrate appropriate clinical decision making					
d. Identify national patient safety goals and quality measures					
e. Use appropriate strategies to reduce reliance on memory					

(continued)

Core Competencies	Midterm			Final	
	S	NI	U	S	U
f. Communicate observations or concerns related to hazards and errors to patient, families, and the health care team					
g. Organize multiple responsibilities and provide care in a timely manner					
VI. Informatics					
a. Navigate the electronic health record for patient information where appropriate for clinical setting					
b. Document clear and concise responses to care in the electronic health record, where appropriate for clinical setting					
c. Identify information and clinical technology using critical thinking to collect, process, and communicate data					
d. Manage data, information, and knowledge of technology in an ethical manner					
e. Protect confidentiality of electronic health records					
VII. Professionalism					
a. Demonstrate core professional values (caring, altruism, autonomy, integrity, human dignity, and social justice)					
b. Maintain professional behavior and appearance					
c. Comply with the Code of Ethics, Standards of Practice, and policies and procedures of Nicholls State University, Department of Nursing, and clinical agencies					
d. Accept constructive criticism and develop plan of action for improvement					
e. Maintain a positive attitude and interact with interprofessional team members, faculty, and fellow students in a positive, professional manner					
f. Provide evidence of preparation for clinical learning experiences					
g. Arrive to clinical experiences at assigned times					
h. Demonstrate expected behaviors and complete tasks in a timely manner					
i. Accept individual responsibility and accountability for nursing interventions, outcomes, and other actions					

(continued)

Core Competencies	Midterm			Final	
	S	NI	U	S	U
j. Engage in self evaluation					
k. Assume responsibility for learning					

Midterm Comments (Address strengths and weaknesses)

Faculty

Student

Student Signature _____   Date _____

Faculty Signature _____   Date _____

Final Comments (Address strengths and weaknesses)

Faculty

Student

Student Signature _____   Date _____

Faculty Signature _____   Date _____

Mid-Clinical Evaluation: Faculty and student *must* complete documentation for remediation of unsatisfactory areas. CPR Tool[a] must be initiated for any unsatisfactory areas.

Unsatisfactory Area	Remediation Strategy

Student Signature _____   Date _____

Faculty Signature _____   Date _____

Developed collaboratively by Nicholls State University Nursing Faculty. Reprinted by permission.

Two copies on file – one for student self evaluation; one for clinical faculty
*Content based upon QSEN Competencies and KSAs.
[a] **Clinical Performance Remediation tool.**

BSN, bachelor of science in nursing; CPR, clinical performance remediation; KSAs, knowledge, skills, and attitudes; NI, needs improvement; QSEN, Quality and Safety Education for Nurses; S, satisfactory; U, unsatisfactory.

©2016 Nicholls State University Department of Nursing, Thibodaux, LA.

Brookhart and Nitko (2015) identified common errors that can occur with rating scales applicable to rating clinical performance. The first three errors can occur with tools that have multiple points on the scale for rating performance, such as 1 to 5 or below average to exceptional. The other errors can occur with any type of clinical performance rating scale.

1. **Leniency error** results when the teacher tends to rate all students toward the high end of the scale.
2. **Severity error** is the opposite of leniency, tending to rate all students toward the low end of the scale.
3. **Central tendency error** is hesitancy to mark either end of the rating scale and instead use only the midpoint of the scale.
4. **Halo effect** is a judgment based on a general impression of the student. With this error, the teacher lets an overall impression of the student influence the ratings of specific aspects of the student's performance. This impression affects the teacher's ability to objectively evaluate and rate specific competencies or behaviors on the tool. The halo may be positive, giving the student a higher rating than is deserved, or negative, letting a general negative impression of the student result in lower ratings of specific aspects of the performance.
5. **Personal bias** occurs when the teacher's biases influence ratings such as favoring nursing students who do not work while attending school over those who are employed while attending school.
6. **Logical error** results when similar ratings are given for items on the scale that are logically related to one another. This is a problem with rating scales that are too long and often too detailed. For example, there may be multiple competencies on communication to be rated. The teacher observes some of these but not all of them. In completing the clinical evaluation form, the teacher gives the same rating to all competencies related to communication on the tool. When this occurs, some of the items on the rating scale can often be combined.
7. **Rater drift** occurs when teachers redefine the competencies to be observed and assessed. Initially, in developing a clinical evaluation form, teachers agree on the competencies or behaviors to be rated and the scale to be used. However, over time, educators may interpret them differently, drifting away from the original intent. For this reason, faculty members, clinical educators, and preceptors in a course should discuss as a group each competency on the clinical evaluation form at the beginning and mid-point in the course. This discussion should include the meaning of the competency and what a student's performance would look like at each rating level in the tool.
8. **Reliability decay** is a similar issue. Brookhart and Nitko (2015) indicated that, immediately following training on using a rating tool, educators tend to use the tool consistently across students and with each other. As the course continues, though, faculty members may become less consistent in their ratings. Discussion of the clinical evaluation tool among course faculty, as indicated earlier, may improve consistency in the use of the tool.

Although there are issues with rating scales, they allow teachers, preceptors, and others to rate performance over time and to note patterns of performance. Exhibit 15.4 provides guidelines for using rating scales for clinical evaluation in nursing.

EXHIBIT 15.4

GUIDELINES FOR USING RATING SCALES FOR CLINICAL EVALUATION

1. Be alert to the possible influence of your own values, attitudes, beliefs, and biases in observing performance and drawing conclusions about it.
2. Use the clinical outcomes or competencies to focus your observations. Give students feedback on other observations made about their performance.
3. Collect sufficient data on students' performance before drawing conclusions about it.
4. Observe the student more than one time before rating performance. Rating scales, when used for clinical evaluation, should represent a pattern of the students' performance over time.
5. If possible, observe students' performance in different clinical situations, either in the patient care or simulated setting. When not possible, develop additional strategies for evaluation so that performance is evaluated with different methods and at different times.
6. Do not rely on first impressions; they may not be accurate.
7. Always discuss observations with students, obtain their perceptions of performance, and be willing to modify judgments and ratings when new data are presented.
8. Review the available clinical learning activities and opportunities in the simulation and learning laboratories. Do they provide sufficient data for completing the rating scale? If not, new learning activities may need to be developed, or the behaviors on the tool may need to be modified to be more realistic considering the clinical teaching circumstances.
9. Avoid using rating scales as the only source of data about a student's performance—use multiple evaluation methods for clinical practice.
10. Rate each outcome or competency individually based on the observations made of performance and conclusions drawn. If you have insufficient information about achievement of a particular competency, do not rate it—leave it blank.
11. Do not let your general impression of the student or personal biases influence your ratings.
12. If the rating form is ineffective for judging student performance, then revise and reevaluate it. Consider these questions: Does the form yield data that can be used to make valid decisions about students' competence? Does the form yield reliable, stable data? Is it easy to use? Is it appropriate considering the types of learning activities that students have in their clinical settings?
13. Discuss as a group (with other educators and preceptors involved in the evaluation) each competency on the rating scale. Come to agreement about the meaning of the competencies and what a student's performance would look like at each rating level in the tool. Share examples of performance, how you would rate them, and your rationale. As a group exercise, observe a video clip or other simulation of a student's performance, rate it with the tool, and come to agreement about the rating. Such exercises and discussions should be held before the course begins and periodically during it to ensure reliability across teachers and settings.

Simulations for Clinical Evaluation

Simulations are not only effective for instruction in nursing, but they are also useful for clinical evaluation. Students can demonstrate procedures and technologies, conduct assessments, analyze clinical scenarios and make decisions about problems and actions to take, carry out nursing interventions, and evaluate the effects of their decisions. Each of these outcomes can be evaluated for feedback to students or for summative grading.

Many nursing education programs have simulation laboratories with human patient simulators, clinically equipped examination rooms, manikins and models for skill practice and assessment, areas for standardized patients, and a wide range of multimedia that facilitate performance evaluations. The rooms can be equipped with two-way mirrors, video cameras, microphones, and other media for observing and rating performance by faculty members and others. Videoconferencing technology can be used to conduct clinical evaluations of students in settings at a distance from the nursing education program, effectively replacing on-site performance evaluations by faculty members.

Incorporating Simulations Into Clinical Evaluation Protocol

The same principles for evaluating student performance in the clinical setting apply to using simulations. The first task is to identify which clinical outcomes will be assessed with a simulation. This decision should be made during the course planning phase as part of the protocol developed for clinical evaluation in the course. It is important to remember when deciding on evaluation methods that assessment can be done for feedback to students and thus remain ungraded, or it can be used for grading purposes.

Once the outcomes or clinical competencies to be evaluated with simulations are identified, the teacher can plan the specifics of the evaluation. Some questions to guide teachers in using simulations for clinical evaluation are:

- What are the specific clinical outcomes or competencies to be evaluated using simulations? These should be designated in the plan or protocol for clinical evaluation in a course.
- What types of simulations are needed to assess the designated outcomes—for example, task trainers or high-fidelity simulators?
- Do the simulations need to be developed, or are they already available in the nursing education program?
- If the simulations need to be developed, who will be responsible for their development? Who will manage their implementation?
- Are the simulations for formative evaluation only? If so, how many practice sessions should be planned? What is the extent of teacher and expert guidance needed? Who will provide that supervision and guidance?
- Are the simulations for summative evaluation (i.e., for high-stakes decisions)? If used for summative clinical evaluation, then faculty members need to determine the process for rating performance and how those ratings will be incorporated into the clinical grade, whether pass–fail or another system for grading. Importantly, the raters need to be trained to ensure consistency in their ratings of performance, and the tools for evaluation must be valid and reliable.
- What tools will be used for rating performance in the simulations, and are they valid and reliable?
- When will the simulations be implemented in the course?
- How will the effectiveness of the simulations be evaluated, and who will be responsible?

These are only a few of the questions for faculty members to consider when planning to use simulations for clinical evaluation.

Standardized Patients

One type of simulation for clinical evaluation uses standardized patients—individuals who have been trained to accurately portray the role of a patient with a specific diagnosis or condition. With simulations using standardized patients, students can be evaluated on a history and physical examination, related skills and procedures, and communication techniques, among other outcomes. Standardized patients are effective for evaluation, because the actors are trained to re-create the same patient condition and clinical situation each time they are with a student, providing for consistency in the performance evaluation.

When standardized patients are used for formative evaluation, they provide feedback to the students on their performance, an important aid to their learning. Standardized patients are trained to provide both written and oral feedback to students and evaluate their performance (McWilliam & Botwinski, 2012). With the transition to distance education, Ballman, Garritano, and Beery (2016) developed interactive case studies using technology to allow students in a distance education program to interact with standardized patients.

Objective Structured Clinical Examination

An Objective Structured Clinical Examination (OSCE) provides a means of evaluating performance in a simulation laboratory rather than in the clinical setting. In an OSCE, students rotate through a series of stations; at each station, they complete an activity or perform a task, which is then evaluated. Some stations assess the student's ability to take a patient's history, perform a physical examination, and implement other interventions while being observed by the teacher or an examiner. The student's performance can then be rated using a rating scale or checklist. At other stations, students might be tested on their knowledge and cognitive skills—they might be asked to analyze data, select interventions and treatments, and manage the patient's condition. OSCEs are typically used for summative clinical evaluation; however, they can also be used formatively to assess performance and provide feedback to students.

Different types of stations can be used in an OSCE. At one type of station the student may interact with a standardized patient to assess the patient, collect a history, and conduct a physical examination. At these stations the teacher or examiner can evaluate students' understanding of varied patient conditions and management of them and can rate the students' performance. At other stations students may demonstrate skills, perform procedures, use technologies, and demonstrate other technical competencies. Performance at those stations is often assessed with checklists. There may also be postencounter stations to facilitate the evaluation of cognitive skills such as interpreting lab results and other data, developing management plans, and making other types of decisions about patient care. Students may be asked to document their findings with the standardized patient, answer questions, and provide evidence for their decisions, among other competencies (Hawkins & Boulet, 2008). At these stations, the teacher or examiner may not be present to observe students.

Media Clips

Media clips—short segments of a digital recording, a video from YouTube, and other forms of multimedia—may be viewed by students as a basis for discussions in post-clinical conferences, in discussion forums, and for other online activities; for small group activities; and for critique and write-up as an assignment. Media clips are often more effective than written descriptions of a scenario, because they allow the student to visualize the patient and clinical situation.

Media clips are appropriate for assessing whether students can apply concepts and content being learned in class to the clinical situation depicted in the media clip, observe and collect data, identify possible problems, identify priority actions and interventions, and evaluate outcomes. Students can answer questions about the media clips as part of a graded learning activity in clinical courses. Media clips are also valuable for formative evaluation, particularly in a group format in which students discuss their ideas and receive feedback from the teacher and peers.

Written Assignments

Written assignments accompanying the clinical experience are effective methods for assessing students' critical thinking and higher-level learning, understanding of content relevant to clinical practice, and ability to express ideas in writing. Many types of written assignments for clinical courses were described in Chapter 14: concept map, short written assignments, nursing care plan, analysis of cases, evidence-based practice paper, teaching plans, reflective journal, group writing projects, and e-portfolio. Chapter 10 provided further information about assessing case scenarios. Written assignments can be included as part of the clinical evaluation. Some will be evaluated formatively, such as reflective journals, while others can be graded.

Conferences

The ability to present ideas orally is an important outcome of clinical practice. Sharing information about a patient, leading others in discussions about clinical practice, presenting ideas in a group format, and giving presentations are skills that students need to develop in a nursing program. Working with nursing staff members and the interprofessional team requires the ability to communicate effectively. Conferences provide a method for developing oral communication skills and for evaluating competency in this area. Discussions also lead to problem solving and higher level thinking if questions are open ended and geared to those outcomes, as discussed in Chapter 11.

Criteria for assessing conferences include the ability of students to:

- Present ideas clearly and in a logical sequence to the group
- Participate actively in the group discussion
- Offer ideas relevant to the topic
- Demonstrate knowledge of the content discussed in the conference
- Offer different perspectives on the topic, engaging the group in critical thinking
- Assume a leadership role, if relevant, in promoting group discussion and arriving at group decisions

Most conferences are evaluated for formative purposes, with the teacher giving feedback to students as a group or to the individual who led the group discussion. When conferences are evaluated as a portion of the clinical or course grade, the teacher should have specific criteria to guide the evaluation and should use a scoring rubric. Exhibit 15.5 provides a sample form that can be used to evaluate how well a student leads a clinical conference or to assess student participation in a conference.

EXHIBIT 15.5

EVALUATION OF PARTICIPATION IN A CLINICAL CONFERENCE

Student's name _____

Conference topic _____

Date _____

Rate the behaviors listed here by circling the appropriate number. Some behaviors will not be applicable depending on the student's role in the conference; mark those as not applicable (na).

Behaviors	Rating					
	Poor				Excellent	
States goals of conference	1	2	3	4	5	na
Leads group in discussion	1	2	3	4	5	na
Asks thought-provoking questions	1	2	3	4	5	na
Uses strategies that encourage all students to participate	1	2	3	4	5	na
Participates actively in discussion	1	2	3	4	5	na
Includes important content	1	2	3	4	5	na
Includes evidence for practice	1	2	3	4	5	na
Offers new perspectives to group	1	2	3	4	5	na
Considers different points of view	1	2	3	4	5	na
Assists group members in recognizing biases and values	1	2	3	4	5	na
Is enthusiastic about topic	1	2	3	4	5	na
Is well prepared for discussion	1	2	3	4	5	na
If leading group, monitors time	1	2	3	4	5	na
Develops quality materials to support discussion	1	2	3	4	5	na
Summarizes major points at end of conference	1	2	3	4	5	na

Group Projects

Most of the clinical evaluation methods presented in this chapter focus on individual student performance, but group projects also can be assessed as part of the clinical evaluation in a course. Some group work is short term—only for the time it takes to develop a product, such as a teaching plan or group presentation. Other groups may be formed for the purpose of cooperative learning, with students working in small groups or teams in clinical practice over a longer period of time. With any of these group formats, both the products developed by the group and the ability of the students to work cooperatively can be assessed.

There are different approaches for grading group projects. The same grade can be given to every student in the group (i.e., a group grade), although this does not take into consideration individual student effort and contribution to the group product. Another approach is for the students to indicate in the finished product the parts to which they contributed, providing a way of assigning individual student grades, with or without a group grade. Students can also provide a self-assessment of how much they contributed to the group project, which can then be integrated into their grade. Alternatively, students can prepare both a group and an individual product.

Rubrics should be used for assessing group projects and should be geared specifically to the project. To assess students' participation and collaboration in the group, the rubric also needs to reflect the goals of group work. With small groups, the teacher can observe and rate individual student cooperation and contributions to the group. However, this is often difficult because the teacher is not a member of the group, and the group dynamics change when the teacher is present. As another approach, students can assess the participation and cooperation of their peers. These peer evaluations can be used for the students' own development and shared among peers but not with the teacher, or they can be incorporated by the teacher in the grade for the group project. Students can also be asked to assess their own participation in the group.

Self-Assessment

Self-assessment is the ability of students to assess their own clinical competencies and identify where further learning is needed. Self-evaluation begins with the first clinical course and develops throughout the nursing program, continuing into professional practice. Through self-evaluation, students examine their clinical performance and identify both strengths and areas for improvement. Using students' own assessments, teachers can develop plans to assist students in gaining the knowledge and skills they need to meet the outcomes of the course. It is important for teachers to establish a positive climate for learning in the course, or students will not be likely to share an honest self-evaluation with them. Self-evaluation is appropriate only for formative evaluation and should never be graded.

In addition to developing a supportive learning environment, the teacher should hold planned conferences with each student to review performance. In these conferences, the teacher can:

- Give specific feedback on performance
- Obtain the student's perceptions of his or her competencies
- Identify strengths and areas for learning from the teacher's and student's perspectives
- Plan with the student learning activities for improving performance, which is critical if the student is not passing the clinical course
- Enhance communication between teacher and student.

CLINICAL EVALUATION IN DISTANCE EDUCATION

Nursing programs use different strategies for offering the clinical component of distance education courses. Often preceptors in the local area guide student learning in the clinical setting and evaluate performance. If cohorts of students are available in an area, adjunct or part-time faculty members might be hired to teach a small group of students in the clinical setting. In other programs, students independently complete clinical learning activities to gain the clinical knowledge and competencies of a course. Regardless of how the clinical component is structured, the course syllabus, competencies to be developed, rating forms, guidelines for clinical practice, and other materials associated with the clinical course need to be available to whomever is providing the instruction and evaluating student learning. Course management systems facilitate communication among students, preceptors, course faculty, and others involved in the students' clinical activities.

The clinical evaluation methods presented in this chapter can be used for distance education. The critical decision for the teacher is to identify which clinical competencies and skills, if any, need to be observed and the performance rated, because that decision suggests different evaluation methods than if the focus of the evaluation is on the cognitive outcomes of the clinical course. In programs in which preceptors or adjunct faculty members are available on site, any of the clinical evaluation methods presented in this chapter can be used as long as they are congruent with the outcomes and competencies. There should be consistency, though, in how the evaluation is done across preceptors and clinical settings.

Strategies should be implemented in the course for preceptors and other educators involved in the performance evaluation to discuss as a group the competencies to be rated, what each competency means, and the performance of those competencies at different levels on the rating scale. This is a critical activity to ensure reliability across preceptors and other evaluators. Preceptor development activities of this type should be done before the course begins and at least once during the course to ensure that evaluators are using the tool as intended and are consistent across students and clinical settings.

Even in clinical courses involving preceptors, faculty members may decide to evaluate clinical skills themselves by reviewing digital recordings of performance or observing students through videoconferencing and other technology. Digitally recording performance is valuable as a strategy for summative evaluation, to assess competencies at the end of a clinical course or another designated point in time, and for review by students for self-assessment and by faculty members to give feedback.

Simulations and standardized patients are other strategies useful in assessing clinical performance in distance education. Performance with standardized patients can be recorded, and students can submit their patient histories and other written documentation that would commonly be done in practice in that situation. Students can also complete case analyses related to the standardized patient encounter for assessing their knowledge base and rationale for their decisions.

Simulations, analyses of cases, case presentations, written assignments, and other strategies presented in this chapter can be used for clinical evaluation in distance education courses. Similar to clinical evaluation in general, a combination of approaches is more effective than one method alone.

GRADING CLINICAL PRACTICE

Grading systems for clinical practice are often two-dimensional, such as pass–fail, satisfactory–unsatisfactory, and met or did not meet the clinical objectives. Some nursing programs add a third category, honors, to acknowledge performance that exceeds the level required. Other grading systems are multidimensional—for example, using letter grades A through F; integers 1 through 5; and percentages. With any of these grading systems, it is not always easy to summarize the multiple types of evaluation data collected about the student's performance into a symbol representing a grade. This is true even in a pass–fail system; it may be difficult to arrive at a judgment to pass or fail based on the evaluation data and the circumstances associated with the student's clinical and simulated practice.

Regardless of the grading system for clinical practice, there are two criteria to be met: (a) the evaluation methods for collecting data about student performance should reflect the clinical competencies and outcomes for which a grade will be assigned, and (b) students must understand how their clinical practice will be evaluated and graded. In planning the course, the teacher needs to decide which of the evaluation methods should be incorporated in the clinical grade. Some of these methods are for summative evaluation, thereby providing a source of information for including in the clinical grade. Other methods, though, are used in clinical practice for feedback only and are not incorporated in the grade.

Categories for grading clinical practice such as pass–fail and satisfactory–unsatisfactory have advantages over a system with multiple levels, although there are some disadvantages as well. Pass–fail places greater emphasis on giving feedback to the learner, because only two categories of performance need to be determined. With a pass–fail grading system, faculty members may be more inclined to provide continual feedback to learners, because they do not have to ultimately differentiate performance according to four or five levels of proficiency such as with a multidimensional system. Performance that exceeds the requirements and expectations, though, is not reflected in the grade for clinical practice unless a third category is included—honors–pass–fail. Pass–fail is used most frequently in nursing programs (Oermann et al., 2009).

A pass–fail system requires only two types of judgment about clinical performance. Do the evaluation data indicate that the student has demonstrated satisfactory performance of the competencies to indicate a pass? Or do the data suggest that the performance of those competencies is not at a satisfactory level? Deciding whether the learner has passed or failed is often easier for the teacher than using the same evaluation information for deciding on multiple levels of performance. A letter system for grading clinical practice, however, acknowledges the different levels of clinical proficiency students may have demonstrated in their clinical practice.

A disadvantage of pass–fail for grading clinical practice is the inability to include a clinical grade into the course grade. One strategy is to separate nursing courses into two components for grading: one for theory and the second for clinical practice (designated as pass–fail), even though the course is considered a whole. Typically, guidelines for the course indicate that the students must pass the clinical component to pass the course. A second mechanism is to offer two separate courses with the clinical course graded on a pass–fail basis.

Methods for Assigning the Clinical Grade

Once the grading system is determined, there are varied ways of using it to arrive at the clinical grade. The grade can be assigned based on the competencies or outcomes achieved by the student. To use this method, the faculty should consider designating some of the competencies or outcomes as critical for achievement in the course. For example, an A might be assigned if all of the clinical competencies or outcomes were met; a B might be assigned if all of the competencies designated by the faculty as critical behaviors and at least half of the others were met.

For pass–fail grading, the faculty can indicate that all of the competencies or outcomes must be met to pass the course or can designate critical ones required for passing the course. For both of these grading systems, the clinical evaluation methods provide the data for determining whether the student's performance reflects achievement of the competencies. These evaluation methods may or may not be graded separately as part of the course grade.

Another way of arriving at the clinical grade is to base it on the evaluation methods. In this system, the clinical evaluation methods become the source of data for the grade. For example,

Paper on analysis of clinical practice issue	10%
Analysis of clinical cases	5%
Conference presentation	10%
Community resource paper	10%
Electronic portfolio	25%
Rating scale (of performance)	40%

In this example, the clinical grade is computed according to the evaluation methods. Observation of performance, and the rating on the clinical evaluation tool, is only a portion of the clinical grade. An advantage of this approach is that it incorporates into the grade the summative evaluation methods completed by students.

If pass–fail is used for grading clinical practice, the grade might be computed as follows:

Paper on analysis of clinical practice issue	10%
Analysis of clinical cases	5%
Conference presentation	10%
Community resource paper	10%
Electronic portfolio	25%
OSCE	40%
Rating scale (of performance) Pass required	

This discussion of grading clinical practice suggests a variety of appropriate mechanisms. The teacher must make it clear to students and others how the evaluation and grading will be carried out in clinical practice, through simulations, and in other settings.

FAILING CLINICAL PRACTICE

Teachers will be faced with determining when students have not met the outcomes of the clinical practicum—that is, when students have not demonstrated sufficient competence to pass the clinical course. There are principles that should be followed in evaluating and grading clinical practice, which are critical if a student fails a clinical course or has the potential for failing it. These principles are discussed later.

Communicate Evaluation and Grading Methods in Writing

The evaluation methods used in a clinical course; how each will be graded, if at all; and how the clinical grade will be assigned should be in writing and communicated to the students. The teacher's practices in evaluating and grading clinical performance must reflect this written information. In courses with adjunct faculty, part-time clinical nurse educators, and preceptors, it is critical that they understand the outcomes of the course, the evaluation methods, how to observe and rate performance, and responsibilities when students are not performing adequately. Preceptors are reluctant to assign failing grades to students whose competence is questionable (Anthony & Wickman, 2015).

There is a need for faculty development, especially for new and part-time clinical teachers. As part of this development, teachers should explore their own beliefs and values about grading clinical performance and come to consensus about what constitutes satisfactory performance in the clinical course.

Identify Effect of Failing Clinical Practicum on Course Grade

If failing clinical practice, whether in a pass–fail or a letter system, means failing the nursing course, this should be stated clearly in the course syllabus and policies. By stating it in the syllabus, which all students receive, they have it in writing before clinical learning activities begin. A sample policy statement for pass–fail clinical grading is:

> The clinical component of NUR XXX is evaluated with a pass or fail. A failing grade in the clinical component results in failure of the course, even if the theory grade is 75% or higher.

In a letter grade system, the policy should include the letter grade representing a failure in clinical practice—for example, below a C grade. A sample policy statement is:

> Students must pass the clinical component of NUR XXX with the grade of C or higher. A grade lower than a C in the clinical component of the course results in failure of the course, even if the theory grade is 75% or higher.

Ask Students to Sign Rating Forms and Evaluation Summaries

Students should sign any written clinical evaluation documents—rating forms (of clinical practicum, clinical examinations, and performance in simulations), notes and any other narrative comments about the student's performance, and summaries of conferences in which performance was discussed. Their signatures do not mean they agree with the ratings or comments, only that they have read them. Students should have an opportunity to write in their own comments. These materials are important, because they document the student's performance and indicate that the teacher provided feedback and shared concerns about that performance. This is critical in situations in which students may be failing the clinical course because of performance problems.

Identify Performance Problems Early and Develop Learning Plans

Students need continuous feedback on their clinical performance. Observations made by the teacher, the preceptor, and others and evaluation data from other sources should be shared with the student. Together they should discuss the data. Students may have different perceptions of their performance and, in some cases, may provide new information that influences the teacher's judgment about clinical competencies.

When the teacher or preceptor identifies performance problems and clinical deficiencies that may affect passing the course, conferences should be held with the student to discuss these areas of concern and develop a plan for remediation. It is critical that these conferences focus on problems in performance combined with specific learning activities for addressing them. The conferences should not be the teacher telling the student everything that is wrong with clinical performance; the student needs an opportunity to respond to the teacher's concerns and identify how to address them.

One of the goals of the conference is to develop a plan with learning activities for the student to correct deficiencies and develop competencies further. The plan should indicate that (a) completing the remedial learning activities does not guarantee that the student will pass the course, (b) one satisfactory performance of the competencies will not constitute a pass clinical grade (the improvement must be sustained), and (c) the student must demonstrate satisfactory performance of the competencies by the end of the course. A template is provided in Exhibit 15.6 that can be used to develop a learning plan for students. It is important to remember that students have until the end of the course to improve their performance unless they are unsafe in the clinical setting. In that case, the student may be removed from the clinical course depending on the policies of the nursing program, which every teacher and student should understand.

Any discussions with students at risk of failing clinical practice should focus on the student's inability to meet the clinical objectives and perform the specified competencies, not on the teacher's perceptions of the student's intelligence and overall ability. In addition, opinions about the student's ability in general should not be discussed with others.

Conferences should be held in private, and a summary of the discussion should be prepared. The summary should include the date and time of the conference, who participated, areas of concern about clinical performance, and the learning plan with a time frame for completion. The summary should be signed by the teacher, the student, and other participants. All clinical teachers should review related policies of the nursing education program, because they might specify other requirements.

Identify Support Services

Students who are at risk of failing clinical practice may have other problems affecting their performance. Teachers should refer students to counseling and other support services and not attempt to provide these resources themselves. Attempting to counsel the student and help the student cope with other problems may bias the teacher and influence judgment of the student's clinical performance.

Document Performance

As the clinical course progresses, the teacher should give feedback to the student about performance and continue to guide learning. It is important to document the

> **EXHIBIT 15.6**
>
> **TEMPLATE OF A LEARNING PLAN**
>
> 1. Identify the knowledge and areas of performance to be improved in clinical practice (specify the related outcomes or competencies).
> 2. For each of the areas to be improved, identify learning activities to be completed by the student with due dates.
> 3. Plan and specify the process to be used for evaluating progress and performance. Include dates for achieving outcomes and developing competencies, and set up specific meeting times for feedback on progress.

observations made, other types of evaluation data collected, and the learning activities completed by the student. The documentation should be shared routinely with students, discussions about performance should be summarized, and students should sign these summaries to confirm that they read them.

The teacher cannot observe and document the performance of only the student at risk of failing the course. There should be a minimum number of observations and documentation of other students in the clinical group, or the student failing the course might believe that he or she was treated differently than others in the group. One strategy is to plan the number of observations of performance to be made for each student in the clinical group to avoid focusing only on the student with performance problems. However, teachers may observe students who are believed to be at risk for failure more closely and document their observations and conferences with those students more thoroughly and frequently than is necessary for the majority of students. When observations result in feedback to students that can be used to improve performance, at-risk students do not usually object to this extra attention.

Follow Policy on Unsafe Clinical Performance

There should be a policy in the nursing program about actions to be taken if a student is unsafe in clinical practice. Students who are not meeting the outcomes of the course or have problems performing some of the competencies can continue in the clinical course as long as they demonstrate safe care. This is because the outcomes and clinical competencies are identified for achievement at the end of the course, not during it.

If the student demonstrates performance that is potentially unsafe, however, the teacher can remove the student from the clinical setting, following the policy of the nursing education program. Specific learning activities outside of the clinical setting need to be offered for students to develop the knowledge and skills they lack; practice in the skills laboratory and in simulation may be valuable in these situations. A learning plan should be prepared and implemented as described earlier.

Follow Policy for Failure of a Clinical Course

In all instances, the teacher must follow the policies of the nursing program. If the student fails the clinical course, the student must be notified of the failure and its consequences as indicated in these policies. In some nursing programs, students are allowed to repeat only one clinical course, and there may be other requirements to be met. If the student will be dismissed from the program because of the failure, the student must be informed of this in writing. Generally, there is a specific time frame for each step in the process, which must be adhered to by the faculty, administrators, and students.

SUMMARY

Through clinical evaluation, a teacher arrives at judgments about students' performance in clinical practice. The teacher's observations of performance should focus on the outcomes to be met or competencies to be developed in the clinical course. These provide the framework for learning in clinical practice and the basis for evaluating performance. Although such a framework is essential in clinical evaluation, teachers also need to examine their own beliefs about the evaluation process and purposes it serves in nursing. Clarifying one's own values, beliefs, attitudes, and biases that may affect evaluation is an important first step.

Many clinical evaluation methods are available for assessing student competencies in clinical practice. The teacher should choose evaluation methods that provide information on how well students are performing the clinical competencies. The teacher also decides whether the evaluation method is intended for formative or summative evaluation. Some of the methods designed for clinical evaluation are strictly to provide feedback to students on areas for improvement and are not graded. Other methods, such as rating forms and certain written assignments, may be used for summative purposes.

The predominant method for clinical evaluation is in observing the performance of students in clinical practice. Although observation is widely used, there are threats to its validity and reliability. Observations of students may be influenced by the teacher's or preceptor's values, attitudes, and biases. In observing clinical performance, there are many aspects of that performance on which the teacher may focus attention. Every observation reflects only a sampling of the learner's performance during a clinical learning activity. Such issues point to the need for a series of observations before drawing conclusions about performance. There are several ways of recording observations of students, including notes about performance, checklists, and rating scales.

Other methods for clinical evaluation are simulations, standardized patients, OSCEs, written assignments, electronic portfolios, conferences, group projects, and self-evaluation. Some methods are appropriate only for formative evaluation and providing feedback to students. Other methods can be used for both formative and summative evaluation (i.e., graded).

Important guidelines for grading clinical practice and working with students who are at risk for failing a clinical course were discussed in the chapter. These guidelines give direction to teachers in establishing sound grading practices and following them when working with students in clinical practice.

NOTE

This chapter was adapted from *Evaluation and Testing in Nursing Education*, 5th ed. (Chapters 13, 14, 15, and 18), by M. H. Oermann and K. B. Gaberson, 2017, New York, NY: Springer Publishing. Copyright ©2017 by Springer Publishing. Adapted with permission.

CNE EXAMINATION TEST BLUEPRINT CORE COMPETENCIES

1. **Use Assessment and Evaluation Strategies**

   A. Provide input for the development of nursing program standards and policies regarding
      1. progression
   B. Enforce nursing program standards related to progression
   C. Use a variety of strategies to assess and evaluate learning in these domains
      1. cognitive
      2. psychomotor
      3. affective
   D. Incorporate current research in assessment and evaluation practices
   E. Analyze available resources for learner assessment and evaluation
   F. Create assessment instruments to evaluate outcomes
   G. Use assessment instruments to evaluate outcomes
   H. Implement evaluation strategies that are appropriate to the learner and learning outcomes
   I. Analyze assessment and evaluation data
   J. Use assessment and evaluation data to enhance the teaching–learning process
   K. Advise learners regarding assessment and evaluation criteria
   L. Provide timely, constructive, and thoughtful feedback to learners

REFERENCES

Altmiller, G. (2016). Strategies for providing constructive feedback to students. *Nurse Educator, 41*(3), 118–119. doi:10.1097/nne.0000000000000227

Anthony, M. L., & Wickman, M. (2015). Precepting challenges: The unsafe student. *Nurse Educator, 40*(3), 113–114. doi:10.1097/nne.0000000000000118

Ballman, K., Garritano, N., & Beery, T. (2016). Broadening the reach of standardized patients in nurse practitioner education to include the distance learner. *Nurse Educator, 41*(5), 230–233. doi:10.1097/nne.0000000000000260

Bonnel, W. (2008). Improving feedback to students in online courses. *Nursing Education Perspectives, 29,* 290–294.

Brookhart, S. M., & Nitko, A. J. (2015). *Educational assessment of students* (7th ed.). Upper Saddle River, NJ: Pearson.

Hall, M. A. (2013). An expanded look at evaluating clinical performance: Faculty use of anecdotal notes in the U.S. and Canada. *Nurse Education in Practice, 13,* 271–276. doi:10.1016/j.nepr.2013.02.001

Hawkins, R. E., & Boulet, J. R. (2008). Direct observation: Standardized patients. In E. S. Holmboe & R. E. Hawkins (Eds.), *Practical guide to the evaluation of clinical competencies* (pp. 102–118). Philadelphia, PA: Mosby.

McWilliam, P. L., & Botwinski, C. A. (2012). Identifying strengths and weaknesses in the utilization of Objective Structured Clinical Examination (OSCE) in a nursing program. *Nursing Education Perspectives, 33,* 35–39.

Oermann, M. H., Yarbrough, S. S., Ard, N., Saewert, K. J., & Charasika, M. (2009). Clinical evaluation and grading practices in schools of nursing: National Survey Findings Part II. *Nursing Education Perspectives, 30,* 274–279.

Quality and Safety Education for Nurses. (2014). Competencies. Retrieved from http://qsen.org/competencies

Sullivan, D. T. (2016). An introduction to curriculum development. In D. M. Billings & J. A. Halstead (Eds.), *Teaching in nursing: A guide for faculty* (5th ed., pp. 89–117). St. Louis, MO: Elsevier.

Certified Nurse Educator (CNE®) Examination Detailed Test Blueprint[1]

1. Facilitate Learning—22%

A. Implement a variety of teaching strategies appropriate to:

1. content
2. setting (i.e., clinical versus classroom)
3. learner needs
4. learning style
5. desired learner outcomes
6. method of delivery (e.g., face-to-face, remote, simulation)

B. Use teaching strategies based on:

1. educational theory
2. evidence-based practices related to education

C. Modify teaching strategies and learning experiences based on consideration of learners':

1. cultural background
2. past clinical experiences
3. past educational and life experiences
4. generational groups (i.e., age)

D. Use information technologies to support the teaching–learning process

E. Practice skilled oral and written (including electronic) communication that reflects an awareness of self and relationships with learners (e.g., evaluation, mentorship, and supervision)

F. Communicate effectively orally and in writing with an ability to convey ideas in a variety of contexts

G. Model reflective thinking practices, including critical thinking

H. Create opportunities for learners to develop their own critical thinking skills

---

[1]Reprinted with permission of the National League for Nursing (NLN), Washington, D.C.

    I. Create a positive learning environment that fosters a free exchange of ideas

    J. Show enthusiasm for teaching, learning, and the nursing profession that inspires and motivates students

    K. Demonstrate personal attributes that facilitate learning (e.g., caring, confidence, patience, integrity, respect, and flexibility)

    L. Respond effectively to unexpected events that affect instruction

    M. Develop collegial working relationships with clinical agency personnel to promote positive learning environments

    N. Use knowledge of evidence-based practice to instruct learners

    O. Demonstrate ability to teach clinical skills

    P. Act as a role model in practice settings

    Q. Foster a safe learning environment

2. Facilitate Learner Development and Socialization—14%

    A. Identify individual learning styles and unique learning needs of learners with these characteristics:

        1. culturally diverse (including international);

        2. English as an additional language

        3. traditional vs. non-traditional (i.e., recent high school graduates vs. those in school later)

        4. at-risk (e.g., educationally disadvantaged, learning and/or physically challenged, social, and economic issues)

        5. previous nursing education

    B. Provide resources for diverse learners to meet their individual learning needs

    C. Advise learners in ways that help them meet their professional goals

    D. Create learning environments that facilitate learners' self-reflection, personal goal setting, and socialization to the role of the nurse

    E. Foster the development of learners in these areas:

        1. cognitive domain

        2. psychomotor domain

        3. affective domain

    F. Assist learners to engage in thoughtful and constructive self- and peer evaluation

    G. Encourage professional development of learners

3. Use Assessment and Evaluation Strategies—17%

    A. Provide input for the development of nursing program standards and policies regarding:

        1. admission

        2. progression

        3. graduation

    B. Enforce nursing program standards related to

        1. admission

        2. progression

        3. graduation

C. Use a variety of strategies to assess and evaluate learning in these domains:
1. cognitive
2. psychomotor
3. affective

D. Incorporate current research in assessment and evaluation practices

E. Analyze available resources for learner assessment and evaluation

F. Create assessment instruments to evaluate outcomes

G. Use assessment instruments to evaluate outcomes

H. Implement evaluation strategies that are appropriate to the learner and learning outcomes

I. Analyze assessment and evaluation data

J. Use assessment and evaluation data to enhance the teaching–learning process

K. Advise learners regarding assessment and evaluation criteria

L. Provide timely, constructive, and thoughtful feedback to learners

4. **Participate in Curriculum Design and Evaluation of Program Outcomes—17%**

A. Demonstrate knowledge of curriculum development including:
1. identifying program outcomes
2. developing competency statements
3. writing course objectives
4. selecting appropriate learning activities
5. selecting appropriate clinical experiences
6. selecting appropriate evaluation strategies

B. Actively participate in the design of the curriculum to reflect:
1. institutional philosophy and mission
2. current nursing and health care trends
3. community and societal needs
4. nursing principles, standards, theory, and research
5. educational principles, theory, and research
6. use of technology

C. Lead the development of curriculum design

D. Lead the development of course design

E. Analyze results of program evaluation

F. Revise the curriculum based on evaluation of:
1. program outcomes
2. learner needs
3. societal and health care trends
4. stakeholder feedback (e.g., from learners, agency personnel, accrediting agencies, advisory boards)

G. Implement curricular revisions using appropriate change theories and strategies

H. Collaborate with community and clinical partners to support educational goals

    I. Design program assessment plans that promote continuous quality improvement

    J. Implement the program assessment plan

    K. Evaluate the program assessment plan

5. **Pursue Systematic Self-Evaluation and Improvement in the Academic Nurse Educator Role—9%**

    A. Engage in activities that promote one's socialization to the role

    B. Maintain membership in professional organizations

    C. Participate actively in professional organizations through committee work and/or leadership roles

    D. Demonstrate a commitment to lifelong learning

    E. Participate in professional development opportunities that increase one's effectiveness in the role

    F. Manage the teaching, scholarship, and service demands as influenced by the requirements of the institutional setting

    G. Use feedback gained from self, peer, learner, and administrative evaluation to improve role effectiveness

    H. Practice according to legal and ethical standards relevant to higher education and nursing education

    I. Mentor and support faculty colleagues in the role of an academic nurse educator

    J. Engage in self-reflection to improve teaching practices

6. **Engage in Scholarship, Service, and Leadership—21%**

    A. Function as a Change Agent and Leader

        1. Function as a change agent and leader
- Model cultural sensitivity when advocating for change
- Evaluate organizational effectiveness in nursing education

        2. Enhance the visibility of nursing and its contributions by providing leadership in the:
- nursing program
- parent institution
- local community
- state or region

        3. Participate in interdisciplinary efforts to address health care and educational needs:
- within the institution
- locally
- regionally

        4. Implement strategies for change within the:
- nursing program
- institution
- local community

        5. Develop leadership skills in others to shape and implement change

6. Adapt to changes created by external factors

7. Create a culture for change within the:
- nursing program
- institution

8. Advocate for nursing, nursing education, and higher education in the political arena

B. Engage in Scholarship of Teaching

1. Exhibit a spirit of inquiry about teaching and learning, student development, and evaluation methods

2. Use evidence-based resources to improve and support teaching

3. Participate in research activities related to nursing education

4. Share teaching expertise with colleagues and others

5. Demonstrate integrity as a scholar

C. Function Effectively within the Institutional Environment and the Academic Community

1. Identify how social, economic, political, and institutional forces influence nursing and higher education

2. Make decisions based on knowledge of historical and current trends and issues in higher education

3. Integrate the values of respect, collegiality, professionalism, and caring to build an organizational climate that fosters the development of learners and colleagues

4. Consider the goals of the nursing program and the mission of the parent institution when proposing change or managing issues

5. Participate on institutional and departmental committees

Resources for Nurse Educators

APPENDIX B.1: CERTIFICATION FOR NURSE EDUCATORS

Mission of Certification Program

The National League for Nursing's Academic Nurse Educator Certification Program "promote[s] excellence in the advanced specialty role of the academic nurse educator."
Goals of Certification:

- Distinguish academic nursing education as a specialty area of practice and an advanced practice role.
- Recognize the academic nurse educator's specialized knowledge, skills, and abilities and excellence in practice.
- Strengthen the use of the core competencies of nurse educator practice.
- Contribute to nurse educators' professional development.

National League for Nursing. (2017). Certification for nurse educators (CNE®). Retrieved from http://www.nln.org/professional-development programs/Certification-for-Nurse-Educators. Reproduced with permission of the National League for Nursing (NLN), Washington, DC.

APPENDIX D.2: SELECTED NURSING AND HIGHER EDUCATION ORGANIZATIONS

American Academy of Nursing	Serves the public and nursing profession by advancing health policy and practice. Academy members, known as Fellows, are nursing's most accomplished leaders in education, practice, administration, and research.	www.aannet .org/about-the -academy

(continued)

American Association of Colleges of Nursing	Represents baccalaureate and higher-degree nursing programs. Promotes quality nursing education. Offers faculty development programs and webinars. Collects data about nursing education programs, faculty, and students, and analyzes trends in nursing education. Publishes position papers.	www.aacn.nche .edu
American Association of Community Colleges	Provides advocacy for community colleges at the national level. Works closely with states on policy.	www.aacc.nche .edu
American Association of University Professors	Focuses on advancing academic freedom and shared governance. Defines fundamental professional values and standards for higher education and faculty.	www.aaup.org
American Association of University Women	Promotes equity and education for women and girls. Advocates for fundamental educational, social, economic, and political issues.	www.aauw.org
American Council on Education	Represents presidents of accredited, degree-granting institutions (2- and 4-year colleges, private and public universities, and nonprofit schools) in the United States. Focuses on higher education challenges, with the goal to improve access and better prepare students.	www.acenet.edu/ Pages/default .aspx
Association of American Colleges and Universities	Focuses on promoting high-quality undergraduate liberal education. Website contains links to resources on liberal education, general education, curriculum, faculty work, assessment, diversity, and others.	www.aacu.org/ about/index.cfm
Association of Black Nursing Faculty, Inc.	Provides a group for Black professional nurses with similar interests and concerns to promote health-related issues and nursing education. Assists members in professional development and provides continuing education.	http://www.abnf .net
Association of Community Health Nursing Educators	Focuses on promoting excellence in community and public health nursing education, research, and practice.	www.achne.org/ i4a/pages/index .cfm?pageid=1
EDUCAUSE	Advances higher education through use of information technology. Focuses on issues and emerging trends and technologies affecting higher education.	www.educause .edu
Interprofessional Education Collaborative (IPEC)	Collaborative of schools of health professions to promote efforts that advance interprofessional learning experiences to prepare future health professionals for team-based care and improved population health outcomes. These organizations that represent higher education in allopathic and osteopathic medicine, dentistry, nursing, pharmacy, and public health created core competencies for interprofessional collaborative practice to guide curricula development across health professions schools.	https:// ipecollaborative .org/About_ IPEC.html

(continued)

Multimedia Educational Resource for Learning and Online Teaching (MERLOT)	Includes repository of resources and information for faculty development and to download for use in teaching. Publishes *Journal of Online Learning and Teaching*.	www.merlot.org
National League for Nursing	Promotes excellence in nursing education at all levels. Offers faculty development programs, webinars, and annual educational conference. Sponsors certification program for nurse educators (CNE). Publishes position papers on nursing education and has a grant program for nursing education research. The NLN Commission for Nursing Education Accreditation (CNEA) accredits nursing programs.	www.nln.org
National Organization of Nurse Practitioner Faculties	Focuses on promoting quality nurse practitioner (NP) education at national and international levels. Leading organization for NP faculty in US and globally.	www.nonpf.com
National Student Nurses Association	Serves as organization for nursing students with goal of enhancing their professional development and promoting transition into the profession.	www.nsna.org
Organization for Associate Degree Nursing (OADN)	Is dedicated to enhancing the quality of Associate Degree (AD) nursing. Advocates for AD nursing and promotes academic progression of AD nursing graduates in furthering their education.	https://www.oadn .org
POD Network	Focuses on faculty, instructional, and organizational development in higher education.	www.podnetwork .org
Quality and Safety Education for Nurses (QSEN)	Collaborative of nurses and other health care professionals focused on education, practice, and scholarship to improve quality and safety of health care. Identified knowledge, skills, and attitudes (KSAs) necessary to continuously improve quality and safety of health care. Website is a central repository of information on core QSEN competencies, KSAs, teaching strategies, and faculty development resources.	http://qsen.org/ about-qsen
Sigma Theta Tau International Honor Society of Nursing	Supports learning and professional development of nurses worldwide. Membership is by invitation to baccalaureate and graduate nursing students with excellence in scholarship and to nurse leaders with exceptional achievements in nursing. Offers conferences for sharing research and publishes *Journal of Nursing Scholarship*, among other resources.	www .nursingsociety .org

Index